Cutaneous Oncology Update

Editor

STANISLAV N. TOLKACHJOV

DERMATOLOGIC CLINICS

www.derm.theclinics.com

Consulting Editor
BRUCE H. THIERS

January 2023 • Volume 41 • Number 1

ELSEVIER

1600 John F. Kennedy Boulevard • Suite 1800 • Philadelphia, Pennsylvania, 19103-2899

http://www.theclinics.com

DERMATOLOGIC CLINICS Volume 41, Number 1
January 2023 ISSN 0733-8635, ISBN-13: 978-0-323-97284-0

Editor: Stacy Eastman
Developmental Editor: Karen Justine Solomon

Dermatologic Clinics (ISSN 0733-8635) is published quarterly by Elsevier Inc., 360 Park Avenue South, New York, NY 10010-1710. Months of publication are January, April, July, and October. Business and editorial offices: 1600 John F. Kennedy Blvd., Suite 1800, Philadelphia, PA 19103-2899. Customer service office: 11830 Westline Drive, St. Louis, MO 63146. Periodicals postage paid at New York, NY, and additional mailing offices. Subscription prices are USD 438.00 per year for US individuals, USD 899.00 per year for US institutions, USD 478.00 per year for Canadian individuals, USD 1,097.00 per year for Canadian institutions, USD 536.00 per year for international individuals, USD 1,097.00 per year for international institutions, USD 100.00 per year for US students/residents, USD 100.00 per year for Canadian students/residents, and USD 240 per year for international students/residents. International air speed delivery is included in all *Clinics* subscription prices. All prices are subject to change without notice. **POSTMASTER:** Send address changes to *Dermatologic Clinics*, Elsevier Health Sciences Division, Subscription Customer Service, 3251 Riverport Lane, Maryland Heights, MO 63043. **Customer Service: 1-800-654-2452 (U.S. and Canada); 314-447-8871 (outside U.S. and Canada). Fax: 314-447-8029. E-mail: journalscustomerservice-usa@elsevier.com (for print support); journalsonlinesupport-usa@elsevier.com (for online support).**

Reprints. For copies of 100 or more, of articles in this publication, please contact the Commercial Reprints Department, Elsevier Inc., 360 Park Avenue South, New York, New York 10010-1710. Tel.: 212-633-3874; Fax: 212-633-3820; Email: reprints@elsevier.com.

The *Dermatologic Clinics* is covered in *MEDLINE/PubMed (Index Medicus)*, *Current Contents/Clinical Medicine*, *Excerpta Medica*, *Chemical Abstracts,* and *ISI/BIOMED*.

Contributors

CONSULTING EDITOR

BRUCE H. THIERS, MD
Professor and Chairman Emeritus, Department
of Dermatology and Dermatologic Surgery,
Medical University of South Carolina,
Charleston, South Carolina

EDITOR

STANISLAV N. TOLKACHJOV, MD, FAAD, FACMS
Director of Mohs Micrographic and
Reconstructive Surgery, Epiphany
Dermatology, Clinical Associate Professor,
Texas A&M College of Medicine, Clinical
Assistant Professor, Department of
Dermatology, University of Texas at
Southwestern, Clinical Core Faculty, Division
of Dermatology, Baylor University Medical
Center, Clinical Faculty, Section of
Dermatology, Veterans Affairs Medical Center,
Dallas, Texas

AUTHORS

NADER ABOUL-FETTOUH, MD
Department of Dermatology, McGovern
Medical School, The University of Texas Health
Science Center at Houston, Houston,
Texas

MURAD ALAM, MD, MBA, MSCI
Departments of Dermatology, Surgery,
Otolaryngology, and Medical Social Sciences,
Feinberg School of Medicine, Northwestern
University, Chicago, Illinois

JANE MARGARET ANDERSON, BSA
Research Department, Moy-Fincher-Chipps
Facial Plastics & Dermatology, Beverly Hills,
California; The University of Texas Health
Science Center San Antonio, San Antonio,
Texas

ANNA BAR, MD
Department of Dermatology, Associate
Professor of Dermatology and Mohs
Micrographic Surgery and Dermatologic
Oncology Program Director, Oregon Health &
Science University, Portland, Oregon

ELLIOT D. BLUE, MD
Postdoctoral Research Fellow, University of
Nebraska Medical Center, Department of
Dermatology, Omaha, Nebraska

DIANA BOLOTIN, MD, PhD
Associate Professor, Chief, Section of
Dermatology, University of Chicago, Chicago,
Illinois

DAVID G. BRODLAND, MD
Assistant Professor, Department of
Dermatology, Assistant Professor, Department
of Otolaryngology, Assistant Professor,
Department of Plastic Surgery, Z & B Skin
Cancer Center, University of Pittsburgh,
Pittsburgh, Pennsylvania

JOI B. CARTER, MD
Associate Professor, Department of
Dermatology,Dartmouth Geisel School of
Medicine, Hanover, New Hampshire, USA

LEON CHEN, MD
US Dermatology Partners, Elite Dermatology,
Houston, Texas

RACHEL E. CHRISTENSEN, BS
Department of Dermatology, Feinberg School of Medicine, Northwestern University, Chicago, Illinois

NNEKA COMFERE, MD
Professor, Departments of Dermatology, and Laboratory Medicine and Pathology, Mayo Clinic, Rochester, Minnesota

JEREMY R. ETZKORN, MD, MS
Department of Dermatology, Hospital of the University of Pennsylvania, Assistant Professor, Department of Dermatology, Perelman Center for Advanced Medicine, University of Pennsylvania, Philadelphia, Pennsylvania

TYLER D. EVANS, MD
Resident, University of Nebraska Medical Center, Department of Dermatology, Omaha, Nebraska

CERRENE N. GIORDANO, MD
Department of Dermatology, Hospital of the University of Pennsylvania, Assistant Professor of Clinical Dermatology, Department of Dermatology, Perelman Center for Advanced Medicine, University of Pennsylvania, Philadelphia, Pennsylvania

NICHOLAS GOLDA, MD, FACMS, FAAD
US Dermatology Partners, Kansas City, Missouri

NIKHIL GOYAL, BS
Perelman School of Medicine, University of Pennsylvania, Philadelphia, Pennsylvania

ANTHONY K. GUZMAN, MD
Department of Dermatology, Brigham and Women's Hospital, Harvard Medical School, Boston, Massachusetts

JENNIFER L. HAND, MD
Associate Professor, Department of Dermatology, Associate Professor, Clinical Genomics, Department of Pediatric and Adolescent Medicine, Mayo Clinic, Rochester, Minnesota

MICHAEL S. HEATH, MD
Department of Dermatology, Physician, Oregon Health & Science University, Portland, Oregon

H. WILLIAM HIGGINS II, MD, MBE
Department of Dermatology, Hospital of the University of Pennsylvania, Lab Director of Pennsylvania Hospital Mohs Micrographic Surgery Unit, Assistant Professor of Clinical Dermatology, Department of Dermatology, Perelman Center for Advanced Medicine, University of Pennsylvania, Philadelphia, Pennsylvania

GEORGE HRUZA, MD, MBA, FACMS, FAAD
Adjunct Professor of Dermatology, Saint Louis University, Laser and Dermatologic Surgery Center, St Louis and Chesterfield, Missouri

NASRO ISAQ, MD
Department of Dermatology, Mayo Clinic, Rochester, Minnesota

BO M. KITRELL, BS
Medical Student, University of Nebraska Medical Center, College of Medicine, Omaha, Nebraska

SHELBY L. KUBICKI, MD
Department of Dermatology, McGovern Medical School, The University of Texas Health Science Center at Houston, Houston, Texas

JAKE LAZAROFF, MD
Section of Dermatology, University of Chicago, Chicago, Illinois

DANIEL J. LEWIS, MD
Department of Dermatology, Hospital of the University of Pennsylvania, Department of Dermatology, University of Pennsylvania, Philadelphia, Pennsylvania

STEPHANIE K. LIN, BA
Donald and Barbara Zucker School of Medicine at Hofstra/Northwell, Hempstead, New York

MARISSA B. LOBL, PhD
Medical Student, University of Nebraska Medical Center, College of Medicine, Omaha, Nebraska

STACY L. MCMURRAY, MD
Department of Dermatology, Hospital of the University of Pennsylvania, Assistant Professor of Clinical Dermatology, Department of Dermatology, Perelman Center for Advanced Medicine, University of Pennsylvania, Philadelphia, Pennsylvania

MICHAEL R. MIGDEN, MD
Professor, Departments of Dermatology and
Head and Neck Surgery, The University of
Texas MD Anderson Cancer Center, Houston,
Texas

CHRISTOPHER J. MILLER, MD
Department of Dermatology, Hospital of the
University of Pennsylvania, Director of Penn
Dermatology Oncology Center, Louis A.
Duhring MD Endowed Professor in
Dermatology, Department of Dermatology,
Perelman Center for Advanced Medicine,
University of Pennsylvania, Philadelphia,
Pennsylvania

LAUREN MOY, MD
Research Department, Moy-Fincher-Chipps
Facial Plastics & Dermatology, Beverly Hills,
California

RONALD L. MOY, MD
Research Department, Moy-Fincher-Chipps
Facial Plastics & Dermatology, Beverly Hills,
California

BRETT C. NEILL, MD
Epiphany Dermatology, Dallas, Texas

RAJIV I. NIJHAWAN, MD
Department of Dermatology, The University of
Texas Southwestern Medical Center, Dallas,
Texas

DANIEL O'LEARY, MD
Assistant Professor, Division of Hematology,
Oncology, andTransplantation, University of
Minnesota, Minneapolis, Minnesota, USA

AMRITA O'LEARY GOYAL, MD
Adjunct Assistant Professor of Dermatology,
Department of Dermatology, University of
Minnesota, Minneapolis, Minnesota

SAREM RASHID, BS
Wellman Center for Photomedicine,
Massachusetts General Hospital, Harvard
Medical School, Boston University School of
Medicine, Boston, Massachusetts

EMILY S. RUIZ, MD, MPH
Department of Dermatology, Brigham and
Women's Hospital, Harvard Medical School,
Boston, Massachusetts

CHRYSALYNE D. SCHMULTS, MD, MSCE
Department of Dermatology, Brigham and
Women's Hospital, Harvard Medical School,
Boston, Massachusetts

EDWARD W. SEGER, MD, MS
Division of Dermatology, University of Kansas
Medical Center, Kansas City, Kansas

KISHAN M. SHAH, MD
Department of Dermatology, The University of
Texas Southwestern Medical Center, Dallas,
Texas

MICHAEL SHAUGHNESSY, MD
Department of Dermatology, Massachusetts
General Hospital, Boston, Massachusetts

KEVIN Y. SHI, MD, PhD
Department of Dermatology, The University of
Texas Southwestern Medical Center, Dallas,
Texas

SERENA SHIMSHAK, BA
Mayo Clinic Alix School of Medicine,
Jacksonville, Florida

THUZAR M. SHIN, MD, PhD
Department of Dermatology, Hospital of the
University of Pennsylvania, Director of High-
Risk Skin Cancer Clinic for Organ Transplant
and Immunosuppressed Patients, Assistant
Professor, Department of Dermatology,
Perelman Center for Advanced Medicine,
University of Pennsylvania, Philadelphia,
Pennsylvania

SIRUNYA SILAPUNT, MD
Department of Dermatology, McGovern
Medical School, The University of Texas Health
Science Center at Houston, Houston, Texas

ALFREDO SILLER Jr, MD
Resident, University of Nebraska Medical
Center, Department of Dermatology, Omaha,
Nebraska

JOSEPH F. SOBANKO, MD
Department of Dermatology, Hospital of the
University of Pennsylvania, Director of
Cosmetic Dermatology and Laser Surgery,
Director of Dermatologic Surgery Education,
Associate Professor, Department of

Dermatology, University of Pennsylvania, Philadelphia, Pennsylvania

OLAYEMI SOKUMBI, MD
Assistant Professor, Departments of Dermatology, and Laboratory Medicine and Pathology, Mayo Clinic, Jacksonville, Florida

DIVYA SRIVASTAVA, MD
Associate Professor, Department of Dermatology, The University of Texas Southwestern Medical Center, Dallas, Texas

CAROLYN M. STULL, MD
Department of Dermatology, Perelman Center for Advanced Medicine, University of Pennsylvania, Philadelphia, Pennsylvania

STANISLAV N. TOLKACHJOV, MD, FAAD, FACMS
Director of Mohs Micrographic and Reconstructive Surgery, Epiphany Dermatology, Clinical Associate Professor, Texas A&M College of Medicine, Clinical Assistant Professor, Department of Dermatology, University of Texas at Southwestern, Clinical Core Faculty, Division of Dermatology, Baylor University Medical Center, Clinical Faculty, Section of Dermatology, Veterans Affairs Medical Center, Dallas, Texas

HENSIN TSAO, MD, PhD
Wellman Center for Photomedicine, Department of Dermatology, Massachusetts General Hospital, Harvard Medical School, Boston, Massachusetts

JACKSON G. TURBEVILLE, MD
Associate Professor, Department of Dermatology, Mayo Clinic, Rochester, Minnesota

JOANNA L. WALKER, MD
Department of Dermatology, Hospital of the University of Pennsylvania, Assistant Professor of Clinical Dermatology, Department of Dermatology, Perelman Center for Advanced Medicine, University of Pennsylvania, Philadelphia, Pennsylvania

FRANCES WALOCKO, MD
Department of Dermatology, Feinberg School of Medicine, Northwestern University, Chicago, Illinois

LEO L. WANG, MD, PhD
Department of Dermatology, Perelman Center for Advanced Medicine, University of Pennsylvania, Philadelphia, Pennsylvania

MELODI JAVID WHITLEY, MD, PhD
Assistant Professor, Director of Transplant Dermatology, University of Nebraska Medical Center, Department of Dermatology, Omaha, Nebraska

BRANDON WORLEY, MD
Florida Dermatology and Skin Cancer Centers, Lake Wales, Florida

ASHLEY WYSONG, MD, MS
Professor and Founding Chair, William W. Bruce MD Distinguished Chair of Dermatology, Director of the Skin Cancer Program, The Fred & Pamela Buffett Cancer Center, University of Nebraska Medical Center, Department of Dermatology, Omaha, Nebraska

JUNQIAN ZHANG, MD
Department of Dermatology, Hospital of the University of Pennsylvania, Assistant Professor of Clinical Dermatology, Department of Dermatology, University of Pennsylvania, Philadelphia, Pennsylvania

Contents

node dissection and radiation therapy. Immune checkpoint inhibitors, such as ave-lumab and pembrolizumab, are first-line agents for metastatic MCC. Monitoring for recurrence can be aided by Merkel cell polyomavirus oncoprotein antibody titers.

Skin cancers represent the most common malignancy worldwide. In children, the diagnosis of skin cancer is rare and raises the possibility of an underlying genetic predisposition. Recent molecular advances have increased understanding of certain genetically determined regulatory pathways that constantly protect the skin from atypical cell growth and cancer. Knowledge about these underlying gene defects aids a dermatologist's ability to recommend confirmatory genetic testing and provides potential targets for future therapies. In this review, we outline genetic conditions important to dermatologists that are associated with skin cancer development and review the current approaches to the management of these patients.

This review of cutaneous B-cell lymphoma (CBCL) is focused on the clinical presentation, treatment, and workup of each type of lymphoma. Part 1 is an overview of each of the CBCLs, including clinical presentation, recent advances in the pathobiology, and evidence regarding treatment strategies. Part 2 is a detailed guide to the steps in diagnosis and workup of a newly diagnosed CBCL according to the International Society for Cutaneous Lymphoma/European Organization for Research and Treatment of Cancer and NCCN guidelines.

Cutaneous T-cell lymphomas are a clinically and histopathologically heterogenous group of disorders, encountered in dermatologic practice. In this article, we provide a detailed practical guide to the evaluation, diagnosis, and management of common cutaneous T-cell lymphomas. Emphasis is placed on the clinical evaluation including the role of the dermatologist in the accurate assessment of body surface area involvement for disease staging, appropriate biopsy techniques, and key considerations, recent advances in the molecular genetic characteristics of disease, and common treatment approaches.

Chemoprophylaxis against nonmelanoma skin cancer (NMSC) should be considered in high-risk populations such as those with certain genetic disorders, immunosuppressive states, chronic radiation, excessive UV exposure, or extensive personal or family history of NMSC. The methods for chemoprevention have progressed beyond traditional sunscreen into more effective strategies including DNA repair enzymes, nicotinamide, systemic retinoids, and nonsteroidal anti-inflammatory drugs. Other therapies are still being investigated and include treatments that target premalignant lesions, capecitabine, hedgehog inhibitors, difluoromethylornithine, metformin, and nutritional factors.

DERMATOLOGIC CLINICS

SERIES OF RELATED INTEREST

Medical Clinics
https://www.medical.theclinics.com/
Immunology and Allergy Clinics
https://www.immunology.theclinics.com/
Clinics in Plastic Surgery
https://www.plasticsurgery.theclinics.com/
Otolaryngologic Clinics
https://www.oto.theclinics.com/

Preface
Cutaneous Oncology
Where We Are and Where We Are Going

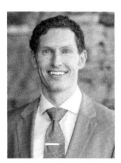

Stanislav N. Tolkachjov, MD, FAAD, FACMS
Editor

Cutaneous malignancies continue to be a cause of morbidity and mortality for patients worldwide. Diagnostic and treatment options for these malignancies have improved, yet our expectations for best patient outcomes continue to drive advancement. The current issue gives a broad overview of the common and uncommon cutaneous malignancies and cutaneous lymphomas, their clinicopathologic characteristics, approaches to diagnosis, and current and future treatment options. New diagnostic and prognostic tools, including gene expression profiling, are discussed for certain malignancies, while targeted treatments and immunotherapies in cutaneous oncology are also reviewed.

The issue also outlines current standard treatments, including Mohs micrographic surgery and nail surgery, with a focus on understanding and executing proper surgical technique, improvements in histopathologic evaluation, and approaches to tumors in special sites, such as the nails and the genitalia. While Mohs surgery has been increasingly used in the treatment of melanoma, this issue provides a discussion of the background to current melanoma treatment guidelines and suggests why these should at least be reevaluated in the context of margins and surgical standards of care.

Tumor-specific articles include squamous cell carcinoma, basal cell carcinoma, melanoma, Merkel cell carcinoma, adnexal and sebaceous carcinomas, mesenchymal tumors, as well as B-cell and T-cell lymphomas. Special populations like patients with immunosuppression and the pediatric age groups are separately discussed with a focus on genodermatoses and skin cancer syndromes. The issue is rounded off by new and established chemoprevention techniques reviewed from a perspective of basic and translational research to clinical use.

The issue is written by a group of highly respected experts in each field presented with a practical approach for clinicians to easily understand and apply to their daily practices. The information is current, referenced, and accompanied by well-designed illustrations and high-quality images allowing readers to reference summarized materials and key points. Readers of the issue should be able to understand current and evolving approaches to cutaneous oncology in the general and special populations, and the issue should serve as a point of reference in the daily clinical practice of managing patients with cutaneous malignancies.

Stanislav N. Tolkachjov, MD, FAAD, FACMS
1640 FM 544, Ste 100
Lewisville, TX 75056, USA

E-mail address:
stan.tolkachjov@gmail.com

Dermatol Clin 41 (2023) xiii
https://doi.org/10.1016/j.det.2022.08.001
0733-8635/23/© 2022 Published by Elsevier Inc.

derm.theclinics.com

Squamous Cell Carcinoma
An Update in Staging, Management, and Postoperative Surveillance Strategies

Anthony K. Guzman, MD*, Chrysalyne D. Schmults, MD, MSCE, Emily S. Ruiz, MD, MPH

KEYWORDS

- Squamous cell carcinoma • Mohs micrographic surgery • SCC • Nonmelanoma skin cancer

KEY POINTS

- Over 1 million new cases of cutaneous squamous cell carcinoma (cSCC) are diagnosed annually in the United States, and there is an alarming overall rising incidence of the disease.
- Although the majority of cSCC are cured by surgical intervention, high-risk tumors may be associated with recurrence, metastasis, or death.
- Patients with high-risk cSCC benefit from a systematic management strategy that encompasses early diagnosis, staging, appropriate intervention based on risk factors, and comprehensive post-treatment surveillance.

INTRODUCTION

Invasive cutaneous squamous cell carcinoma (cSCC) represents the second-most prevalent cutaneous malignancy, with over 1 million estimated new cases diagnosed annually in the United States.[1] Despite the clear association of cSCC with modifiable risk factors—notably cumulative ultraviolet radiation exposure[2]—an increasing overall incidence is observed.[1,3,4] Systemic immunosuppression also constitutes an important risk factor in the rising incidence of cSCC; iatrogenic etiologies include solid organ transplantation,[5–7] as well as long-term immunomodulatory therapy for inflammatory conditions like rheumatoid arthritis,[8] and inflammatory bowel disease.[9] Patients with hematologic malignancies also have an elevated risk of developing cSCC and more aggressive disease.[10,11]

The majority of cSCCs have an excellent prognosis,[12,13] largely owing to high rates of cure after wide local excision (WLE)[14] or Mohs micrographic surgery (MMS).[15] However, up to 3.7% and 1.5% of cSCC cases will lead to metastatic disease and death from disease, respectively.[1] Given the number of tumors diagnosed annually, it is important to stratify cSCCs to identify those with an elevated risk of developing a poor outcome; such high-risk tumors benefit from a structured diagnostic strategy, therapeutic plan, and surveillance. In the following review, we provide a comprehensive, evidence-based update on the diagnostic approach, staging paradigm, management recommendations, and post-treatment surveillance of cSCC.

Initial Diagnosis

A definitive diagnosis of cSCC is ascertained with a histopathologic specimen, most commonly acquired by punch or shave biopsy to at least the level of the deep reticular dermis; specimens confined to the epidermis may preclude the ability to diagnose invasive disease. When deep invasion, recurrent tumor, or other aggressive features are suspected, deeper sampling or scouting biopsies may be needed if more superficial methods are insufficient.[16] Initial histopathology may also

Department of Dermatology, Brigham and Women's Hospital, Harvard Medical School, Boston, MA, USA
* Corresponding author. 1153 Centre Street, Suite 4J (Mohs and Dermatologic Surgery), Jamaica Plain, MA 02130.
E-mail address: aguzman7@bwh.harvard.edu

Dermatol Clin 41 (2023) 1–11
https://doi.org/10.1016/j.det.2022.07.004
0733-8635/23/© 2022 Elsevier Inc. All rights reserved.

allow for the preliminary identification of key prognostic features associated with high-risk disease, such as the degree of differentiation, the presence of perineural invasion (PNI) and/or lymphovascular invasion (LVI), and the anatomic level of invasion; however, complete tumor removal is frequently required for a full prognostic evaluation.[17] Clinicians should have a low threshold for rebiopsy in cases in which there is strong clinical suspicion for cSCC despite discordant or equivocal histopathology.

A dedicated lymph node (LN) examination should be performed in patients with high-stage tumors or those that demonstrate aggressive behavior, with greatest attention to the lymphatic draining basin of the cSCC. The manual palpation of suspicious LN has been shown to have a high specificity [96%, 95% confidence interval (CI) (93%–98%)] in excluding underlying metastatic disease.[18] Notably, this critical component of the clinical examination is often overlooked by clinicians, even in anatomic locations at higher risk for metastasis.[19]

Risk Stratification

The 2022 version of the National Comprehensive Cancer Network (NCCN) stratifies cSCCs into low-risk, high-risk, and very high-risk for the purpose of guiding the appropriate choice of therapeutic intervention and surveillance[20]; importantly, these guidelines do not suggest prognostic information, in contrast to the American Joint Committee on Cancer Staging Manual, 8th Edition cSCC staging system (AJCC8) and the Brigham and Women's Hospital (BWH) T staging system. The NCCN includes key features identifiable by clinical examination (location, size, clinical border), patient history (primary/recurrent tumor status, immunosuppression, prior radiation therapy, chronic inflammatory skin disease, rapid growth, neurologic symptoms), and histopathology (tumor differentiation, aggressive histologic features, depth, level of invasion, PNI, LVI) (**Table 1**).[20]

Prognostic Staging

The two most widely used prognostic staging systems for cSCC are BWH and the AJCC8 staging systems, both of which categorize tumors by the preoperative size of the tumor and the presence of other key prognostic risk factors (**Table 2**).[17] In the AJCC8 system, T1 and T2 are based solely on tumor diameter. Only one risk factor—a diameter of 4 cm, PNI, tumor thickness greater than 6 mm, invasion deep into the subcutaneous fat, or minor bone erosion—is required to progress to AJCC8 T3. AJCC8 T4 tumors have more

significant bone involvement. In contrast, the risk factors for the BWH system include poorly differentiated histology, depth of invasion beyond subcutaneous fat, and large-caliber nerve invasion (LCNI), defined as nerves measuring ≥ 0.1 mm in caliber.[12] Low-stage tumors have ≤ 1 risk factor, whereas BWH T2b tumors have 2 to 3 high-risk factors. BWH T3 tumors either have bone invasion or all 4 high-risk factors.

A number of studies has been published comparing the two staging systems. Validated in both retrospective cohorts as well as in external independent systematic literature reviews,[21,22] the BWH cSCC staging system outperforms the AJCC8 system in terms of prognostic tumor risk stratification.[17,23] Importantly, in contrast to the AJCC8 system, which demonstrates similar rates of poor outcomes between T2 and T3 tumors, the BWH system demonstrates higher specificity (93%) and positive predictive value (30%) for identifying cases at risk for metastasis or death, thus minimizing the inappropriate upstaging of low-risk disease.[17] Furthermore, in a nested case-control study, the BWH system similarly outperformed AJCC8, showing increased risk of metastatic disease with increasing stage; in this population-based study, the BWH system estimated odds ratios for metastasis were 4.6 [95% CI (2.23–9.49)] and 21.3 [95% CI (6.07–74.88)] for the T2a and T2b categories, respectively.[24] These findings were further corroborated in the largest external validation to date; the BWH system demonstrated the highest specificity [92.8%, 95% CI (90.8%–94.3%)] and positive predictive value [13.2%, 95% CI (10.6%–16.2%)] of the existing staging systems in a population-based nationwide cohort study.[25]

Published studies have attempted to further refine the prognostic ability of both staging systems. Although the majority of poor outcomes occur in BWH T2b/T3 tumors, almost a third of nodal metastases occur in BWH T2a tumors.[17] A recent retrospective multi-institutional cohort study has shown that BWH T2a tumors with 1 major criterion (ie, primary tumor diameter ≥ 40 mm, invasion depth beyond subcutaneous fat, poor differentiation, or LCNI) and ≥ 1 minor criterion (ie, invasion depth in subcutaneous fat, moderate differentiation, small-caliber PNI, or LVI) are thrice more likely to lead to a poor outcome compared with those that do not meet these criteria.[26] Similarly, the Salamanca refinement further stratifies the relatively heterogeneous AJCC8 T3 category on the basis of the presence of PNI, invasion beyond the subcutaneous fat, or ≥ 3 AJCC8 risk factors combined; in a retrospective cohort of 196 primary head and neck cSCCs, 28.8% of

Table 1
NCCN risk stratification to determine treatment options and surveillance for local cutaneous squamous cell carcinoma

Risk Groups	Low Risk	High Risk	Very High Risk
Clinical Features			
Location/Size	Trunk, extremities ≤ 2 cm	Trunk, extremities >2 cm–≤4 cm Head, neck, hands, feet, pretibia, anogenital (any size)	>4 cm (any location)
Borders	Well defined	Poorly defined	
Primary vs. recurrent	Primary	Recurrent	
Immunosuppression	No	Yes	
Site of prior radiotherapy or chronic inflammatory process	No	Yes	
Rapidly growing tumor	No	Yes	
Neurologic symptoms	No	Yes	
Histopathology			
Degree of differentiation	Well or moderately differentiated		Poorly differentiated
Histologic features [acantholytic (adenoid), adenosquamous, or metaplastic (carcinosarcomatous)] subtypes	No	Yes	Desmoplastic
Thickness or level of invasion	≤6 mm and no invasion beyond subcutaneous fat		>6 mm or invasion beyond subcutaneous fat
Perineural involvement	No	Yes	Tumor cells within the nerve sheath of a nerve lying deeper than the dermis or measuring ≥0.1 mm
Lymphovascular involvement	No	No	Yes

disease-specific poor outcomes occurred in the low-risk T3a category, in contrast to 71.2% in the high-risk T3b/T3c categories.[27] In addition to further intracategory risk stratification based on clinical and histopathologic features, genetic profiling of cSCC may also represent an important future avenue to identify tumors at the highest risk of poor outcomes.

Baseline Radiologic Imaging

There are currently no consensus guidelines that specify which cSCC tumors should undergo routine radiologic imaging at the time of diagnosis or following treatment. However, recent data support the role of imaging in mitigating the incidence of poor outcomes in high-risk diseases. In a retrospective analysis, among a cohort of 83 patients with high-risk cSCC that underwent either structural and/or functional baseline or surveillance imaging, 30% of cases imaged demonstrated metastatic disease, 69% of which was not detected on physical examination alone; these positive findings were most often discovered during the first two years of post-treatment surveillance.[28] Furthermore, a retrospective analysis of 108 BWH T2b/T3 cSCCs showed that tumors that did not undergo imaging at the time of diagnosis were twice as likely to develop a poor outcome (ie, local recurrence, nodal metastasis, or death from disease) compared with those that did receive imaging.[29] This risk difference was

Table 2
AJCC8 and BWH T staging systems

AJCC 8th Edition

T1	<2 cm in greatest diameter
T2	≥2 cm, but <4 cm in greatest diameter
T3	Tumor ≥4 cm in greatest diameter or minor bone invasion or perineural invasion or deep invasion[a]
T4a	Tumor with gross cortical bone and/or marrow invasion
T4b	Tumor with skull bone invasion and/or skull base foramen involvement

BWH

T1	0 high-risk factors[b]
T2a	1 high-risk factors
T2b	2–3 high-risk factors
T3	4 high-risk factors or bone invasion

[a] Deep invasion defined as invasion beyond the subcutaneous far or >6 mm (as measured from the granular layer of adjacent normal epidermis to the base of the tumor), perineural invasion defined as tumor cells in the nerve sheath of a nerve lying deeper than the dermis or measuring 0.1 mm or larger in caliber or presenting with clinical or radiographic involvement of named nerves without skull base invasion or transgression.
[b] BWH high-risk factors include tumor diameter ≥2 cm, poorly differentiated histology, perineural invasion of nerves ≥0.1 mm in caliber, or tumor invasion beyond subcutaneous fat (excluding bone invasion, which upgrades tumor to BWH stage T3).

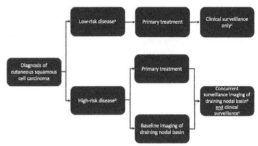

Fig. 1. Baseline and surveillance diagnostic imaging algorithm for local cSCC. [a]Low-risk disease: BWH stage T1 or T2a tumors. [b]High-risk disease: BWH stage T2b or T3 tumors, tumors with extensive PNI, recurrent tumors, and/or in immunocompromised patients with a history of aggressive tumor formation. [c]For low-risk patients: every 6 months for 2 years, then every 6–12 months for 3 years, then annually for life. For high-risk patients: every 3–6 months for 2 years, then every 6–12 months for 3 years, then annually for life. For very high-risk patients: every 3–6 months for 2 years, then every 6 months for 3 years, then every 6–12 months for life. [d]Every 4–6 months for 3 years after primary treatment of the tumor.

attributed to earlier identification and more proactive management of local and metastatic disease, which has been previously shown to impact outcomes.[30] On the basis of imaging findings, a change in treatment was made in 33% of cases; among these, a modification in surgical approach was made in 56% of cases, chemotherapy was added in 25%, and radiation was added in 69%.[29]

A recommended algorithm outlining the use of diagnostic imaging for local cSCC is shown in **Fig. 1**. When there is clinical concern for deep structural involvement of underlying tissue deep to the adipose, such as fascia, muscle, bone, and/or nerves, or when there is a higher risk of metastatic spread, baseline imaging is an important adjunct to clinical examination in BWH T2b/T3 tumors. In addition, concern for involvement of underlying complex structures (such as the parotid or orbital bone) should also prompt imaging as a component of preoperative planning. MRI delineates bone erosion and marrow involvement

and provides superior resolution for defining the extent of soft tissue disease, including PNI. Symptoms that prompt clinical concern for the involvement of named nerves—such as facial nerve motor deficits—should prompt further characterization by MRI; imaging-positive patients have been shown to have worse survival, warranting more aggressive adjuvant therapy.[31,32] In contrast, other tumors with incidental or large-caliber PNI alone do not necessarily require MRI. The authors also recommend that BWH T2b/T3 tumors undergo baseline computed tomography (CT) with contrast for nodal staging; alternatively, MRI or PET may be considered in patients with documented contrast media reactions or allergies.

Given the risk of metastasis after treatment, repeat surveillance scans that encompass the draining nodal basin should be considered for BWH T2b/T3 tumors. The authors performed imaging every 3 to 6 months for 2 to 3 years, depending on tumor and patient risk factors. Although CT, PET/CT, and ultrasound (US) may be used to image the nodal basin, there is limited data directly comparing the different modalities in cSCC. In a recent retrospective study of 246 high-risk cSCCs,[18] the US demonstrated superior sensitivity [91%, 95% CI (71%–99%)] in the detection of nodal metastatic disease compared to clinical examination alone [50%, 95% CI (28%–72%)] and may facilitate the earlier detection of subclinical disease.[28] PET/CT can be used in patients who have clinical concerns about nodal or distant metastatic disease; in a small, five-patient series, this modality demonstrated high specificity (99.6%, 95% CI [98%-100%]) in the detection of cSCC nodal metastases in CLL patients.[33] The comparison of the various imaging modalities is primarily derived from head and neck cancers; a meta-analysis comparing CT, MRI, PET/CT, and US in detecting lymphadenopathy associated with oronasopharyngeal cSCC found no difference in sensitivity between the modalities; specifically, the pooled sensitivity estimates were 52% [95% (CI) 39%–65%], 65% [95% (CI) 34%–87%] 66% [95% (CI) 47%–80%] and 66% [95% (CI) 45%–77%], respectively, for CT, MRI, PET/CT, and US.[34]

Ultimately, owing to the lack of coherent consensus guidelines for imaging in cSCC, the choice of diagnostic modality is case dependent and varies depending on several intrinsic factors of the modality. CT with intravenous contrast is widely accessible and clearly delineates primary tumor margins and abnormal LN; it is the primary imaging examination for the staging and restaging of most cancers in the head and neck.[35] Although PET/CT is more expensive and less widely available than CT, its sensitivity for the detection of local residual or recurrent nasopharyngeal carcinoma (95%) was shown to be significantly higher than CT (76%) ($P < 0.001$) and MRI (78%) ($P < 0.001$) in a systematic review.[36] US is low-cost, widely available, and does not expose patients to ionizing radiation; however, image quality and the identification of abnormalities are highly dependent on the clinician and available equipment.[35] Finally, although MRI with gadolinium-based contrast provides exceptional characterization of soft tissue, including PNI, the modality may be unavailable in many geographic locations and is highly dependent on the ability of local radiologists modify the scanner protocols to optimize the resolution for head and neck imaging.[35] Regardless of the modality chosen, any radiologic findings concerning for metastatic lymphadenopathy should be confirmed with biopsy via core biopsy, fine needle aspiration, or surgical excision.

Management of Squamous Cell Carcinoma in Situ

In patients with SCC in situ (SCCIS) (full thickness epidermal atypia without dermal invasion), nonsurgical superficial destructive modalities are often prioritized. Although standard excision and MMS have the lowest post-treatment recurrence rates,[37,38] treatment with a combination of 5-fluorouracil (5-FU)/calcipotriene,[39] cryotherapy,[40,41] 5-FU monotherapy,[42] imiquimod,[43] or photodynamic therapy (PDT)[42,44] also has a high response rate.[45] Moreover, a trial of less invasive therapy does not preclude subsequent surgery should the lesion persist or recur.

The authors most frequently recommend combination treatment with topical 5% 5-FU and 0.005% calcipotriene for the treatment of cSCCIS. Although this formulation has not been studied for this indication, it likely has similar efficacy to 5-FU monotherapy but with a shorter treatment course that may improve patient compliance. The synergistic effect elicited through the induction of CD4+ T cells results in a marked reduction in actinic damage compared with placebo (87.8% vs 26.3%, $P < 0.0001$).[39] The combination treatment may also be associated with a reduced long-term risk of developing subsequent cSCC. In a blinded prospective cohort study of 86 subjects of a randomized double-blind clinical trial, those treated with topical 5-FU/calcipotriene developed significantly fewer cSCC on the treated face and scalp within three years compared with control subjects [7% vs 28%, hazard ratio (HR) 0.215, 95% CI (0.048–0.972), $P = 0.032$].[46] In the authors' experience, patients typically achieve an optimal treatment response after treating twice daily for 4 days (head and neck) or for 10 days (trunk and extremities).

Management of Low-Risk Invasive Cutaneous Squamous Cell Carcinoma

Surgical removal is the primary first-line treatment for most low-risk invasive cSCC. Depending on the tumor location and histology, this can be achieved with either a standard excision or MMS. A circumferential clinical margin of 4 mm to 6 mm with depth to mid-adipose is advised for standard excisions. A 6 mm margin is indicated if a standard excision is utilized for cSCCs that have any of the following characteristics: ≥2 cm in diameter, on a high-risk location (lips, nose, eyelids, ears, scalp), with high histologic grade, and/or with invasion into subcutaneous tissue[14]; in these cases, the defect should either be reconstructed primarily or delayed until histologic confirmation of negative margins. Standard excision results in a clear surgical margin in approximately 95% of low-risk tumors.[14,47] Positive histologic margins should be managed with re-excision or MMS.

MMS is indicated for cSCC located on anatomic locations in which surgical margins would result in significant functional and/or cosmetic compromise (head, neck, hands, feet, lower legs, genitals, and peri-areolar skin) or those arising in immunosuppressed patients.[48] Furthermore, MMS or other forms of surgery with complete circumferential peripheral and deep margin assessment are indicated in higher-risk tumors that are large, recurrent, or with aggressive features.[48,49] MMS confers the specific advantage of the ability to assess 100% of the peripheral and deep margins intraoperatively; in contrast, only 1% to 2% of the specimen margins are evaluated to assess for complete tumor extirpation in standard excisions.[50] When used appropriately, MMS is associated with decreased reconstruction complexity, reduced risk of positive histologic margins, and lower cost when compared with standard excision.[51] The specific indications, techniques, and outcomes associated with MMS are discussed in detail in a dedicated review article in this volume.

Although there is some observational data that supports the use of electrodessication and curettage (ED&C) in dermally invasive cSCC,[52] this intervention should be reserved for in situ disease given the lack of histologic margin control and inferior cosmetic outcomes compared with surgery.[53] ED&C is contraindicated in tumors on the central midface, terminal hair-bearing areas, or those associated with recurrent disease, high-risk features, and/or poorly defined deep or superficial clinical margins.

Management of High-Risk Invasive Cutaneous Squamous Cell Carcinoma

Multidisciplinary management is essential to the management of high-risk cSCCs and should include representation from dermatology, surgical oncology/head and neck surgery, radiation oncology, medical oncology, and nursing. Complete surgical removal is the gold standard for the treatment of high-risk cSCC. In contrast to low-risk invasive cSCC, complete margin assessment is imperative, and therefore, MMS or other forms of peripheral and deep en face margin assessment are the preferred surgical modality per the NCCN guidelines.[20] In large tumors with deep invasion or with extensive LVI or PNI, MMS can be utilized to demarcate the peripheral superficial margin and identify areas of deep tumor involvement before further resection in an operating room. If this is not feasible, then WLE with en face processing to ensure complete margin assessment can be performed, but reconstruction should be delayed pending clear histologic margins.[54]

There are no consensus indications for adjuvant radiation therapy (ART) in the setting of negative postsurgical margins due to a lack of long-term prospective data. Consequently, practice patterns are highly variable. The NCCN endorses ART after surgical excision of cSCC to reduce the risk of tumor recurrence in cases of extensive PNI or large nerve involvement.[20,55,56] Clinical data is limited on the benefits of ART. A retrospective analysis demonstrated improved overall survival for a cohort of cSCCs of the head and neck treated with surgery that received ART [HR, 0.59; 95% CI (0.38–0.90)], with additional benefit to those with PNI [HR, 0.44; 95% CI (0.24–0.86)].[57] A study from two academic centers of ART following clear margin surgery found half the rate of locoregional recurrence in BWH T2b/T3 tumors treated with ART compared with surgery monotherapy (unpublished data). The decision to recommend ART depends on tumor risk as well as patient factors; therefore, a multidisciplinary evaluation should be considered for high-stage tumors for this purpose. Prospective studies are needed to further elucidate which patients are most likely to benefit from ART.

Chemosensitizers, such as cisplatin or cetuximab, can be added to ART regimens to augment the effects; however, data in cSCC is limited. A retrospective cohort study of patients with cSCC of the head and neck demonstrated that adjuvant chemoradiation with a platinum agent was associated with greater median recurrence-free survival that ART alone (40.3 months vs 15.4 months); however, no difference in overall survival was found.[58] Moreover, the optimal chemosensitization agent and regimen have not been defined in cSCC. In a small series of 23 patients that underwent cetuximab or cisplatin chemoradiation for locally advanced cSCC, no significant differences in 2-year disease-free survival (50% vs 30%, $P = 0.25$), nor overall survival (73% vs 40%, $P = 0.32$) were seen, respectively.[59] Additional prospective data is needed to identify patients that will most benefit from this treatment approach.

The appropriate role of sentinel lymph node biopsy (SLNB) in the management of cSCC is also unclear. Foremost, there is a lack of a clear definition of which patients are most likely to benefit from the procedure. Limited evidence suggests that the presence of high-risk disease factors (tumor diameter ≥ 2 cm, tumor depth >6 mm, invasion below subcutaneous fat, PNI of nerves with a diameter ≥ 0.1 mm, moderate or poor histologic differentiation, LVI, immunosuppression) may predict SLNB positivity.[60] Corroborating these findings, in a recent retrospective cohort of 58 patients in whom lymphoscintigraphy was performed and a sentinel node identified, 4 (6.9%) had a positive SLNB; all 4 of the patients had BWH T2b tumors, and 3 of them were immunosuppressed.[61] A separate systematic review of studies of patients with cSCC who underwent SLNB demonstrated a 29.8% positivity rate among BWH T2b tumors.[62] Of note, a retrospective review of 53 patients who were diagnosed with high-risk cSCC of the head and neck that underwent WLE and SLNB showed a false omission rate of 7.1% [95% CI (2%–19%)][63]; this may be in part because of the large size of many high-risk cSCC and different lymphatic draining patterns compared with melanoma, in which SLNB has a clearer role. The prognostic significance of positive SLNB findings is not definitively established. A systematic review of the available literature showed that relapse-free survival and overall survival were not affected by sentinel SLN status.[64]

There is no standard of care regarding the use of immunotherapy in the adjuvant or neoadjuvant setting for cSCC. In a pilot phase II clinical trial, 20 subjects with locoregionally advanced, resectable cSCC of the head and neck were treated with neoadjuvant cemiplimab; 14 [70%, 95% CI (45.7%–88.1%)] demonstrated a complete (no viable tumor remaining) or major ($\leq$10% viable tumor) pathologic response in the post-treatment surgical specimens.[65] In the same study, the 12-month disease-free survival and overall survival rates were 89.5% [95% CI (76.7%–100%)] and 95% [95% CI (85.9%–100%)], respectively.[65] Data from a larger phase II multi-institutional study should be available later this year. Other systemic agents are not used in the neoadjuvant setting.

Post-Treatment Follow-up

The diagnosis of a patient's first cSCC may often herald the development of new primary tumors; regardless of tumor stage, the 5-year probability of subsequent nonmelanoma skin cancer after a diagnosis of a first is 40.7% [95% CI (36.5%–45.2%)], and after a second the probability is 82.0% [95% CI (80.2%–83.7%)].[66] Of note, up to 80% of recurrences or metastases manifest within 2 years after treatment, and approximately 95% occur within 5 years.[15] The 2-year post-treatment window, therefore, constitutes the most crucial time for follow-up of high-stage tumors. For low-risk cSCC, patients should undergo routine skin surveillance every 6 to 12 months. Patients with a history of a high-stage cSCC should undergo more frequent clinical examinations every 3 to 6 months for the first 2 to 3 years after diagnosis. As previously discussed, diagnostic imaging surveillance should be considered for appropriate patients every 6 months for 2 to 3 years.

Skin Cancer Risk Reduction and Prophylaxis

The diagnosis of a patient's first cSCC is a risk factor for the development of subsequent tumors.[66] Consequently, in addition to regular in-office surveillance and screening, clinicians must advocate for lifestyle modifications that reduce the incidence of further disease. In addition to counseling patients on the importance of at-home self-examinations, behaviors to reduce the damaging exposure of ultraviolet light—including the use of high sun protection factor (SPF) sunscreen,[67] ultraviolet protection factor (UPF) protective clothing,[68] and the avoidance of peak exposure hours—should be emphasized.

A multitude of oral and topical forms of skin cancer prophylaxis have been suggested with varying levels of evidence.[16] Oral nicotinamide is an inexpensive and widely available over-the-counter vitamin that has been shown to reduce the incidence of subsequent nonmelanoma skin cancers by 20% to 30%.[69] Acitretin is another oral chemo-preventative agent that is associated with a 54% reduction in the incidence of cSCC in renal transplant patients.[70] However, excessively high costs, the need for frequent laboratory monitoring (complete blood count, liver function tests, and lipid panel), and side effects[71] (headaches, myalgias, and hyperlipidemia[72]) are common causes of withdrawal from treatment that likely limit its widespread adoption.[70] However, this therapy should be considered for patients who have developed 3 to 5 new cSCCs annually or have a history of a high-risk cSCC.

SUMMARY

The rising incidence of cSCC constitutes a public health crisis. Although most cases of cSCC are cured with surgical excision alone, the high-risk disease requires multidisciplinary management, encompassing complete tumor staging, possible multimodal therapy, appropriate use of clinical and radiologic surveillance, and the encouragement of lifestyle modifications that reduce the risk of future disease. Promising avenues for future prospective research include the further optimization of existing cSCC staging systems and the characterization of the patient populations most likely to benefit from adjuvant therapy.

FUNDING/SUPPORT

None.

ROLE OF THE FUNDER/SPONSOR

The funding sources had no role in the design and conduct of the study; collection, management, analysis, and interpretation of the data; preparation, review, or approval of the manuscript; and decision to submit the manuscript for publication.

CLINICS CARE POINTS

- High-risk cSCC requires a coordinated, multidisciplinary treatment approach to mitigate the risk of poor outcomes.
- Radiologic surveillance plays an important role in the postoperative follow-up of high-risk tumors.
- Oral skin cancer prophylaxis, such as nicotinamide and acitretin, should be considered in patients who have a history of multiple cSCC and in those at risk of developing a high-risk tumor.

DISCLOSURE

None.

REFERENCES

1. Karia PS, Han J, Schmults CD. Cutaneous squamous cell carcinoma: estimated incidence of disease, nodal metastasis, and deaths from disease in the United States, 2012. J Am Acad Dermatol 2013;68(6):957–66.
2. D'Orazio J, Jarrett S, Amaro-Ortiz A, et al. UV radiation and the skin. Int J Mol Sci 2013;14(6):12222–48.
3. Demers AA, Nugent Z, Mihalcioiu C, et al. Trends of nonmelanoma skin cancer from 1960 through 2000 in a Canadian population. J Am Acad Dermatol 2005;53(2):320–8.
4. Rogers HW, Weinstock MA, Feldman SR, et al. Incidence Estimate of Nonmelanoma Skin Cancer (Keratinocyte Carcinomas) in the U.S. Population, 2012. JAMA Dermatol 2015;151(10):1081–6.
5. Mudigonda T, Levender MM, O'Neill JL, et al. Incidence, risk factors, and preventative management of skin cancers in organ transplant recipients: a review of single- and multicenter retrospective studies from 2006 to 2010. Dermatol Surg 2013;39(3 Pt 1):345–64.
6. Scott JF, Brough KR, Grigoryan KV, et al. Risk Factors for Keratinocyte Carcinoma in Recipients of Allogeneic Hematopoietic Cell Transplants. JAMA Dermatol 2020;156(6):631–9.
7. O'Reilly Zwald F, Brown M. Skin cancer in solid organ transplant recipients: advances in therapy and management: part I. Epidemiology of skin cancer in solid organ transplant recipients. J Am Acad Dermatol 2011;65(2):253–61.
8. Krathen MS, Gottlieb AB, Mease PJ. Pharmacologic immunomodulation and cutaneous malignancy in rheumatoid arthritis, psoriasis, and psoriatic arthritis. J Rheumatol 2010;37(11):2205–15.
9. Hagen JW, Pugliano-Mauro MA. Nonmelanoma Skin Cancer Risk in Patients With Inflammatory Bowel Disease Undergoing Thiopurine Therapy: A Systematic Review of the Literature. Dermatol Surg 2018;44(4):469–80.
10. Lai M, Pampena R, Cornacchia L, et al. Cutaneous squamous cell carcinoma in patients with chronic lymphocytic leukemia: a systematic review of the literature. Int J Dermatol 2021. https://doi.org/10.1111/ijd.15813.
11. Brewer JD, Shanafelt TD, Khezri F, et al. Increased incidence and recurrence rates of nonmelanoma skin cancer in patients with non-Hodgkin lymphoma: a Rochester Epidemiology Project population-based study in Minnesota. J Am Acad Dermatol 2015;72(2):302–9.
12. Jambusaria-Pahlajani A, Kanetsky PA, Karia PS, et al. Evaluation of AJCC tumor staging for cutaneous squamous cell carcinoma and a proposed alternative tumor staging system. JAMA Dermatol 2013;149(4):402–10.
13. Brougham ND, Dennett ER, Cameron R, et al. The incidence of metastasis from cutaneous squamous cell carcinoma and the impact of its risk factors. J Surg Oncol 2012;106(7):811–5.
14. Brodland DG, Zitelli JA. Surgical margins for excision of primary cutaneous squamous cell carcinoma. J Am Acad Dermatol 1992;27(2 Pt 1):241–8. https://doi.org/10.1016/0190-9622(92)70178-i.
15. Rowe DE, Carroll RJ, Day CL Jr. Prognostic factors for local recurrence, metastasis, and survival rates in squamous cell carcinoma of the skin, ear, and lip. Implications for treatment modality selection. J Am Acad Dermatol 1992;26(6):976–90. https://doi.org/10.1016/0190-9622(92)70144-5.
16. Work G, Invited R, Kim JYS, et al. Guidelines of care for the management of cutaneous squamous cell carcinoma. J Am Acad Dermatol 2018;78(3):560–78. https://doi.org/10.1016/j.jaad.2017.10.007.
17. Ruiz ES, Karia PS, Besaw R, et al. Performance of the American Joint Committee on Cancer Staging Manual, 8th Edition vs the Brigham and Women's Hospital Tumor Classification System for Cutaneous Squamous Cell Carcinoma. JAMA Dermatol 2019;155(7):819–25.
18. Tokez S, Koekelkoren FHJ, Baatenburg de Jong RJ, et al. Assessment of the Diagnostic Accuracy of Baseline Clinical Examination and Ultrasonographic Imaging for the Detection of Lymph Node Metastasis in Patients With High-Risk Cutaneous Squamous Cell Carcinoma of the Head and Neck. JAMA Dermatol 2021. https://doi.org/10.1001/jamadermatol.2021.4990.
19. Eickstaedt JB, Fancher W, Havighurst T, et al. Lack of documentation of lymph node examination in patients with squamous cell carcinoma of the lower lip. Arch Dermatol Res 2021. https://doi.org/10.1007/s00403-021-02281-4.
20. National Comprehensive Cancer Network. Squamous Cell Skin Cancer (Version 1.2022). Available

at: https://www.nccn.org/professionals/physician_gls/pdf/squamous.pdf. Accessed January 2, 2022.

21. Karia PS, Jambusaria-Pahlajani A, Harrington DP, et al. Evaluation of American Joint Committee on Cancer, International Union Against Cancer, and Brigham and Women's Hospital tumor staging for cutaneous squamous cell carcinoma. J Clin Oncol 2014;32(4):327–34. https://doi.org/10.1200/JCO.2012.48.5326.

22. Schmitt AR, Brewer JD, Bordeaux JS, et al. Staging for cutaneous squamous cell carcinoma as a predictor of sentinel lymph node biopsy results: meta-analysis of American Joint Committee on Cancer criteria and a proposed alternative system. JAMA Dermatol 2014;150(1):19–24. https://doi.org/10.1001/jamadermatol.2013.6675.

23. Karia PS, Morgan FC, Califano JA, et al. Comparison of Tumor Classifications for Cutaneous Squamous Cell Carcinoma of the Head and Neck in the 7th vs 8th Edition of the AJCC Cancer Staging Manual. JAMA Dermatol 2018;154(2):175–81. https://doi.org/10.1001/jamadermatol.2017.3960.

24. Roscher I, Falk RS, Vos L, et al. Validating 4 Staging Systems for Cutaneous Squamous Cell Carcinoma Using Population-Based Data: A Nested Case-Control Study. JAMA Dermatol 2018;154(4):428–34. https://doi.org/10.1001/jamadermatol.2017.6428.

25. Venables ZC, Tokez S, Hollestein LM, et al. Validation of Four Cutaneous Squamous Cell Carcinoma Staging Systems Using Nationwide Data. Br J Dermatol 2021. https://doi.org/10.1111/bjd.20909.

26. Gupta N, Weitzman RE, Murad F, et al. Identifying Brigham and Women's Hospital stage T2a cutaneous squamous cell carcinomas at risk of poor outcomes. J Am Acad Dermatol 2021. https://doi.org/10.1016/j.jaad.2021.11.046.

27. Puebla-Tornero L, Corchete-Sanchez LA, Conde-Ferreiros A, et al. Performance of Salamanca refinement of the T3-AJCC8 versus the Brigham and Women's Hospital and Tubingen alternative staging systems for high-risk cutaneous squamous cell carcinoma. J Am Acad Dermatol 2021;84(4):938–45. https://doi.org/10.1016/j.jaad.2020.12.020.

28. Maher JM, Schmults CD, Murad F, et al. Detection of subclinical disease with baseline and surveillance imaging in high-risk cutaneous squamous cell carcinomas. J Am Acad Dermatol 2020;82(4):920–6. https://doi.org/10.1016/j.jaad.2019.10.067.

29. Ruiz ES, Karia PS, Morgan FC, et al. The positive impact of radiologic imaging on high-stage cutaneous squamous cell carcinoma management. J Am Acad Dermatol 2017;76(2):217–25. https://doi.org/10.1016/j.jaad.2016.08.051.

30. Oddone N, Morgan GJ, Palme CE, et al. Metastatic cutaneous squamous cell carcinoma of the head and neck: the Immunosuppression, Treatment, Extranodal spread, and Margin status (ITEM) prognostic score to predict outcome and the need to improve survival. Cancer 2009;115(9):1883–91. https://doi.org/10.1002/cncr.24208.

31. Williams LS, Mancuso AA, Mendenhall WM. Perineural spread of cutaneous squamous and basal cell carcinoma: CT and MR detection and its impact on patient management and prognosis. Int J Radiat Oncol Biol Phys 2001;49(4):1061–9. https://doi.org/10.1016/s0360-3016(00)01407-3.

32. Balamucki CJ, DeJesus R, Galloway TJ, et al. Impact of radiographic findings on for prognosis skin cancer with perineural invasion. Am J Clin Oncol 2015;38(3):248–51. https://doi.org/10.1097/COC.0b013e3182940ddf.

33. Tomaszewski JM, Lau E, Corry J. Utility of positron emission tomography/computed tomography for nodal staging of cutaneous squamous cell carcinoma in patients with chronic lymphocytic leukemia. Am J Otolaryngol 2014;35(1):66–9. https://doi.org/10.1016/j.amjoto.2013.08.014.

34. Liao LJ, Lo WC, Hsu WL, et al. Detection of cervical lymph node metastasis in head and neck cancer patients with clinically N0 neck-a meta-analysis comparing different imaging modalities. BMC Cancer 2012;12:236. https://doi.org/10.1186/1471-2407-12-236.

35. Guenette JP. Radiologic Evaluation of the Head and Neck Cancer Patient. Hematol Oncol Clin North Am 2021;35(5):863–73. https://doi.org/10.1016/j.hoc.2021.05.001.

36. Liu T, Xu W, Yan WL, et al. MRI for diagnosis of local residual or recurrent nasopharyngeal carcinoma, which one is the best? A systematic review. Radiother Oncol 2007;85(3):327–35. https://doi.org/10.1016/j.radonc.2007.11.002.

37. Overmark M, Koskenmies S, Pitkanen S. A Retrospective Study of Treatment of Squamous Cell Carcinoma In situ. Acta Derm Venereol 2016;96(1):64–7. https://doi.org/10.2340/00015555-2175.

38. Hansen JP, Drake AL, Walling HW. Bowen's Disease: a four-year retrospective review of epidemiology and treatment at a university center. Dermatol Surg 2008;34(7):878–83. https://doi.org/10.1111/j.1524-4725.2008.34172.x.

39. Cunningham TJ, Tabacchi M, Eliane JP, et al. Randomized trial of calcipotriol combined with 5-fluorouracil for skin cancer precursor immunotherapy. J Clin Invest 2017;127(1):106–16. https://doi.org/10.1172/JCI89820.

40. Kuflik EG, Gage AA. The five-year cure rate achieved by cryosurgery for skin cancer. J Am Acad Dermatol 1991;24(6 Pt 1):1002–4. https://doi.org/10.1016/0190-9622(91)70160-4.

41. Holt PJ. Cryotherapy for skin cancer: results over a 5-year period using liquid nitrogen spray

cryosurgery. Br J Dermatol 1988;119(2):231–40. https://doi.org/10.1111/j.1365-2133.1988.tb03205.x.

42. Salim A, Leman JA, McColl JH, et al. Randomized comparison of photodynamic therapy with topical 5-fluorouracil in Bowen's disease. Br J Dermatol 2003;148(3):539–43. https://doi.org/10.1046/j.1365-2133.2003.05033.x.

43. Patel GK, Goodwin R, Chawla M, et al. Imiquimod 5% cream monotherapy for cutaneous squamous cell carcinoma in situ (Bowen's disease): a randomized, double-blind, placebo-controlled trial. J Am Acad Dermatol 2006;54(6):1025–32. https://doi.org/10.1016/j.jaad.2006.01.055.

44. Fink-Puches R, Soyer HP, Hofer A, et al. Long-term follow-up and histological changes of superficial nonmelanoma skin cancers treated with topical delta-aminolevulinic acid photodynamic therapy. Arch Dermatol 1998;134(7):821–6. https://doi.org/10.1001/archderm.134.7.821.

45. Cornejo CM, Jambusaria-Pahlajani A, Willenbrink TJ, et al. Field cancerization: Treatment. J Am Acad Dermatol 2020;83(3):719–30. https://doi.org/10.1016/j.jaad.2020.03.127.

46. Rosenberg AR, Tabacchi M, Ngo KH, et al. Skin cancer precursor immunotherapy for squamous cell carcinoma prevention. JCI Insight 2019;4(6). https://doi.org/10.1172/jci.insight.125476.

47. Lansbury L, Leonardi-Bee J, Perkins W, et al. Bath-Hextall FJ. Interventions for non-metastatic squamous cell carcinoma of the skin. Cochrane Database Syst Rev 2010;(4):CD007869.

48. Ad Hoc Task F, Connolly SM, Baker DR, et al. AAD/ACMS/ASDSA/ASMS 2012 appropriate use criteria for Mohs micrographic surgery: a report of the American Academy of Dermatology, American College of Mohs Surgery, American Society for Dermatologic Surgery Association, and the American Society for Mohs Surgery. J Am Acad Dermatol 2012;67(4):531–50.

49. Stancut E, Melvin OG, Griffin RL, et al. Institutional Adherence to Current Mohs Surgery Appropriate Use Criteria With Reasons for Nonadherence and Recommendations for Future Versions. Dermatol Surg 2022. https://doi.org/10.1097/DSS.0000000000003369.

50. Tolkachjov SN, Brodland DG, Coldiron BM, et al. Understanding Mohs Micrographic Surgery: A Review and Practical Guide for the Nondermatologist. Mayo Clin Proc 2017;92(8):1261–71.

51. Massey PR, Gupta S, Rothstein BE, et al. Total Margin-Controlled Excision is Superior to Standard Excision for Keratinocyte Carcinoma on the Nose: A Veterans Affairs Nested Cohort Study. Ann Surg Onco 2021;28(7):3656–63.

52. Stewart JR, Lang ME, Brewer JD. Efficacy of nonexcisional treatment modalities for superficially invasive and in situ squamous cell carcinoma: A systematic review and meta-analysis. J Am Acad Dermatol 2021. https://doi.org/10.1016/j.jaad.2021.07.067.

53. Galles E, Parvataneni R, Stuart SE, et al. Patient-reported outcomes of electrodessication and curettage for treatment of nonmelanoma skin cancer. J Am Acad Dermatol 2014;71(5):1026–8.

54. Stratigos AJ, Garbe C, Dessinioti C, et al. European interdisciplinary guideline on invasive squamous cell carcinoma of the skin: Part 2. Treatment. Eur J Cancer\ 2020;128:83–102. https://doi.org/10.1016/j.ejca.2020.01.008.

55. Geist DE, Garcia-Moliner M, Fitzek MM, et al. Perineural invasion of cutaneous squamous cell carcinoma and basal cell carcinoma: raising awareness and optimizing management. Dermatol Surg 2008;34(12):1642–51.

56. Jambusaria-Pahlajani A, Miller CJ, Quon H, et al. Surgical monotherapy versus surgery plus adjuvant radiotherapy in high-risk cutaneous squamous cell carcinoma: a systematic review of outcomes. Dermatol Surg 2009;35(4):574–85.

57. Harris BN, Pipkorn P, Nguyen KNB, et al. Association of Adjuvant Radiation Therapy With Survival in Patients With Advanced Cutaneous Squamous Cell Carcinoma of the Head and Neck. JAMA Otolaryngol Head Neck Surg 2019;145(2):153–8.

58. Tanvetyanon T, Padhya T, McCaffrey J, et al. Postoperative concurrent chemotherapy and radiotherapy for high-risk cutaneous squamous cell carcinoma of the head and neck. Head Neck 2015;37(6):840–5.

59. Lu SM, Lien WW. Concurrent Radiotherapy With Cetuximab or Platinum-based Chemotherapy for Locally Advanced Cutaneous Squamous Cell Carcinoma of the Head and Neck. Am J Clin Oncol 2018;41(1):95–9.

60. Tremblay-Abel V, Poulin MA, Blouin MM, et al. Sentinel Lymph Node Biopsy in High-Risk Cutaneous Squamous Cell Carcinoma: Analysis of a Large Size Retrospective Series. Dermatol Surg 2021;47(7):908–13.

61. Pride RLD, Lopez JJ, Brewer JD, et al. Outcomes of Sentinel Lymph Node Biopsy for Primary Cutaneous Squamous Cell Carcinoma of the Head and Neck. Dermatol Surg 2022;48(2):157–61.

62. Tejera-Vaquerizo A, Canueto J, Llombart B, et al. Predictive Value of Sentinel Lymph Node Biopsy in Cutaneous Squamous Cell Carcinoma Based on the AJCC-8 and Brigham and Women's Hospital Staging Criteria. Dermatol Surg 2020;46(7):857–62.

63. Durham AB, Lowe L, Malloy KM, et al. Sentinel Lymph Node Biopsy for Cutaneous Squamous Cell Carcinoma on the Head and Neck. JAMA Otolaryngol Head Neck Surg 2016;142(12):1171–6.

64. Lhote R, Lambert J, Lejeune J, et al. Sentinel Lymph Node Biopsy in Cutaneous Squamous Cell Carcinoma Series of 37 Cases and Systematic Review

of the Literature. Acta Derm Venereol 2018;98(7): 671–6.

65. Ferrarotto R, Amit M, Nagarajan P, et al. Pilot Phase II Trial of Neoadjuvant Immunotherapy in Locoregionally Advanced, Resectable Cutaneous Squamous Cell Carcinoma of the Head and Neck. Clin Cancer Res 2021;27(16):4557–65.

66. Wehner MR, Linos E, Parvataneni R, et al. Timing of subsequent new tumors in patients who present with basal cell carcinoma or cutaneous squamous cell carcinoma. JAMA Dermatol 2015;151(4):382–8.

67. Kohli I, Nicholson CL, Williams JD, et al. Greater efficacy of SPF 100+ sunscreen compared with SPF 50+ in sunburn prevention during 5 consecutive days of sunlight exposure: A randomized, double-blind clinical trial. J Am Acad Dermatol 2020;82(4): 869–77.

68. Igoe DP, Amar A, Schouten P, et al. Assessment of Biologically Effective Solar Ultraviolet Exposures for Court Staff and Competitors During a Major Australian Tennis Tournament. Photochem Photobiol 2019;95(6):1461–7.

69. Chen AC, Martin AJ, Choy B, et al. A Phase 3 Randomized Trial of Nicotinamide for Skin-Cancer Chemoprevention. N Engl J Med 2015;373(17):1618–26.

70. Badri O, Schmults CD, Karia PS, et al. Efficacy and Cost Analysis for Acitretin for Basal and Squamous Cell Carcinoma Prophylaxis in Renal Transplant Recipients. Dermatol Surg 2021;47(1):125–6.

71. Chen K, Craig JC, Shumack S. Oral retinoids for the prevention of skin cancers in solid organ transplant recipients: a systematic review of randomized controlled trials. Br J Dermatol 2005;152(3): 518–23.

72. Bavinck JN, Tieben LM, Van der Woude FJ, et al. Prevention of skin cancer and reduction of keratotic skin lesions during acitretin therapy in renal transplant recipients: a double-blind, placebo-controlled study. J Clin Oncol 1995;13(8):1933–8. https://doi. org/10.1200/JCO.1995.13.8.1933.

Basal Cell Carcinoma

Michael S. Heath, MD*, Anna Bar, MD

KEYWORDS

- Basal cell carcinoma • Diagnosis • Treatment • Management • Prevention

KEY POINTS

- Basal cell carcinoma incidence is increasing globally.
- Diagnosis is made using clinical recognition, emerging imaging techniques, and gold standard histopathologic evaluation.
- Surgical management including Mohs micrographic surgery in high-risk tumors is the most effective treatment, although alternatives including radiation, systemic, and topical therapies exist for specific situations.
- Systemic treatments for locally advanced and metastatic basal cell carcinoma include Hedgehog pathway inhibitors, targeted checkpoint therapy, among others.

INTRODUCTION
Epidemiology

Basal cell carcinoma (BCC) is the most common type of cancer in the world. In the United States, the 2012 annual estimated incidence ranged from 2.7 to 4.3 million cases.[1,2] Lifetime risk of developing BCC in the United States is 20% or greater overall, and 30% or greater for whites.[3,4] Age-adjusted BCC incidence rates in the United States have more than doubled during 2 decades.[5] Increasing annual incidence of BCC has additionally been reported globally.[6–9]

PATIENT EVALUATION OVERVIEW
Determining Patient Risk Factors

The probability of developing a BCC varies considerably based on a patient's phenotype, environmental exposures, and genetic predisposition. Many of these risk factors are intertwined by a common pathogenic link, which is exposure and susceptibility to ultraviolet radiation (UVR).

Phenotypic risk factors include male sex, red or blond hair, fair skin, pale eyes, skin that burns and never tans, and higher number of moles.[5,10–12] Multiple studies have shown that those with Fitzpatrick type I or type II skin types have relative risks of developing BCC between 2 and 4.[13–15] Type III skin alone is only a risk factor if the patient additionally has a history of severe sunburns.

Significant exposures that should be part of assessing an individual's risk include higher number of severe or blistering sunburns and higher levels of cumulative UVR, especially if it occurs during childhood or adolescence.[5,10,16] The risk for BCC may be more strongly linked to intermittent sun exposure as compared with squamous cell carcinoma (SCC), which is more heavily influenced by chronic regular sun exposure.[11,15,16] Indoor tanning bed use is a dose-related risk factor, especially for early-onset BCC.[17–19]

Occupational and iatrogenic ionizing radiations are risk factors for the development of BCC.[20] Younger age of radiation therapy (RT) and higher doses both correlate with increasing risk of BCC as well as total number of BCC.[20–22] RT for childhood malignancy such as lymphoma is a significant risk factor for developing BCC. When compared with pediatric patients with cancer who did not undergo RT, patients who received 35 Gy or greater had 40-fold increased risk of BCC.[23] Solid organ transplant and psoralen and ultraviolet A (UVA) are additional iatrogenic risks factors for BCC, although to a lesser extent than SCC.[24,25]

Department of Dermatology, Oregon Health & Science University, 3303 Southwest Bond Avenue CH16D, Portland, OR 97239, USA
* Corresponding author.
E-mail address: heatmi@ohsu.edu

Dermatol Clin 41 (2023) 13–21
https://doi.org/10.1016/j.det.2022.07.005
0733-8635/23/

Clinical Evaluation

Despite the description of more than 26 different BCC subtypes, most tumors can be classified into 4 distinct clinicopathologic subtypes: nodular, superficial, morpheaform, and fibroepithelial (fibroepithelioma of Pinkus).[26] Nodular BCC is the most common subtype, and it presents as a pearly papule with rolled borders and arborizing vessels. Superficial BCC is more common in younger patients and on the trunk.[27,28] Morpheaform BCC have a sclerotic or indurated appearance and are often poorly demarcated. Fibroepithelioma of Pinkus is a rare but unique variant, which can seem as a smooth flat plaque or pedunculated papule on the lower trunk; some debate whether it is a trichoblastoma subtype given its relatively indolent course.

High-Risk Basal Cell Carcinomas

Most BCC have a low risk of recurrence or metastasis and are treated conservatively with destructive procedures or surgery.[29] Both patient and tumor characteristics are used to risk stratify patients to guide management.

The National Comprehensive Cancer Network guidelines have indicated that a BCC should be considered high-risk if any of the factors listed in **Table 1** are present.

Staging of Basal Cell Carcinoma

The American Joint Committee on Cancer (AJCC) eighth edition tumor staging for BCC located on the head and neck include the following[30]:

- T1—Less than 2 cm in greatest diameter
- T2—2 cm or greater but less than 4 cm in greatest diameter
- T3—4 cm or greater in greatest diameter or minor bone invasion or perineural invasion or deep invasion
- T4a—Tumor with gross cortical bone and/or marrow invasion
- T4b—Tumor with skull bone invasion and/or skull base foramen involvement

The Brigham and Women's Hospital (BWH) tumor classification system for BCC was developed as a more specific staging system.[31] BWH prioritized significant risk of metastasis and/or death and determined the following tumor stages:

- T1—Tumor diameter of less than 2 cm or tumor diameter of 2 cm or greater with 0 or 1 risk factor*
- T2—Tumor diameter of 2 cm or greater with 2 or 3 risk factors*

Table 1
National Comprehensive Cancer Network guidelines high-risk basal cell carcinomas [29]

Tumor factors	• ≥2 cm on trunk or extremities • Any size lesion located on head, neck, feet, pretibial leg, or anogenital region • Recurrent tumor • Poorly defined tumor • Perineural involvement • Aggressive histopathologic subtype (infiltrative, micronodular, morpheaform, basosquamous, sclerosing, or carcinosarcomatous differentiation)
Patient factors	• Prior RT to area • Solid organ or hematopoietic transplant • Immune deficiencies (congenital, HIV/AIDS, or autoimmune) • Treatment with immunosuppressive therapies • Patients with cancer on immunotherapies or checkpoint inhibitors

Abbreviations: HIV/AIDS, human immunodeficiency virus (HIV) / acquired immunodeficiency syndrome (AIDS)
Original table using previously published information.

*Risk factors: Tumor diameter of 4 cm or greater, head and neck location, and depth beyond fat.

Within the BWH cohort of high-grade tumors the AJCC eighth edition and BWH tumor staging had equal sensitivity but BWH had higher specificity (92% vs 80%) and higher positive predictive value (24% vs 11%) for recognizing tumors at risk for metastasis and/or death.[31] The risk of metastasis or death in the BWH T1 cohort was 0%, which was significant compared with the 37% risk in the T2 cohort.[31]

Metastatic Basal Cell Carcinoma

Metastatic BCC (mBCC) is exceedingly rare, and unfortunately, not well documented in registries. The most common sites of metastasis in descending order are lymph nodes (LN; 53%), lung (33%), bone (20%), skin/subcutaneous (11%), and liver (4%).[32–35] Average time to death after diagnosis of LN metastasis is 3.6 to 7.3 years, whereas extranodal metastases survival is 8 to 24 months, although advances in therapy likely increase survival.[32,34–36]

There is an estimated 1.9% to 6.5% risk of metastasis and/or death in patients with primary tumors 2 cm or greater in diameter.[34,37] Primary tumors 4 cm or greater are 11.9 times more likely to lead to metastasis and/or death compared with tumors 2 to 3.9 cm in diameter.[34,37] The strongest predictor of metastasis and/or death in primary tumors 2 cm or greater is extension beyond fat, which independently increased the risk by a factor of 28.6.[37] Head and neck locations were nearly 12 times more likely to have metastasis or lead to death.[32,35,37] In patients with BCC 2 cm or greater, the risk of metastasis and death in those with underlying nevoid basal cell carcinoma syndrome (NBCCS) is 50%, and in nonsyndromic patients with prior RT, the risk is 22%.[37]

Noninvasive Diagnostics

Dermoscopy
Dermoscopy is a common clinical tool to aid in the identification of BCC. Some highly predictive BCC features seen with dermoscopy include arborizing vessels, blue and pink stromal hue, translucency, blue/gray ovoid nests, and if pigmented, leaf-like and spoke-wheel structures. Systematic review and meta-analysis of the reported accuracy of dermoscopy for BCC show a pooled sensitivity of 89% to 91% and specificity of 95%.[38] The combination of clinical examination in conjunction with dermoscopy outperforms clinical examination alone, with a sensitivity of 85% compared with 67%.[38] As with any diagnostic test, there are limitations to dermoscopy, most notably the skill level of the user.[38]

Reflectance confocal microscopy
Reflectance confocal microscopy (RCM) focuses a beam of near infrared light at specific target within the skin, which is then reflected through a pinhole, to a highly sensitive detector. Multiple captured points within the tissue are combined to produce high-resolution images of in vivo skin.[39]

RCM requires highly specialized training for accurate diagnosis. Experienced providers using RCM can diagnosis BCC with a sensitivity of 91.7% and specificity of 91.3%.[40] A randomized controlled trial designed in real-world application compared RCM versus punch biopsy in the diagnosis and subtyping of BCC. This trial showed equivalent sensitivity in BCC diagnosis (99%) but RCM had inferior specificity (59% vs 100%) and was less sensitive in detecting aggressive BCC subtypes compared with standard of care punch biopsy (33.3% vs 77.3%).[41] RCM is limited by required training, high cost, and limitations of only viewing the upper dermis.

Optical coherence tomography
Optical coherence tomography (OCT) takes advantage of the differences in optical properties exhibited by structures in the skin. An image is produced by using the summation of refracted infrared light. OCT images have relatively less resolution than RCM but can reach a much greater depth (1.5 mm vs 200 μm). Prospective cohort studies evaluating OCT accuracy of BCC diagnosis with in vivo tissue demonstrated a sensitivity ranging from 79% to 94% and specificity ranging from 85% to 96%.[42–44] OCT has exhibited utility in delineating surgical margins but real-world clinical use is limited by poor resolution, expense, and required training.[45]

BASAL CELL CARCINOMA TREATMENT
Low-Risk Basal Cell Carcinoma Treatment

Although treatments should be individualized, in general low-risk BCC are denoted by the absence of any high-risk features (see **Table 1**).

Curette and electrodesiccation
Curette and electrodesiccation (C&E) involves using a curette to delineate tumor margins and removing tumor down to level of dermis. Electrodessication is then used to destroy residual neoplastic cells. This is traditionally performed with 3 cycles of alternating C&E. Problems include the lack of histopathologic margin assessment; hence, it is recommended only for superficial lesions lacking terminal hair follicles. Treatment efficacy is largely based on observational and retrospective data, which is additionally limited by inadequate follow-up. Reported C&E recurrence rates vary from 4% to 27%.[46–50] If during C&E the clinician reaches subcutaneous tissue, the contrast in tumor and surrounding stroma is lost, and the procedure should be discontinued and substituted for treatment that will provide a surgical margin evaluation.

Standard excision
Low-risk tumors are often treated with excision with 4-mm clinical margins. This standard excision technique has shown recurrence rates less than 5% in low-risk BCC.[47,51,52] In facial BCC, which by location alone are considered high-risk, the recurrence rate at 10 years is 12.2%.[53] Postoperative margin assessment is required. Intraoperative surgical margin assessment should be obtained if surgical closure will require tissue rearrangement or skin graft, due to concern for residual tumor seeding and risk of higher risk recurrence.[29,54]

Table 2
Alternative basal cell carcinoma treatments

Treatment	Dosing	Efficacy	Side Effects
Imiquimod 5% cream	Apply daily 3–5 d per week, for 6 wk[a]	70%–85% clearance in sBCC[55–58]	Local sclerosis, ulceration, vesiculation, flu-like symptoms
5-FU cream	Apply twice daily for 6 wk	64% 5-y clearance rate in sBCC[57,58]	Local crusting, pruritus, edema, pain
Cryosurgery[b]	Two freeze cycles of 25–30 s each, separated by 2–4-min thaw period	Recurrence rates vary from 19% to 39% in prospective trials[59–61]	Poor cosmetic outcomes, ulceration, pain, scarring, pigment changes
PDT	Topical application of photosensitizer (5-ALA or MAL) followed hours after by exposure with blue, red, or broadband light irradiation. Treatment repeated for incomplete response	86.4% complete clearance rate and 10.3% 1-y recurrence rate[62]	Local pain, burning, pruritus, crusting, bleeding

Abbreviations: 5-ALA, 5-aminolevulinic acid; 5-FU, 5-Fluorouracil; MAL, methylaminolevulinic acid; PDT, Photodynamic therapy; sBCC, superficial basal cell carcinoma.
  [a] Frequency dependent on patient tolerability.
  [b] High variability reliant on provider experience and tumor characteristics.

Alternative treatments

Due to lower efficacy, alternative treatments are reserved for extenuating situations when standard of care treatment is not feasible. Treatments are summarized in **Table 2**.

High-Risk Basal Cell Carcinoma Treatment

Mohs micrographic surgery

High-risk BCCs have propensity to extend beyond the clinical margins, penetrate deeper tissues, or are in areas critical to function or cosmesis, where standard excision margins are not possible. For these reasons, Mohs micrographic surgery (MMS) is the most effective treatment because intraoperative complete margin evaluation before reconstruction is required. In the treatment of primary BCC, MMS provides lower 5-year recurrence rates compared with standard excision (1.0% vs 10.1%).[63] Similar benefit is seen when comparing recurrence rates in the treatment of recurrent BCC (5.6% vs 17.4%).[64] **Fig.** 1A demonstrates the initial clinically identified BCC. **Fig.** 1B demonstrates the subclinical extent of the tumor identified on MMS. **Fig.** 1C, D demonstrates the same day surgical repair followed by 6-month follow-up.

Radiation therapy

RT is most often used as an alternative when patient or tumor factors preclude surgical treatment.

Treatments take place over a series of weeks. Randomized controlled studies comparing radiotherapy versus excision show greater than 10-fold higher failure rates and significantly worse cosmetic outcomes in those who received radiation as judged by both clinicians and patients.[65,66]

Postoperative RT is recommended for tumors with either clinical or radiologic perineural extension or following surgical lymphadenectomy for nodal metastasis.[29,67] RT can be considered in the setting of positive surgical margins not amendable to surgery, BCC recurrence, and locally advanced BCC (LaBCC) with bone or muscle infiltration.[67]

Considerations for RT include age due to the risk of long-term sequelae of radiation. Additionally, genetic syndromes that predispose patients to developing skin cancer should avoid RT. A history of connective tissue disease is an additional relative contraindication.

Locally Advanced and Metastatic Basal Cell Carcinoma Treatment

In rare circumstances in which BCC spreads beyond the cure of surgery or RT, systemic treatments are needed. The Hedgehog (HH) pathway is normally quiescent in adulthood but in embryonic development plays a role in cell proliferation and differentiation.[68,69] HH ligands are extracellular signaling molecules that interact with protein

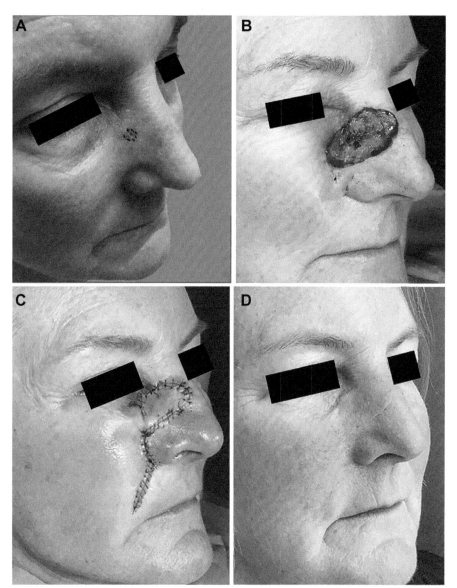

Fig. 1. (A) The initial clinically identified BCC. (B) The subclinical extent of the tumor identified on MMS. (C) Same day reconstruction. (D) Follow up 6 months after surgery.

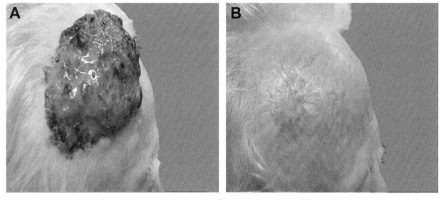

Fig. 2. Shows a LaBCC at initial presentation (A) and after treatment with SMO antagonist (B).

Table 3
Systemic treatments for locally advanced and metastatic basal cell carcinoma

Drug (Class)	LaBCC Response	mBCC Response	Side Effects and Considerations
Vismodegib (selective SMO antagonist)	• 31%–32% complete[a] • 29%–35% partial • 24%–37% stable • 2%–10% progression	• 0%–4% complete • 30%–48% partial • 42%–48% stable • 6%–11% progression	• Muscle spasms • Alopecia • Taste disturbances • Weight loss • Fatigue
Sonidegib (selective SMO inhibitor)	• 3% complete • 54% partial • 42% stable • 1% progression	• 0% complete • 15% partial • 82% stable • 3% progression	• Gastrointestinal disturbance • Embryofetal toxicity Note: Nearly one-third of patient discontinue therapy due to side effect
Cemiplimab (PD-1 inhibitor)	• 6% complete • 25% partial • 49% stable • 22% progression	• 0% complete • 21% partial • 36% stable • 25% progression	• Fatigue • Hypertension • Pruritus • Colitis • Pneumonitis • Endocrinopathy

[a] Patients with NBCCS have improved response (46% with complete response).

patched homolog 1 (PTCH1) receptor. The interaction of HH ligand and PTCH1 receptor results in activation of smoothened (SMO), ultimately leading to the activation of downstream proteins and gene transcription.[69] Abnormal HH signaling is present in 95% of BCC including the loss of PTCH1 function or activating mutation of SMO leading to constitutionally activated HH pathway.[68,69] In NBCCS, germline mutations of *PTCH1* gene are prototypical. HH pathway inhibitors are first-line treatments in LaBCC and mBCC. **Fig. 2** shows a LaBCC at initial presentation (2A) and after treatment with SMO antagonist (2B). Systemic treatments for advanced disease are summarized in **Table 3**.

Additional treatments: Itraconazole, which has HH signaling inhibitory properties, and combination carboplatin and paclitaxel have both been reported in the treatment of mBCC, although conclusions are limited to small reports and exploratory trials.[70,71]

Prevention

Sun protection is highly recommended for the prevention of skin cancers. Surprisingly, results from a randomized controlled trial evaluating daily sunscreen use in Australia compared with discretionary use of sunscreen found no difference in BCC diagnoses.[72,73] Although the strength of sunscreen (sun protection factor 15), the length of follow-up (4.5 years), among other factors may have diluted the results. Regardless, sun protection starting at a young age is still recommended.

Nicotinamide successfully reduces nonmelanoma skin cancers and actinic keratoses. When isolating BCC alone, nicotinamide reduced the rate of diagnosis by 20% although this was not statistically significant.[74] With nicotinamide dosing of 500 mg twice daily, there are minimal safety concerns; thus, it may be recommended due to potential benefit.

BASAL CELL CARCINOMA FOLLOW-UP

Patients diagnosed with BCC are at increased risk of developing additional BCC, as well as developing SCC and melanoma.[75–77] Estimates suggest within 3 years of BCC diagnosis there is a nearly 30-fold risk of subsequent BCC and 14-fold risk of SCC. For these reasons, after BCC diagnosis, we recommend a total body skin examination 1 to 2 times annually with subsequent changes in frequency based on additional skin cancer diagnosis. In high-risk patients or patients with high-risk tumors, increased skin surveillance may be warranted.

SUMMARY

BCC is the most common cancer globally and the rate of incidence is increasing. Patient risk factors for BCC include susceptibility to and high exposures to UVR. Identification can be made on clinical examination, which is enhanced with dermoscopy. Several novel imaging techniques have been studied, although utility and justification for widespread clinical use is unproven. Tumors can be delineated into low-risk or high-risk BCC, which guides appropriate treatment. Surgical management including MMS for high-risk tumors is the most effective treatment. RT can be considered in patients not amendable to surgery. SMO inhibitors are first-line treatment of LaBCC and mBCC. Future directions should be aimed at prevention, earlier detection, and treatment of advanced disease.

CLINICS CARE POINTS

- Clinical examination aided by dermoscopy increases recognition and diagnosis of BCC
- Margin assessment is essential: in low-risk BCC, postoperative margin assessment should be obtained, and in high-risk BCC, intraoperative margin assessment is indicated
- Newer oral (vismodegib, sonidegib) or intravenous agents (cemiplimab) are the recommended treatment in LaBCC and mBCC

ACKNOWLEDGMENTS

There is no funding sources related to this article. Dr. Anna Bar has the following disclosures: Consultant to Regeneron, Castle Biosciences, PellePharm, Polynoma, and Pulse Biosciences.

DISCLOSURE

Dr A. Bar is a consultant for Regeneron.

REFERENCES

1. Rogers HW, Weinstock MA, Feldman SR, et al. Incidence Estimate of Nonmelanoma Skin Cancer (Keratinocyte Carcinomas) in the U.S. Population, 2012. JAMA Dermatol 2015;151(10):1081–6.
2. American Cancer Society. Cancer Statistics Center. Available at: http://cancerstatisticscenter.cancer.org. Accessed January 2.
3. Lear JT, Smith AG. Basal cell carcinoma. Postgrad Med J 1997;73(863):538–42.
4. Rigel DS, Friedman RJ, Kopf AW. Lifetime risk for development of skin cancer in the U.S. population: current estimate is now 1 in 5. J Am Acad Dermatol 1996;35(6):1012–3.
5. Wu S, Han J, Li WQ, et al. Basal-cell carcinoma incidence and associated risk factors in U.S. women and men. Am J Epidemiol 2013;178(6):890–7.
6. Abarca JF, Casiccia CC. Skin cancer and ultraviolet-B radiation under the Antarctic ozone hole: southern Chile, 1987-2000. Photodermatol Photoimmunol Photomed 2002;18(6):294–302.
7. Sng J, Koh D, Siong WC, et al. Skin cancer trends among Asians living in Singapore from 1968 to 2006. J Am Acad Dermatol 2009;61(3):426–32.
8. Bath-Hextall F, Leonardi-Bee J, Smith C, et al. Trends in incidence of skin basal cell carcinoma. Additional evidence from a UK primary care database study. Int J Cancer 2007;121(9):2105–8.
9. Staples MP, Elwood M, Burton RC, et al. Non-melanoma skin cancer in Australia: the 2002 national survey and trends since 1985. Med J Aust 2006;184(1):6–10.
10. Khalesi M, Whiteman DC, Tran B, et al. A meta-analysis of pigmentary characteristics, sun sensitivity, freckling and melanocytic nevi and risk of basal cell carcinoma of the skin. Cancer Epidemiol 2013; 37(5):534–43.
11. Zanetti R, Rosso S, Martinez C, et al. Comparison of risk patterns in carcinoma and melanoma of the skin in men: a multi-centre case-case-control study. Br J Cancer 2006;94(5):743–51.
12. van Dam RM, Huang Z, Rimm EB, et al. Risk factors for basal cell carcinoma of the skin in men: results from the health professionals follow-up study. Am J Epidemiol 1999;150(5):459–68.
13. Lear JT, Tan BB, Smith AG, et al. Risk factors for basal cell carcinoma in the UK: case-control study in 806 patients. J R Soc Med 1997;90(7):371–4.
14. Kricker A, Armstrong BK, English DR, et al. Pigmentary and cutaneous risk factors for non-melanocytic skin cancer–a case-control study. Int J Cancer 1991;48(5):650–62.
15. Maia M, Proença NG, de Moraes JC. Risk factors for basal cell carcinoma: a case-control study. Rev Saude Publica 1995;29(1):27–37.
16. Gallagher RP, Hill GB, Bajdik CD, et al. Sunlight exposure, pigmentary factors, and risk of nonmelanocytic skin cancer. I. Basal cell carcinoma. Arch Dermatol 1995;131(2):157–63.
17. Karagas MR, Zens MS, Li Z, et al. Early-onset basal cell carcinoma and indoor tanning: a population-based study. Pediatrics 2014;134(1):e4–12.
18. Gandini S, Doré JF, Autier P, et al. Epidemiological evidence of carcinogenicity of sunbed use and of efficacy of preventive measures. J Eur Acad Dermatol Venereol 2019;33(Suppl 2):57–62.
19. Wehner MR, Shive ML, Chren MM, et al. Indoor tanning and non-melanoma skin cancer: systematic review and meta-analysis. Bmj 2012;345:e5909.
20. Karagas MR, McDonald JA, Greenberg ER, et al. Risk of basal cell and squamous cell skin cancers after ionizing radiation therapy. For The Skin Cancer Prevention Study Group. J Natl Cancer Inst 1996; 88(24):1848–53.
21. Preston DL, Ron E, Tokuoka S, et al. Solid cancer incidence in atomic bomb survivors: 1958-1998. Radiat Res 2007;168(1):1–64.
22. Lichter MD, Karagas MR, Mott LA, et al. Therapeutic ionizing radiation and the incidence of basal cell

carcinoma and squamous cell carcinoma. The New Hampshire Skin Cancer Study Group. Arch Dermatol 2000;136(8):1007–11.

23. Watt TC, Inskip PD, Stratton K, et al. Radiation-related risk of basal cell carcinoma: a report from the Childhood Cancer Survivor Study. J Natl Cancer Inst 2012;104(16):1240–50.

24. Hartevelt MM, Bavinck JN, Kootte AM, et al. Incidence of skin cancer after renal transplantation in The Netherlands. Transplantation 1990;49(3):506–9.

25. Stern RS. The risk of squamous cell and basal cell cancer associated with psoralen and ultraviolet A therapy: a 30-year prospective study. J Am Acad Dermatol 2012;66(4):553–62.

26. Wade TR, Ackerman AB. The many faces of basal-cell carcinoma. J Dermatol Surg Oncol 1978;4(1):23–8.

27. McCormack CJ, Kelly JW, Dorevitch AP. Differences in age and body site distribution of the histological subtypes of basal cell carcinoma. A possible indicator of differing causes. Arch Dermatol 1997;133(5):593–6.

28. Scrivener Y, Grosshans E, Cribier B. Variations of basal cell carcinomas according to gender, age, location and histopathological subtype. Br J Dermatol 2002;147(1):41–7.

29. NCCN. Basal Cell Skin Cancer (Version 1.2022). Available at: https://www.nccn.org/professionals/physician_gls/pdf/nmsc.pdf. Accessed January 8, 2022.

30. Amin M, Edge S, Greene F, et al. AJCC cancer staging manual. 8th edition. New York: Springer Publishing; 2017.

31. Morgan FC, Ruiz ES, Karia PS, et al. Brigham and Women's Hospital tumor classification system for basal cell carcinoma identifies patients with risk of metastasis and death. J Am Acad Dermatol 2021;85(3):582–7.

32. Domarus HV, Stevens PJ. Metastatic basal cell carcinoma: Report of five cases and review of 170 cases in the literature. J Am Acad Dermatol 1984;10(6):1043–60.

33. Lo JS, Snow SN, Reizner GT, et al. Metastatic basal cell carcinoma: Report of twelve cases with a review of the literature. J Am Acad Dermatol 1991;24(5, Part 1):715–9.

34. Snow SN, Sahl W, Lo JS, et al. Metastatic basal cell carcinoma. Report of five cases. Article. Cancer 1994;73(2):328–35.

35. Wysong A, Aasi SZ, Tang JY. Update on Metastatic Basal Cell Carcinoma: A Summary of Published Cases From 1981 Through 2011. JAMA Dermatol 2013;149(5):615–6.

36. McCusker M, Basset-Seguin N, Dummer R, et al. Metastatic basal cell carcinoma: Prognosis dependent on anatomic site and spread of disease. Eur J Cancer 2014;50(4):774–83.

37. Morgan FC, Ruiz ES, Karia PS, et al. Factors predictive of recurrence, metastasis, and death from primary basal cell carcinoma 2 cm or larger in diameter. J Am Acad Dermatol 2020;83(3):832–8.

38. Reiter O, Mimouni I, Gdalevich M, et al. The diagnostic accuracy of dermoscopy for basal cell carcinoma: A systematic review and meta-analysis. J Am Acad Dermatol 2019;80(5):1380–8.

39. Nwaneshiudu A, Kuschal C, Sakamoto FH, et al. Introduction to Confocal Microscopy. J Invest Dermatol 2012;132(12):1–5.

40. Xiong YD, Ma S, Li X, et al. A meta-analysis of reflectance confocal microscopy for the diagnosis of malignant skin tumours. J Eur Acad Dermatol Venereol 2016;30(8):1295–302.

41. Woliner-van der Weg W, Peppelman M, Elshot YS, et al. Biopsy outperforms reflectance confocal microscopy in diagnosing and subtyping basal cell carcinoma: results and experiences from a randomized controlled multicentre trial. Br J Dermatol 2021;184(4):663–71.

42. Ulrich M, von Braunmuehl T, Kurzen H, et al. The sensitivity and specificity of optical coherence tomography for the assisted diagnosis of nonpigmented basal cell carcinoma: an observational study. Br J Dermatol 2015;173(2):428–35.

43. Jørgensen TM, Tycho A, Mogensen M, et al. Machine-learning classification of non-melanoma skin cancers from image features obtained by optical coherence tomography. Skin Res Technol 2008;14(3):364–9.

44. Mogensen M, Joergensen TM, Nürnberg BM, et al. Assessment of optical coherence tomography imaging in the diagnosis of non-melanoma skin cancer and benign lesions versus normal skin: observer-blinded evaluation by dermatologists and pathologists. Dermatol Surg 2009;35(6):965–72.

45. Parashar K, Torres AE, Boothby-Shoemaker W, et al. Imaging Technologies for Pre-surgical Margin Assessment of Basal Cell Carcinoma. J Am Acad Dermatol 2021. https://doi.org/10.1016/j.jaad.2021.11.010.

46. Barlow JO, Zalla MJ, Kyle A, et al. Treatment of basal cell carcinoma with curettage alone. J Am Acad Dermatol 2006;54(6):1039–45.

47. Thissen MRTM, Neumann MHA, Schouten LJ. A Systematic Review of Treatment Modalities for Primary Basal Cell Carcinomas. Arch Dermatol 1999;135(10):1177–83.

48. Blixt E, Nelsen D, Stratman E. Recurrence rates of aggressive histologic types of basal cell carcinoma after treatment with electrodesiccation and curettage alone. Dermatol Surg 2013;39(5):719–25.

49. Rodriguez-Vigil T, Vázquez-López F, Perez-Oliva N. Recurrence rates of primary basal cell carcinoma in facial risk areas treated with curettage and electrodesiccation. J Am Acad Dermatol 2007;56(1):91–5.

50. Kopf AW, Bart RS, Schrager D, et al. Curettage-electrodesiccation treatment of basal cell carcinomas. Arch Dermatol 1977;113(4):439–43.
51. Armstrong LTD, Magnusson MR, Guppy MPB. Risk factors for recurrence of facial basal cell carcinoma after surgical excision: A follow-up analysis. J Plast Reconstr Aesthet Surg 2017;70(12):1738–45.
52. Wolf DJ, Zitelli JA. Surgical margins for basal cell carcinoma. Arch Dermatol 1987;123(3):340–4.
53. van Loo E, Mosterd K, Krekels GA, et al. Surgical excision versus Mohs' micrographic surgery for basal cell carcinoma of the face: A randomised clinical trial with 10 year follow-up. Eur J Cancer 2014; 50(17):3011–20.
54. Kondo RN, Gon ADS, Pontello Junior R. Recurrence rate of basal cell carcinoma in patients submitted to skin flaps or grafts. An Bras Dermatol 2019;94(4): 442–5.
55. Quirk C, Gebauer K, De'Ambrosis B, et al. Sustained clearance of superficial basal cell carcinomas treated with imiquimod cream 5%: results of a prospective 5-year study. Cutis 2010;85(6):318–24.
56. Schulze HJ, Cribier B, Requena L, et al. Imiquimod 5% cream for the treatment of superficial basal cell carcinoma: results from a randomized vehicle-controlled phase III study in Europe. Br J Dermatol 2005;152(5):939–47.
57. Arits AH, Mosterd K, Essers BA, et al. Photodynamic therapy versus topical imiquimod versus topical fluorouracil for treatment of superficial basal-cell carcinoma: a single blind, non-inferiority, randomised controlled trial. Lancet Oncol 2013;14(7):647–54.
58. Roozeboom MH, Arits A, Mosterd K, et al. Three-Year Follow-Up Results of Photodynamic Therapy vs. Imiquimod vs. Fluorouracil for Treatment of Superficial Basal Cell Carcinoma: A Single-Blind, Non-inferiority, Randomized Controlled Trial. J Invest Dermatol 2016;136(8):1568–74.
59. Wang I, Bendsoe N, Klinteberg CA, et al. Photodynamic therapy vs. cryosurgery of basal cell carcinomas: results of a phase III clinical trial. Br J Dermatol 2001;144(4):832–40.
60. Basset-Seguin N, Ibbotson SH, Emtestam L, et al. Topical methyl aminolaevulinate photodynamic therapy versus cryotherapy for superficial basal cell carcinoma: a 5 year randomized trial. Eur J Dermatol 2008;18(5):547–53.
61. Hall VL, Leppard BJ, McGill J, et al. Treatment of basal-cell carcinoma: comparison of radiotherapy and cryotherapy. Clin Radiol 1986;37(1):33–4.
62. Wang H, Xu Y, Shi J, et al. Photodynamic therapy in the treatment of basal cell carcinoma: a systematic review and meta-analysis. Photodermatol Photoimmunol Photomed 2015;31(1):44–53.
63. Rowe DE, Carroll RJ, Day CL Jr. Long-term recurrence rates in previously untreated (primary) basal cell carcinoma: implications for patient follow-up. J Dermatol Surg Oncol 1989;15(3):315–28.
64. Rowe DE, Carroll RJ, Day CL Jr. Mohs surgery is the treatment of choice for recurrent (previously treated) basal cell carcinoma. J Dermatol Surg Oncol 1989; 15(4):424–31.
65. Avril MF, Auperin A, Margulis A, et al. Basal cell carcinoma of the face: surgery or radiotherapy? Results of a randomized study. Br J Cancer 1997;76(1):100–6.
66. Thomson J, Hogan S, Leonardi-Bee J, et al. Bath-Hextall FJ. Interventions for basal cell carcinoma: abridged Cochrane systematic review and GRADE assessments. Br J Dermatol 2021;185(3):499–511.
67. Likhacheva A, Awan M, Barker CA, et al. Definitive and Postoperative Radiation Therapy for Basal and Squamous Cell Cancers of the Skin: Executive Summary of an American Society for Radiation Oncology Clinical Practice Guideline. Pract Radiat Oncol 2020;10(1):8–20.
68. Epstein EH. Basal cell carcinomas: attack of the hedgehog. Nat Rev Cancer 2008;8(10):743–54.
69. Campione E, Di Prete M, Lozzi F, et al. High-Risk Recurrence Basal Cell Carcinoma: Focus on Hedgehog Pathway Inhibitors and Review of the Literature. Chemotherapy 2020;65(1–2):2–10.
70. Kim DJ, Kim J, Spaunhurst K, et al. Open-label, exploratory phase II trial of oral itraconazole for the treatment of basal cell carcinoma. J Clin Oncol 2014;32(8):745–51.
71. Moeholt K, Aagaard H, Pfeiffer P, et al. Platinum-based cytotoxic therapy in basal cell carcinoma–a review of the literature. Acta Oncol 1996;35(6): 677–82.
72. Green A, Williams G, Neale R, et al. Daily sunscreen application and betacarotene supplementation in prevention of basal-cell and squamous-cell carcinomas of the skin: a randomised controlled trial. Lancet 1999;354(9180):723–9.
73. Sánchez G, Nova J, Rodriguez-Hernandez AE, et al. Sun protection for preventing basal cell and squamous cell skin cancers. Cochrane Database Syst Rev 2016;7(7):Cd011161.
74. Chen AC, Martin AJ, Choy B, et al. A Phase 3 Randomized Trial of Nicotinamide for Skin-Cancer Chemoprevention. N Engl J Med 2015;373(17):1618–26.
75. Wu S, Cho E, Li WQ, et al. History of Keratinocyte Carcinoma and Risk of Melanoma: A Prospective Cohort Study. J Natl Cancer Inst 2017;109(4).
76. Wehner MR, Linos E, Parvataneni R, et al. Timing of subsequent new tumors in patients who present with basal cell carcinoma or cutaneous squamous cell carcinoma. JAMA Dermatol 2015;151(4):382–8.
77. Revenga F, Paricio JF, Vázquez MM, et al. Risk of subsequent non-melanoma skin cancer in a cohort of patients with primary basal cell carcinoma. J Eur Acad Dermatol Venereol 2004;18(4):514–5.

Targeted Therapy and Immunotherapy in Nonmelanoma Skin Cancer

Nader Aboul-Fettouh, MD[a], Shelby L. Kubicki, MD[a], Leon Chen, MD[b,c], Sirunya Silapunt, MD[a], Michael R. Migden, MD[d,e],*

KEYWORDS

- Basal cell carcinoma ● Squamous cell carcinoma ● Immunotherapy ● Targeted therapy
- PD-1 inhibitors ● Hedgehog pathway inhibitors ● Systemic therapy

KEY POINTS

- Advanced nonmelanoma skin cancers include tumors that are poor candidates for surgery, radiation, or a combination of the two.
- Hedgehog pathway inhibitors and programmed death-1 inhibitors have found the most success in systemic treatment of advanced nonmelanoma skin cancers within the last decade.
- Future directions include intralesional therapy and combination therapy with other systemic medications or oncolytic viral therapy.

INTRODUCTION

The increase in worldwide incidence of nonmelanoma skin cancer (NMSC), including cutaneous squamous cell carcinoma (cSCC) and basal cell carcinoma (BCC), has led to a search for new and effective therapies.[1] Although the majority of early-stage NMSC is treated with surgery or other localized therapies (eg, curettage and electrodesiccation, topical therapy, laser therapy), treating advanced NMSC continues to be a challenge. Recent advancements in systemic therapies, including hedgehog-pathway inhibitors (HPIs) and programmed death-1 (PD-1) inhibitors, have been tremendously useful in decreasing morbidity and mortality associated with advanced NMSC.

PATIENT SELECTION AND DEFINING ADVANCED TUMORS

There are currently no definitive objective criteria for advanced NMSC. In this review, advanced NMSC will refer to locally advanced or metastatic disease. Patients with locally advanced tumors tend to be poor candidates for surgery and/or radiation. At times, resecting locally advanced tumors may be technically feasible; however, it may result in significant morbidity and/or disfigurement for the patient. Even if feasible, some patients may be unwilling to endure extensive surgery for a locally advanced tumor. These patients should be considered for systemic therapies.

Targeted Therapy

Epidermal growth factor receptor inhibitors

The epidermal growth factor receptor (EGFR) protein is a member of the ErbB family of tyrosine kinase (TK) receptors.[2] In keratinocytes, EGFR is involved in several cellular regulatory functions, including cellular proliferation, adhesion and migration, survival, and differentiation.[3] EGFR overexpression is common in cSCC and

[a] Department of Dermatology, McGovern Medical School at the University of Texas Health Science Center at Houston, 6655 Travis St., #980 Houston, TX 77030, USA; [b] US Dermatology Partners, 1213 Hermann Dr #650, Houston, TX 77004, USA; [c] Elite Dermatology, 20326, TX-249 Ste 400, Houston, TX 77070, USA; [d] Department of Dermatology, The University of Texas MD Anderson Cancer Center, 1400 Pressler Street., 1452, Houston, TX 77030, USA; [e] Department of Head and Neck Surgery, The University of Texas MD Anderson Cancer Center, 1400 Pressler Street, 1452, Houston, TX 77030, USA
* Corresponding author. Department of Head and Neck Surgery, The University of Texas MD Anderson Cancer Center, 1400 Pressler Street, 1452, Houston, TX 77030.
E-mail address: mrmigden@mdanderson.org

Dermatol Clin 41 (2023) 23–37
https://doi.org/10.1016/j.det.2022.07.009

associated with a more aggressive phenotype and poorer prognosis.[4] EGFR inhibitors (EGFRIs) were an early attempt at using targeted therapy in the treatment of advanced cSCC. Cutaneous and gastrointestinal adverse events (AEs) are the most frequently reported with EGFRIs. AEs can cause significant morbidity and decreased quality of life, often necessitating drug interruptions or cessation.[5] Cetuximab, a human/mouse chimeric monoclonal antibody that binds and inhibits the ligand-binding domain of EGFR, is one of several EGFRIs used to treat NMSC.

Hedgehog-pathway inhibitors

The Hedgehog (Hh) signaling pathway contributes significantly to normal embryonic development but is largely inactive in adults.[6] Three proteins are involved in the Hh signaling cascade: Hh ligand, cell surface receptor patched (Ptch), and G-protein-coupled receptor smoothened (Smo). When Hh ligand is not present, Ptch suppresses Smo activity. On Hh ligand binding to Ptch, release of Smo inhibition allows the transcription factor Gli to enter the cell nucleus, increasing cell proliferation and tumor formation. Sporadic BCCs may develop due to loss-of-function mutations in Ptch (70–80% of occurrences) or gain-of-function in Smo (6–21% of occurrences).[7] Vismodegib and sonidegib are small-molecule inhibitors of Smo that block Hh signaling activation and are used to treat advanced BCC. Below are the key United States Food and Drug Administration (USFDA) approvals for HPIs as of February 11, 2022.

- Vismodegib: Adults with metastatic or locally advanced BCC who have tumor recurrence following surgery or are not candidates for surgery or radiation.
- Sonidegib: Adults with locally advanced BCC that has recurred following surgery or radiation or for those who are not candidates for surgery or radiation.

HPIs are typically well-tolerated. The most common AEs include muscle spasms, alopecia, and dysgeusia.[8]

Programmed death-1 inhibitors

Immunotherapies enhance the immune system's recognition of tumor cells. The PD-1 protein is a T-cell surface receptor that, when bound to its ligands PD-L1 or PD-L2, transduces a signal that inhibits T-cell proliferation, cytokine production, and cytolytic function.[9] Tumor cells or tumor-infiltrating lymphocytes may express PD-L1 to prevent the activation of new cytotoxic T-cells in the lymph nodes and subsequent recruitment to the tumor.[10]

This enables the tumor to escape immune system surveillance (**Fig. 1**).

PD-1 inhibitors are immune checkpoint inhibitors (ICIs) that bind PD-1, reversing T-cell suppression and enhancing endogenous antitumor immunity to unleash long-term antitumor responses.[11] PD-1 inhibitors such as cemiplimab, pembrolizumab, and nivolumab have emerged as ICIs for the treatment of a variety of cancers, including advanced NMSC.[12] Below are the key USFDA approvals for PD-1 inhibitors as of February 11, 2022.

- Cemiplimab: Adults with metastatic or locally advanced cSCC who are not candidates for surgery or radiation.
- Pembrolizumab: Adults with recurrent, metastatic, or locally advanced cSCC who are not candidates for surgery or radiation.
- Cemiplimab: Adults with locally advanced BCC previously treated with an HPI or for whom an HPI is not appropriate. Accelerated approval for adults with metastatic BCC previously treated with an HPI or for whom an HPI is not appropriate.

Although PD-1 inhibitors are generally well-tolerated, patients are at risk of immune-related AEs (irAEs) including pneumonitis, hepatitis, colitis, adrenal insufficiency, hypothyroidism and hyperthyroidism, diabetes mellitus, nephritis, and infusion reactions. Other common AEs include fatigue, musculoskeletal pain, and rash.[13]

BASAL CELL CARCINOMA

BCC is the most common NMSC with an estimated age-adjusted incidence of 1488 and 1019 cases per 100,000 person-years for men and women, respectively.[14] BCC has an estimated metastasis rate of 0.0028% to 0.55%.[15,16] For locally advanced or metastatic BCC, systemic therapies should be considered. The sections below, **Table 1** and **Table 2** describe the systemic therapies used for the treatment of BCC.

Cytotoxic Agents for Treatment of Advanced Basal Cell Carcinoma

Cytotoxic chemotherapies were the original systemic agents used to treat advanced BCC. Pfeiffer and colleagues and Moeholt and colleagues published retrospective reviews of 93 patients with advanced BCC treated with these agents.[17,18] Objective response rates (ORRs) differed greatly between studies at 38% and 83%, respectively. However, because many responders received combination systemic therapy with surgery or radiation, the data is not representative of responses to

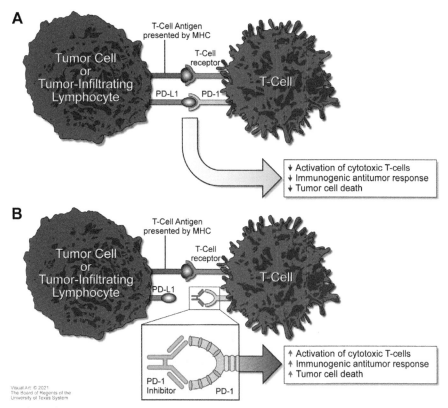

Fig. 1. (*A*) Binding of PD ligand-1 (PD-L1) on the tumor cell or tumor-infiltrating lymphocyte and the corresponding receptor, Program death-1 (PD-1), on T-cells allows cancer cells to escape from the immune system by preventing activation of cytotoxic T-cells and attenuating the antitumor response. (*B*) Binding of a PD-1 inhibitor to PD-1 inhibits the formation of the PD-1/PD-L1 complex. Subsequently, cytotoxic T-cells are upregulated and a more robust immunogenic antitumor effect can be observed. MHC: major histocompatibility complex. (© 2022 The Board of Regents of the University of Texas System.)

systemic therapy alone. Although the Moeholt article provides a high ORR, the authors admit the reported ORR is bound to be optimistic due to publication bias in this highly selected group of patients. In the Pfeiffer study, median survival was 8 months (range 2–36 months) in the non-cis-platinum-containing regimen group and 16+ months (3–51+ months) in the group receiving cis-platinum-containing regimens.[17] Jefford and colleagues described a patient with metastatic BCC with initial response to cisplatin and paclitaxel, then recurrence and progression after 3 months.[19] In addition to suboptimal response rates and median survival, cytotoxic agents are associated with significant AEs. These agents have a narrow therapeutic index, with AEs including significant hematological toxicity, fatigue, nausea, and alopecia.[20]

Hedgehog-Pathway Inhibitors for Treatment of Advanced Basal Cell Carcinoma

HPIs are considered the first-line therapy for advanced BCC. Vismodegib was the first HPI approved in 2012 after initial data published from the ERIVANCE BCC study. This phase II, international, multicenter, nonrandomized clinical trial evaluated the efficacy and safety of vismodegib in patients with locally advanced or metastatic BCC.[21] The final update at 39 months showed an investigator-assessed ORR of 48.5% in the metastatic group (all with partial response [PR]) and 60.3% in the locally advanced group (N = 20 with complete response [CR] and N = 18 with PR). Median duration of response (DOR) for the metastatic and locally advanced groups was 14.8 and 26.2 months, respectively. Median overall survival (OS) was only estimable in the metastatic cohort (33.4 months). Notably, no deaths were reported as related to vismodegib. The efficacy and safety of vismodegib was further reinforced with the Safety Events in Vismodegib (STEVIE) and MIKIE trials.[22,23]

The STEVIE trial evaluated 147 patients with advanced BCC treated with vismodegib with safety as a primary endpoint.[22] Ninety-eight

Table 1
Sampling of published reports of cytotoxic chemotherapy for basal cell carcinoma

Authors, Year	Regimen	Line of Therapy	Patients (N)	Response Rate	DOR (Months)	Notes/Limitations
Cytotoxic and platinum-based agents						
Pfeiffer et al,[17] 1990	Methotrexate, 5-FU, cyclophosphamide, doxorubicin, bleomycin, vinblastine, cisplatin[a]	First/second+	47	38% (4% in nonplatinum containing, 77% in platinum containing)	Not evaluable	Review of BCC treated with systemic chemotherapy. 2/47 received concurrent RT
Moeholt et al,[18] 1996	Platinum-based chemotherapy[a]	First/second+	46	83%	Not evaluable	Review of BCC treated with platinum-based cytotoxic therapy. 15/26 had subsequent RT or surgery
Jaal et al,[70] 2012	A) cisplatin and doxorubicin B) cisplatin and doxorubicin	First	2	100%	A) 16, B) 3	Locally advanced BCC treated with induction chemotherapy followed by radiotherapy

Abbreviations: 5-FU, 5-fluorouracil; BCC, basal cell carcinoma; DOR, duration of response; RT, radiation therapy.
[a] Monotherapy or combination therapy with other systemic agents.

Major clinical trials of targeted therapy and immunotherapy for basal cell carcinoma

Authors, Year	Regimen	Line of Therapy	Patients (N)	Response Rate	DOR (Months)	Notes/Limitations
Targeted Therapy						
ERIVANCE study, Sekulic et al,[21] 2017	Vismodegib 150 mg daily	First/second+	63 (laBCC), 33 (mBCC)	60.3% (laBCC), 48.5% (mBCC)	26.2 (laBCC), 14.8 (mBCC)	Investigator-assessed response rate
STEVIE study. Basset-Seguin et al,[22] 2017	Vismodegib 150 mg daily	First/second+	1077 (laBCC), 84 (mBCC)	68.5% (laBCC), 36.9% (mBCC)	23.0 (laBCC), 13.9 (mBCC)	Primary endpoint safety, investigator-assessed response rate
MIKIE study. Dreno et al,[23] 2017	Vismodegib A) 150 mg daily × 12 weeks followed by 3 cycles placebo daily × 8 weeks, then vismodegib 150 mg daily × 12 weeks; or B) 150 mg daily × 24 weeks followed by 3 cycles placebo daily × 8 weeks, then vismodegib 150 mg daily × 8 weeks	First/second+	A) 116 B) 113	A) 62.7% B) 54.0%	Not evaluable	Patients with multiple BCC, response rate listed is mean relative reduction in number of BCC
BOLT study. Dummer et al.,[24]2021	Sonidegib 200 mg A) 200 mg daily or B) 800 mg daily		66 (A/laBCC), 13 (A/mBCC), 128 (B/laBCC), 23 (B/mBCC)	56% (A/laBCC) 8% (A/mBCC) 46.1% (B/laBCC) 17% (B/mBCC)	26.1 (A/laBCC) 24.0 (A/mBCC) 23.3 (B/laBCC)	Central assessment of response rate. In the B/mBCC group, response duration was not estimable
Immunotherapy						
Chang et al,[34] 2019	Pembrolizumab 200 mg q3w with or without vismodegib 150 mg daily	First/second+	16	38%	16.8	Proof of concept study indicating that pembrolizumab has activity against BCC
STUDY 1620 Stratigos et al,[33] 2021	Cemiplimab 350 mg q3w	Second+	84	31%	2–21	
Aboul-Fettouh et al,[32] 2021	Cemiplimab, nivolumab, or pembrolizumab; excludes STUDY1620	First/second+	19	6 SD (32%) 6 PR (32%) 2 near CR (11%) 2 CR (11%) 2 MR (11%) 1 PD (5%).	-	Review of largely case reports

Note that this is a limited sampling of published reports.

Abbreviations: BCC, basal cell carcinoma; CR, complete response; DOR, duration of response; laBCC, locally advanced BCC; mBCC, metastatic BCC; MR, mixed response; PD, progressive disease; PR, partial response; SD, stable disease.

percent of patients experienced at least 1 treatment-emergent AE (TEAE), with the most common being muscle spasms, alopecia, dysgeusia, and decreased weight. Serious TEAEs were reported in 23.8% of patients. No grade 3 TEAEs were reported at 10+ events per 100 patient-years. Grade 5 (fatal) TEAEs were considered related to vismodegib in 7 (3.8%) patients; however, after Data Safety Monitoring Board review, all cases were determined to be unrelated to vismodegib (N = 6) or not assessable due to insufficient clinical data (N = 1). This is in stark contrast to the morbidity and mortality associated with AEs secondary to cytotoxic chemotherapy.

Sonidegib was USFDA-approved in 2015 for the treatment of patients with advanced BCC based on results from the phase II BOLT trial.[24] The BOLT trial randomized patients in a 1:2 ratio between treatment arms that differed in sonidegib dosing (200 mg vs 800 mg). Results from this trial are listed in **Table 1**. An update at 42 months showed that per central review, ORRs were 48% and 41.7% for the 200 mg and 800 mg groups, respectively. AEs and treatment discontinuation were less common in the 200 mg cohort, with a similar ORR. These studies suggest that HPIs are an effective and tolerable first-line therapy for patients with advanced BCC. Unfortunately, some patients have shown resistance to HPIs.[25]

Programmed Death-1 Inhibitors for Treatment of Advanced Basal Cell Carcinoma

In 2016, Ikeda and colleagues reported one of the first cases of metastatic BCC with near-complete regression after off-label treatment with PD-1 inhibitor nivolumab.[26] This treatment success aligns with current understanding of the interaction between our immune system and BCC.[27] BCC has a higher tumor mutational burden (TMB) compared with other malignancies, including cSCC.[28] In BCC, infiltrating lymphocytes are commonly observed adjacent to the tumor nests or within the stroma between tumor nests.[29] This suggests that BCC may induce an immune response by the host immediately adjacent to the tumor.[30] In the setting of organ transplantation, the risk of BCC increases roughly 10-fold because long-term immunosuppression is a high-risk factor for tumorigenesis.[31] Several additional cases of BCC responsive to PD-1 inhibitors led to an open-label, multicenter, single-arm phase 2 trial of cemiplimab in locally advanced BCC after HPI therapy (Study 1620 [NCT03132636]).[32]

Study 1620 enrolled patients with advanced BCC who had progressed during HPI therapy, failed to demonstrate objective response after 9 months on HPI therapy, or were intolerant of a prior HPI.[33] Patients received cemiplimab-rwlc for up to 93 weeks until disease progression, intolerable toxicity, or completion of planned treatment. Confirmed ORR was 31%. Median DOR had not been reached at time of data cutoff (range 2–21+ months). Grade 3-4 TEAEs occurred in 48% of patients; of those only 11% (N = 9) discontinued treatment. Initial results from Study 1620 led to USFDA approval of cemiplimab for locally advanced BCC and accelerated approval for metastatic BCC.

Chang and colleagues reported the first proof-of-concept trial in the treatment of 16 patients having advanced BCC with pembrolizumab with or without vismodegib.[34] The ORR at 18 weeks was 44% (4/9) for the pembrolizumab monotherapy group and 29% (2/7) for the combination therapy group. The pembrolizumab monotherapy group reported 11% CR, 33% PR, 44% stable disease (SD), and 11% progressive disease (PD), whereas the pembrolizumab-vismodegib dual therapy group reported 29% CR, 14% PR, and 57% SD. There were no life-threatening irAEs, and the most reported irAEs were dermatitis and fatigue. Although the 2 small groups were not directly compared, the authors proposed that pembrolizumab monotherapy is not definitively inferior to combination therapy with vismodegib. Future trials are needed to confirm the efficacy and tolerability of PD-1 inhibitors for advanced BCC.

CUTANEOUS SQUAMOUS CELL CARCINOMA

cSCC represents a significant health crisis for patients at high risk of NMSC because they have increased the incidence of cSCC and are at higher risk for aggressive and metastatic disease.[35] Approximately 5% of tumors progress to advanced cSCC, an alarming percentage for a disease with an incidence between 9 and 96 per 100,000 men and 56 and 68 per 100,000 women in areas such as the United Kingdom, Sweden, and Germany.[36–38] Although the majority of early cSCC are treated with surgery, advanced cSCC often necessitates the use of systemic agents. **Tables 3** and **4** display the use of several systemic agents in advanced cSCC.

Cytotoxic Agents for Treatment of Advanced Cutaneous Squamous Cell Carcinoma

Similar to their use in BCC, cytotoxic agents for advanced cSCC are limited by their narrow therapeutic index. Early trials rarely used cytotoxic agents as monotherapy, and rather combined their use with radiation or surgery to attempt complete

Table 3
Reports of cytotoxic chemotherapy for treatment of cutaneous squamous cell carcinoma

Authors, Year	Regimen	Line of Treatment	Patients (N)	ORR	DOR (Months)	Notes/Limitations
Guthrie et al,[41] 1985	Cisplatin + doxorubicin	First/second+	4	75%	3–24	One underwent subsequent surgery
Sadek et al,[40] 1990	Cisplatin + 5-FU + bleomycin	First/second+	12	84%	NE	Most underwent subsequent surgery/RT
Shin et al,[71] 2002	IFN-alpha + 13-cis-retinoic acid + cisplatin	First/second+	39	34%	9	None with distant metastases.
Nottage et al,[72] 2017	Cisplatin or carboplatin	First	19	100%	NE	All underwent concomitant RT

Abbreviations: 5-FU, 5-fluorouracil; DOR, duration of response; IFN, interferon; N, number; NE, not evaluable; ORR, objective response rate; RT, radiation therapy.

tumor clearance.[39–41] However, these treatments lacked adequate response, DOR, and tolerability.

Epidermal Growth Factor Receptor Inhibitors for Treatment of Advanced Cutaneous Squamous Cell Carcinoma

EGFRIs cetuximab and panitumumab were among early modern targeted therapies for advanced cSCC. A phase II study of cetuximab as first-line monotherapy for patients with advanced cSCC showed a suboptimal ORR of 28% and a mean OS of 8.1 months.[42] A retrospective report by Montaudié and colleagues demonstrated more promising results with an ORR of 42%, DOR of 70% at 12 weeks, and median OS of 17.5 months. However, the study included large proportion of patients with only locally advanced disease (66%).[43] Gefitinib and erolitinib are 2 small TK inhibitors (TKIs) that also demonstrated low ORRs (16% and 10%, respectively).[44,45] In addition to suboptimal responses, both intrinsic and acquired resistance are barriers to the efficacy of EGFR inhibitors, limiting their use as monotherapy in advanced cSCC.[46]

Programmed Death-1 Inhibitors for Treatment of Advanced Cutaneous Squamous Cell Carcinoma

cSCC occurs 65 to 250 times more frequently in immunosuppressed patients and has a higher TMB than most neoplasms, making immunotherapy a mechanistically reasonable treatment of advanced cSCC.[47,48] Further support comes from studies indicating that TMB has predictive value for tumor response when using ICIs in advanced malignancies.[49] Compared with BCC where lymphocytes generated by the host immune response are found adjacent to tumor nests, lymphocytes in cSCC are observed both at the periphery of and infiltrating within the tumor.[50]

The first USFDA approval for cemiplimab came after registration trials by Migden and colleagues showed ORRs of 41.1% to 50% in phase I and II studies for patients with either locally advanced or metastatic cSCC. Disease control rate (DCR) ranged from 62% to 71.2%.[51] The majority of reported AEs were diarrhea and fatigue, reported by 25% of enrolled patients. Most patients in these cohorts were elderly with several comorbidities, and AEs were reported regardless of attribution. Patients should be closely monitored for life-threatening irAEs such as colitis, pneumonitis, and hepatitis.

Pembrolizumab was USFDA-approved for advanced cSCC in 2020 based on results of KEYNOTE-629, a single arm phase II trial that treated 105 patients. Patients had a 40.3% ORR with a 56.6% DCR, lower than the cemiplimab trial, although the majority of patients received pembrolizumab as at least second-line therapy (64.8%).[52] These studies indicate that PD-1 inhibitors represent a well-tolerated, effective treatment option for patients with advanced cSCC. Additional studies reporting the use of PD-1 inhibitors for advanced cSCC are listed in **Table 4**. Unfortunately, there is a chance of developing acquired resistance during or after immunotherapy, although it has not been well-characterized in NMSC. In metastatic melanoma, mechanisms of resistance to PD-1/PD-L1 blockade continue to be characterized but are believed to be

Table 4
Major clinical trials and retrospective studies of targeted therapy and immunotherapy for treatment of cSCC

Authors, Year	Regimen	Line of Treatment	Patients (N)	Response Rate	DOR (Months)	Notes/ Limitations
Targeted Therapy						
Maubec et al,[42] 2011	Cetuximab 250 mg/kg q1w[a]	First/ second+	36	28%	6.8	
Montauedie et al,[43] 2020	Cetuximab 250 mg/kg q1w[a]	First/ second+	58	42%	NE	Retrospective study
Foote et al,[71] 2014	Panitumumab 6 mg/kg q2w	First/ second+	16	31%	5	
William et al,[44] 2017	Gefitinib 250 mg daily	Second+	37	16%	31.4	
Gold et al,[45] 2018	Erlotinib 150 mg daily	Second+	29	10%	NE	
Immunotherapy						
Migden et al,[51] 2018	Cemiplimab 3 mg/kg q2w	First/ second+	26	50%	NE	Phase I study of expansion cohorts of patients with locally advanced or metastatic cSCC
Rischin et al,[74] 2020	Cemiplimab A) 3 mg/kg q2w, B) 350 mg q3w	First/ second+	59 (A) 56 (B)	49.2% (A) 41.1% (B)	NE	Phase II study of cemiplimab in patients with metastatic cSCC at weight-based vs fixed doses
Migden et al. 2020[73]	Cemiplimab 3 mg/kg q2w	First/ second+	78	44%	NE	Phase II study of cemiplimab in patients with locally advanced cSCC
Grob et al. 2020[74]	Pembrolizumab 200 mg q3w	First/ second+	105	34%	NE	
CARSKIN study. Maubec et al,[42] 2020	Pembrolizumab 200 mg q3w	First/ second+	57	41%	NE	
KEYNOTE-629 study. Hughes et al,[52] 2021	Pembrolizumab 200 mg q3w	First/ second+	54 (lacSCC) 105 (mcSCC)	59.0% (lacSCC) 35.2% (mcSCC)	NE	

Note that this is a limited sampling of published reports.

Abbreviations: cSCC, cutaneous squamous cell carcinoma; DOR, duration of response; lacSCC, locally advanced cSCC; mcSCC, metastatic cSCC; N, number; NE, not evaluable; q1w, once every 1 week; q2w, once every 2 weeks; q3w, once every 3 weeks; RT, radiation therapy.

[a] One dose of cetuximab 400 mg/kg was administered before starting listed dose.

multifaceted, with mechanisms including loss of T-cell function, disruption of antigen presentation, and evolution of interferon resistance.[53]

COMBINATION THERAPY

Although this review focuses on monotherapy, it is worth noting that combination therapy with multiple systemic agents may increase response rates in a synergistic fashion. The percentage of clinical trials evaluating monotherapy with PD-1/PD-L1 inhibitors has decreased in recent years compared with an overall increase in those investigating combination therapy.[54] When treating other types of advanced malignancies, PD-1 inhibitors are often combined with vascular endothelial growth factor targeted therapy, chemotherapy, and ICIs, including cytotoxic T-lymphocyte-associated protein 4 inhibitors such as ipilimumab. In addition, novel intralesional immunotherapies are an appealing approach due to the theoretical advantages of a higher local concentration with limited systemic exposure. Intralesional oncolytic virus therapy talimogene-laherparepvec (Imlygic, Amgen) is USFDA-approved for advanced melanoma and when combined with ipilimumab, demonstrates an ORR of 41%.[55] A study investigating intralesional PD-1 inhibitor therapy for recurrent cSCC is currently underway.[56] The IGNYTE open-label, single-arm phase II clinical trial is currently investigating the oncolytic RPI herpes simplex virus in combination with nivolumab and has shown promising early results.[57]

Combining systemic therapies with radiation or surgery has been in clinical practice since the early days of cytotoxic chemotherapy. Locally advanced tumors may be deemed resectable after tumor shrinkage using systemic therapies. When treating advanced tumors, a multidisciplinary approach, including a medical oncologist, dermatologic oncologist, surgical oncologist, and radiation oncologist, among others, is vital.

RARE TUMORS (MERKEL CELL CARCINOMA, SEBACEOUS CARCINOMA, DERMATOFIBROSARCOMA PROTUBERANS)

Merkel cell carcinoma (MCC) is a rare, aggressive, cutaneous neoplasm associated with Merkel cell polyoma virus. It has a high rate of nodal and distant metastases. PD-L1 inhibitor avelumab and PD-1 inhibitor pembrolizumab are USFDA-approved for advanced MCC. Major clinical trials investigating these agents as well as additional reports of immunotherapy for MCC are outlined in **Table 5.**[58–63]

Table 5 Systemic therapy for treatment of MCC						
Authors, Year	Regimen	Line of Therapy	Patients (N)	Response Rate	DOR (Weeks)	Notes/Limitations
D'Angelo et al,[58] 2018	Avelumab 10 mg/kg q2w	First	29	62.1%	NE	
D'Angelo et al,[59] 2020	Avelumab 10 mg/kg q2w	Second+	88	33%	40.5	
Nghiem et al,[60] 2021	Pembrolizumab 2 mg/kg q3w	First	50	58%	1–51.8+	
POD1UM-201 study. Grignani et al,[62] 2021	Retifanlimab 500 mg q4w	First	65	46.2%	NE	
Glutsch et al,[63] 2021	Ipilimumab plus nivolumab (various doses)	Second+	5	60%	NE	Case series of patients with avelumab-refractory metastatic MCC

Note that this is a limited sampling of published reports.
Abbreviations: DOR, duration of response; MCC, Merkel cell carcinoma; NE, not evaluable; q2w, once every 2 weeks; q3w, once every 3 weeks; q4w, once every 4 weeks.

Table 6
Systemic therapy for treatment of rare cutaneous neoplasms

Authors, Year	Age (Years), Sex	Primary Tumor Location	Metastases	Prior Treatments	Regimen	Response	DOR	Notes/Side Effects
Sebaceous Carcinoma								
Ota et al,[64] 2019	69, F	Right eyelid	Lung, subcutaneous	Surgery	1) Paclitaxel 200 mg/m^2 and carboplatin AUC 5 q3w x21w 2) docetaxel 60 mg/m^2 q3w × 18w	1) PR then developed brain metastases 2) PR	1) 10 months 2) 4 months	Received whole-brain irradiation prior to starting docetaxel
Kodali et al,[66] 2018	72, F	Right orbit	Lymph nodes	Surgery, subcutaneous methotrexate, cyclophosphamide, rituximab, subconjunctival mitomycin-C	Pembrolizumab 2 mg/kg q3w with carboplatin × 18 weeks, followed by maintenance pembrolizumab × 24 months	CR	44 months	Initially diagnosed and treated as ocular cicatricial pemphigoid
Banerjee et al,[67] 2021	54, M	Right chest wall	Chest wall	Surgery	Pembrolizumab 200 mg q3w × 15 weeks	CR	28 weeks	
DFSP								
Chen et al,[68] 2019	29, F	Left orbit	Lung	Surgery, RT	Ifosfamide, cisplatin, apatinib ×6 cycles, then maintenance apatinib	PR	6 months	Refused imatinib due to cost

| Rutkowski[69] 2010 | 23.8–69.6 (n = 24) | Locally advanced or metastatic disease | - | Varies | Imatinib 400–800 mg daily | 11 (45.9%) PR, 6 (25%) SD, 4 (16.6%) PD | - | 1-year OS rate 87.5%. Response rate did not differ between 400 mg daily and 400 mg twice daily |

Note that this is a limited sampling of published reports.

Abbreviations: 5-FU, 5-fluorouracil; DFSP, dermatofibrosarcoma protuberans; DOR, duration of response; F, female; M, male; OS, overall survival; PD, progressive disease; PR, partial response; q3w, once every 3 weeks; RT, radiation treatment; SD, stable disease.

Sebaceous carcinoma (SC) rarely metastasizes, and there is no established first-line treatment of affected patients. Most reports of metastatic SC describe systemic therapy as second-line treatment after failure of surgery and/or radiation. Existing reports outline treatment with cytotoxic chemotherapy and PD-1 inhibitors.[64–67]

Dermatofibrosarcoma protruberans (DFSP) is a rare cutaneous soft tissue sarcoma that is often locally aggressive. Imatinib, a TKI, was USFDA-approved to treat advanced DFSP in 2005 based on the results of 2 phase II trials conducted in Europe. Imatinib is first-line for treatment of metastatic DFSP, whereas Mohs surgery remains first-line for locally advanced disease. Systemic treatment of other rare forms of NMSC is mostly described in case reports outlined in **Table 6**.[68,69]

DISCUSSION

Compared with traditional cytotoxic chemotherapy, modern targeted therapies and immunotherapies have AE profiles better suited for the elderly population that presents with the majority of advanced cSCC. For advanced BCC, first-line HPIs and second-line PD-1 inhibitors have replaced antiquated cytotoxic agents. For advanced cSCC, PD-1 inhibitors are first-line based on their high benefit-to-risk ratio. PD-1 inhibitors demonstrate a higher ORR in advanced cSCC compared with BCC. Although both tumors generate a host immune response, cSCC may show more tumor-associated lymphocytes that infiltrate within tumor nests. Although a causative mechanism has not been established between these differences, the architectural variations noted may help explain the difference noted in ORR. Exciting new therapies are currently undergoing clinical trials, including intralesional PD-1 inhibitor trials and those that combine immunotherapy with the oncolytic viral therapy RP1. Combining systemic therapies with surgery and/or radiation allows for a much higher rate of tumor clearance than seen in prior decades. This is an exciting era for cutaneous oncology because we continue to discover more effective treatment options for advanced NMSC.

CLINICS CARE POINTS

- A multidisciplinary approach to advanced NMSC is vital because a combination of systemic, surgical, and radiation treatment options may be necessary to optimize treatment outcomes.

- For advanced BCC, HPIs, including vismodegib and sonidegib, are first-line therapy with suitable response rates and tolerability. PD-1 inhibitor cemiplimab was recently approved as second-line therapy for those who failed or are intolerant of an HPI.

- For advanced cSCC, PD-1 inhibitors cemiplimab and pembrolizumab are first-line therapy because they are well-tolerated and demonstrate good response rates.

DISCLOSURE OF INTEREST

M. R Migden has participated on advisory boards and received honoraria from Regeneron Pharmaceuticals, Inc., Sun Pharmaceuticals, and Sanofi; advisory role with Rakuten Medical. The authors have no other relevant affiliations or financial involvement with any organization or entity with a financial interest in or financial conflict with the subject matter or materials discussed in the article apart from those disclosed.

REFERENCES

1. Leiter U, Eigentler T, Garbe C. Epidemiology of skin cancer. Adv Exp Med Biol 2014;810:120–40.
2. Oda K, Matsuoka Y, Funahashi A, et al. A comprehensive pathway map of epidermal growth factor receptor signaling. Mol Syst Biol 2005;1:2005. 0010.
3. Tran QT, Kennedy LH, Leon Carrion S, et al. EGFR regulation of epidermal barrier function. Physiol Genomics 2012;44(8):455–69.
4. Cañueto J, Cardeñoso E, García JL, et al. Epidermal growth factor receptor expression is associated with poor outcome in cutaneous squamous cell carcinoma. Br J Dermatol 2017;176(5):1279–87.
5. Chanprapaph K, Vachiramon V, Rattanakaemakorn P. Epidermal growth factor receptor inhibitors: a review of cutaneous adverse events and management. Dermatol Res Pract 2014;2014:734249.
6. Skoda AM, Simovic D, Karin V, et al. The role of the Hedgehog signaling pathway in cancer: a comprehensive review. Bosn J Basic Med Sci 2018;18(1): 8–20.
7. Stecca B, Pandolfi S. Hedgehog-Gli signaling in basal cell carcinoma and other skin cancers: prospects for therapy. Res Rep Biol 2015;6:55–71.
8. Carpenter RL, Ray H. Safety and tolerability of sonic hedgehog pathway inhibitors in cancer. Drug Saf 2019;42(2):263–79.
9. Riley JL. PD-1 signaling in primary T cells. Immunol Rev 2009;229(1):114–25.
10. Robainas M, Otano R, Bueno S, et al. Understanding the role of PD-L1/PD1 pathway blockade and

autophagy in cancer therapy. Onco Targets Ther 2017;10:1803–7.

11. Akinleye A, Rasool Z. Immune checkpoint inhibitors of PD-L1 as cancer therapeutics. Hematol Oncol 2019;12(1):92.

12. Brahmer JR, Tykodi SS, Chow LQM, et al. Safety and activity of anti-PD-L1 antibody in patients with advanced cancer. N Engl J Med 2012;366(26): 2455–65.

13. Baraibar I, Melero I, Ponz-Sarvise M, et al. Safety and tolerability of immune checkpoint inhibitors (Pd-1 and pd-l1) in cancer. Drug Saf 2019;42(2): 281–94.

14. Wu S, Han J, Li W-Q, et al. Basal-cell carcinoma incidence and associated risk factors in U.S. women and men. Am J Epidemiol 2013;178(6):890–7.

15. Lo JS, Snow SN, Reizner GT, et al. Metastatic basal cell carcinoma: report of twelve cases with a review of the literature. J Am Acad Dermatol 1991;24(5 Pt 1):715–9.

16. Seo S-H, Shim W-H, Shin D-H, et al. Pulmonary metastasis of Basal cell carcinoma. Ann Dermatol 2011;23(2):213–6.

17. Pfeiffer P, Hansen O, Rose C. Systemic cytotoxic therapy of basal cell carcinoma. A review of the literature. Eur J Cancer 1990;26(1):73–7.

18. Moeholt K, Aagaard H, Pfeiffer P, et al. Platinum-Based Cytotoxic Therapy in Basal Cell Carcinoma a review of the literature. Acta Oncol 1996;35(6): 677–82.

19. Jefford M, Kiffer JD, Somers G, et al. Metastatic basal cell carcinoma: rapid symptomatic response to cisplatin and paclitaxel. ANZ J Surg 2004;74(8): 704–5.

20. Chatelut E, Delord J-P, Canal P. Toxicity patterns of cytotoxic drugs. Invest New Drugs 2003;21(2):141–8.

21. Sekulic A, Migden MR, Basset-Seguin N, et al. Long-term safety and efficacy of vismodegib in patients with advanced basal cell carcinoma: final update of the pivotal ERIVANCE BCC study. BMC cancer 2017;17(1):332.

22. Basset-Séguin N, Hauschild A, Kunstfeld R, et al. Vismodegib in patients with advanced basal cell carcinoma: Primary analysis of STEVIE, an international, open-label trial. Eur J Cancer 2017;86: 334–48.

23. Dréno B, Kunstfeld R, Hauschild A, et al. Two intermittent vismodegib dosing regimens in patients with multiple basal-cell carcinomas (Mikie): a randomised, regimen-controlled, double-blind, phase 2 trial. Lancet Oncol 2017;18(3):404–12.

24. Dummer R, Lear JT, Guminski A, et al. Efficacy of sonidegib in histologic subtypes of advanced basal cell carcinoma: Results from the final analysis of the randomized phase 2 Basal Cell Carcinoma Outcomes With LDE225 Treatment (BOLT) trial at 42 months. J Am Acad Dermatol 2021;84(4):1162–4.

25. Pricl S, Cortelazzi B, Dal Col V, et al. Smoothened (Smo) receptor mutations dictate resistance to vismodegib in basal cell carcinoma. Mol Oncol 2015; 9(2):389–97.

26. Ikeda S, Goodman AM, Cohen PR, et al. Metastatic basal cell carcinoma with amplification of PD-L1: exceptional response to anti-PD1 therapy. NPJ Genom Med 2016;1:16037.

27. Omland SH, Nielsen PS, Gjerdrum LMR, et al. Immunosuppressive environment in basal cell carcinoma: the role of regulatory t cells. Acta Derm Venereol 2016;96(7):917–21.

28. Jayaraman SS, Rayhan DJ, Hazany S, et al. Mutational landscape of basal cell carcinomas by whole-exome sequencing. J Invest Dermatol 2014; 134(1):213–20.

29. Deng JS, Brod BA, Saito R, et al. Immune-associated cells in basal cell carcinomas of skin. J Cutan Pathol 1996;23(2):140–6.

30. Urosevic M, Dummer R. Immunotherapy for nonmelanoma skin cancer: does it have a future? Cancer 2002;94(2):477–85.

31. Berg D, Otley CC. Skin cancer in organ transplant recipients: Epidemiology, pathogenesis, and management. J Am Acad Dermatol 2002;47(1):1–17 [quiz: 18-20].

32. Aboul-Fettouh N, Chen L, Silapunt S, et al. Use of pd-1 inhibitors in the treatment of advanced basal cell carcinoma. Dermatol Surg 2021;47(11):1511–2.

33. Stratigos AJ, Sekulic A, Peris K, et al. Cemiplimab in locally advanced basal cell carcinoma after hedgehog inhibitor therapy: an open-label, multi-centre, single-arm, phase 2 trial. Lancet Oncol 2021;22(6): 848–57.

34. Chang ALS, Tran DC, Cannon JGD, et al. Pembrolizumab for advanced basal cell carcinoma: An investigator-initiated, proof-of-concept study. J Am Acad Dermatol 2019;80(2):564–6.

35. Schmults CD, Karia PS, Carter JB, et al. Factors predictive of recurrence and death from cutaneous squamous cell carcinoma: a 10-year, single-institution cohort study. JAMA Dermatol 2013; 149(5):541–7.

36. Brewster DH, Bhatti LA, Inglis JHC, et al. Recent trends in incidence of nonmelanoma skin cancers in the East of Scotland, 1992-2003. Br J Dermatol 2007;156(6):1295–300.

37. Andersson EM, Paoli J, Wastensson G. Incidence of cutaneous squamous cell carcinoma in coastal and inland areas of Western Sweden. Cancer Epidemiol 2011;35(6):e69–74.

38. Katalinic A, Kunze U, Schäfer T. Epidemiology of cutaneous melanoma and non-melanoma skin cancer in Schleswig-Holstein, Germany: incidence, clinical subtypes, tumour stages and localization (Epidemiology of skin cancer). Br J Dermatol 2003; 149(6):1200–6.

39. DeConti RC. Chemotherapy of squamous cell carcinoma of the skin. Semin Oncol 2012;39(2):145–9.

40. Sadek H, Azli N, Wendling JL, et al. Treatment of advanced squamous cell carcinoma of the skin with cisplatin, 5-fluorouracil, and bleomycin. Cancer 1990;66(8):1692–6.

41. Guthrie TH, McElveen LJ, Porubsky ES, et al. Cisplatin and doxorubicin. An effective chemotherapy combination in the treatment of advanced basal cell and squamous carcinoma of the skin. Cancer 1985;55(8):1629–32.

42. Maubec E, Boubaya M, Petrow P, et al. Phase ii study of pembrolizumab as first-line, single-drug therapy for patients with unresectable cutaneous squamous cell carcinomas. J Clin Oncol 2020; 38(26):3051–61.

43. Montaudié H, Viotti J, Combemale P, et al. Cetuximab is efficient and safe in patients with advanced cutaneous squamous cell carcinoma: a retrospective, multicentre study. Oncotarget 2020;11(4): 378–85.

44. William WN, Feng L, Ferrarotto R, et al. Gefitinib for patients with incurable cutaneous squamous cell carcinoma: A single-arm phase II clinical trial. J Am Acad Dermatol 2017;77(6):1110–3.e2.

45. Gold KA, Kies MS, William WN, et al. Erlotinib in the treatment of recurrent or metastatic cutaneous squamous cell carcinoma: A single-arm phase 2 clinical trial. Cancer 2018;124(10):2169–73.

46. Wheeler DL, Dunn EF, Harari PM. Understanding resistance to EGFR inhibitors-impact on future treatment strategies. Nat Rev Clin Oncol 2010;7(9): 493–507.

47. Pickering CR, Zhou JH, Lee JJ, et al. Mutational landscape of aggressive cutaneous squamous cell carcinoma. Clin Cancer Res 2014;20(24):6582–92.

48. Euvrard S, Kanitakis J, Claudy A. Skin cancers after organ transplantation. N Engl J Med 2003;348(17): 1681–91.

49. Wu Y, Xu J, Du C, et al. The predictive value of tumor mutation burden on efficacy of immune checkpoint inhibitors in cancers: a systematic review and meta-analysis. Front Oncol 2019;9:1161.

50. Amoils M, Kim J, Lee C, et al. Pd-l1 expression and tumor-infiltrating lymphocytes in high-risk and metastatic cutaneous squamous cell carcinoma. Otolaryngol Head Neck Surg 2019;160(1):93–9.

51. Migden MR, Rischin D, Schmults CD, et al. PD-1 Blockade with Cemiplimab in Advanced Cutaneous Squamous-Cell Carcinoma. N Engl J Med 2018; 379(4):341–51.

52. Hughes BGM, Munoz-Couselo E, Mortier L, et al. Pembrolizumab for locally advanced and recurrent/ metastatic cutaneous squamous cell carcinoma (KEYNOTE-629 study): an open-label, nonrandomized, multicenter, phase II trial. Ann Oncol 2021; 32(10):1276–85.

53. Nowicki TS, Hu-Lieskovan S, Ribas A. Mechanisms of resistance to pd-1 and pd-l1 blockade. Cancer J 2018;24(1):47–53.

54. Upadhaya S, Neftelino ST, Hodge JP, et al. Combinations take centre stage in PD1/PDL1 inhibitor clinical trials. Nat Rev Drug Discov 2021;20(3):168–9.

55. Puzanov I, Milhem MM, Andtbacka RHI, et al. Primary analysis of a phase 1b multicenter trial to evaluate safety and efficacy of talimogene laherparepvec (T-vec) and ipilimumab (Ipi) in previously untreated, unresected stage IIIB-IV melanoma. J Clin Oncol 2014;32(15_suppl):9029.

56. Regeneron P. A phase 1 study of pre-operative cemiplimab (Regn2810), administered intralesionally, for patients with recurrent cutaneous squamous cell carcinoma(Cscc). Clinical trial registration. 2021. NCT03889912. Available at: https:// clinicaltrials.gov/ct2/show/NCT03889912. Accessed July 15, 2021.

57. Middleton MR, Sacco JJ, Merchan JR, et al. An open label, multicenter, phase I/II study of RP1 as a single agent and in combination with PD1 blockade in patients with solid tumors. J Clin Oncol 2019;37(15_ suppl):TPS2671.

58. D'Angelo SP, Russell J, Lebbé C, et al. Efficacy and safety of first-line avelumab treatment in patients with stage iv metastatic merkel cell carcinoma: a preplanned interim analysis of a clinical trial. JAMA Oncol 2018;4(9):e180077.

59. D'Angelo SP, Bhatia S, Brohl AS, et al. Avelumab in patients with previously treated metastatic Merkel cell carcinoma: long-term data and biomarker analyses from the single-arm phase 2 JAVELIN Merkel 200 trial. J Immunother Cancer 2020;8(1):e000674.

60. Nghiem P, Bhatia S, Lipson EJ, et al. Three-year survival, correlates and salvage therapies in patients receiving first-line pembrolizumab for advanced Merkel cell carcinoma. J Immunother Cancer 2021; 9(4):e002478.

61. Grignani G, Rutkowski P, Lebbe C, et al. 545 A phase 2 study of retifanlimab in patients with advanced or metastatic merkel cell carcinoma (Mcc) (POD1UM-201). J Immunother Cancer 2021; 9(Suppl 2):A574–5.

62. Glutsch V, Kneitz H, Gesierich A, et al. Activity of ipilimumab plus nivolumab in avelumab-refractory Merkel cell carcinoma. Cancer Immunol Immunother 2021;70(7):2087–93.

63. Ota S, Sakamoto T, Ochiai R, et al. Successful treatment with taxane-based chemotherapy in advanced sebaceous carcinoma: a case report and literature review. Case Rep Oncol 2019;12(1):47–52.

64. Kodali S, Tipirneni E, Gibson PC, et al. Carboplatin and Pembrolizumab Chemoimmunotherapy Achieves Remission in Recurrent, Metastatic Sebaceous Carcinoma. Ophthalmic Plast Reconstr Surg 2018;34(5):e149–51.

65. Banerjee N, Hossain F, Wirtschafter E, et al. Pembrolizumab in the treatment of microsatellite instability-high sebaceous carcinoma: a case report with review of the literature. JCO Precis Oncol 2020;4:61–5.

66. Chen H, Liu Y, Peng F, et al. Pulmonary metastases of fibrosarcomatous dermatofibrosarcoma protuberans respond to apatinib-based angiogenesis and chemotherapy: a case report. Ann Transl Med 2019;7(7):149.

67. Rutkowski P, Van Glabbeke M, Rankin CJ, et al. Imatinib mesylate in advanced dermatofibrosarcoma protuberans: pooled analysis of two phase II clinical trials. J Clin Oncol 2010;28(10):1772–9.

68. Jaal J, Putnik K. Induction cisplatin-based chemotherapy and following radiotherapy in locally advanced basal cell carcinoma of the skin. Acta Oncol 2012;51(7):952–4.

69. Shin DM, Glisson BS, Myers J, et al. Phase II and biologic study of interferon alfa, retinoic acid, and cisplatin in advanced squamous skin cancer. J Clin Oncol 2002;20(2):364–70.

70. Nottage MK, Lin C, Hughes BGM, et al. Prospective study of definitive chemoradiation in locally or regionally advanced squamous cell carcinoma of the skin. Head Neck 2017;39(4):679–83.

71. Foote MC, McGrath M, Guminski A, et al. Phase II study of single-agent panitumumab in patients with incurable cutaneous squamous cell carcinoma. Ann Oncol 2014;25(10):2047–52.

72. Rischin D, Migden MR, Lim AM, et al. Phase 2 study of cemiplimab in patients with metastatic cutaneous squamous cell carcinoma: primary analysis of fixed-dosing, long-term outcome of weight-based dosing. J Immunother Cancer 2020;8(1):e000775. Original research.

73. Migden MR, Khushalani NI, Chang ALS, et al. Cemiplimab in locally advanced cutaneous squamous cell carcinoma: results from an open-label, phase 2, single-arm trial. Lancet Oncol 2020;21(2):294–305.

74. Grob J-J, Gonzalez R, Basset-Seguin N, et al. Pembrolizumab monotherapy for recurrent or metastatic cutaneous squamous cell carcinoma: a single-arm phase II trial (KEYNOTE-629). J Clin Oncol 2020;38(25):2916–25.

Mohs Micrographic Surgery

Nicholas Golda, MD[a],*, George Hruza, MD, MBA[b]

KEYWORDS

- Mohs surgery • Micrographic surgery • Skin cancer treatment
- Complete circumferential peripheral and deep margin assessment

KEY POINTS

- Mohs surgery is the most effective treatment of skin cancer and offers maximum tissue conservation.
- The procedure requires refined surgical technique and careful laboratory processes in order to achieve the best possible patient outcomes.
- The treatment of melanoma and melanoma in situ by Mohs micrographic surgery has undergone significant refinement and wider acceptance, with cure rates equal to or superior to conventional excision.

INTRODUCTION

Mohs micrographic surgery (MMS) is a specialized technique for the surgical management of skin cancer. Since the first patient was treated by Dr Mohs in 1936, Mohs surgeons have established themselves as leading contributors to the science of cutaneous oncology, innovators in laboratory techniques for the microscopic assessment of skin cancer specimens, and expert providers of reconstruction following the surgical removal of skin cancer. MMS, nearly 90 years following its first use, remains the gold standard for skin cancer cure and is one of the most tissue-conserving and cost-effective options for skin cancer care when used appropriately and when recurrences and prevention of advanced disease are accounted for.

INITIAL PATIENT EVALUATION

Although MMS is the most effective and often the most conservative treatment of skin cancer, there are many situations where less technically demanding and lower cost treatment options may be a superior option for a given clinical scenario. To this end, the American Academy of Dermatology (AAD) developed the appropriate use criteria (AUC) for Mohs surgery.[1] This tool can assist physicians in determining whether MMS is appropriate for a given skin cancer. As a decision aid, the AUC does not serve to mandate a particular treatment over another. Tumors that are deemed appropriate for MMS by the AUC may still be treated with other techniques based on specific patient factors, and tumors that are uncertain or inappropriate may occasionally be treated with MMS if there are patient factors unaccounted for by the AUC that compel this decision. In general, however, MMS is considered appropriate in the following scenarios[2]:

- Where there is risk of disfigurement or functional impairment
- Recurrence
- Most cancers in immunosuppressed patients
- Large malignancies
- Poorly defined clinical borders
- Aggressive histologic features
- Sites where healing is difficult and tissue conservation will facilitate wound healing
- Patients with genetic skin cancer predisposition syndromes

[a] US Dermatology Partners, 3265 NE Ralph Powell Rd, Lee's Summit, MO 64064, USA; [b] Saint Louis University, Laser and Dermatologic Surgery Center, 1001 Chesterfield Pkwy E #101, Chesterfield, MO 6301, USA
* Corresponding author.
E-mail address: nicholas.golda@gmail.com

Dermatol Clin 41 (2023) 39–47
https://doi.org/10.1016/j.det.2022.07.006
0733-8635/23/© 2022 Elsevier Inc. All rights reserved.

derm.theclinics.com

- Cancers in previously irradiated skin, traumatic scars, sites of osteomyelitis, and chronically inflamed skin.

In order for MMS to be successful, the tumor being treated must grow in a contiguous manner. This includes most cutaneous malignancies such as basal cell carcinoma, squamous cell carcinoma, cutaneous adnexal malignancies, melanoma and melanoma in situ/lentigo maligna, dermatofibrosarcoma protuberans, cutaneous leiomyosarcoma, extramammary Paget disease, atypical fibroxanthoma/pleomorphic dermal sarcoma, Merkel cell carcinoma, and other less common cutaneous malignancies.[3] Cutaneous malignancies typically not amenable to treatment with MMS include angiosarcoma and Kaposi sarcoma. A patient must also be able to tolerate the procedure with the use of local anesthesia and possibly oral anxiolysis only.

PROCEDURE OVERVIEW
Preoperative Considerations

Identifying the correct site for surgery is important because wrong site surgery is a common cause of legal action against dermatologic surgeons.[4] Patients are often unable to accurately recall the correct site of a biopsy. Utilizing photographs taken at the time of biopsy is a best practice for avoiding wrong site surgery.[5] When no photograph of the biopsy site is available, Mohs surgeons can often identify the biopsy site clinically but may also confirm their site selection with the patient and any family that are present who may have assisted the patient with wound care for the biopsy site.

Photography and clinical documentation of the patient's state before initiating surgery can be helpful in both illustrating for the patient and documenting for medicolegal purposes any existing asymmetries, scars, palsies, or other anatomic irregularities that the patient may not be aware of to avoid attribution of these to the surgical procedure. Before injecting local anesthetic, mark relevant anatomic boundaries or features that may be helpful in reconstruction planning because the edema from injected anesthesia can make landmarks more challenging to identify.

Initiating the Procedure

Mohs surgery, in most cases, is carried out as a clean (nonsterile) procedure utilizing sterile instruments in a nonsterile clinical setting, nonsterile gloves, and clean drapes. Surgeons generally prepare for surgery using handwashing or alcohol hand sanitizers, and the surgical site is made antiseptic by the use of chlorhexidine gluconate or povidone iodine.

Some surgeons will then proceed to take the first Mohs stage, whereas others will first debulk the tumor by either curettage or scalpel. Curettage can grossly define the size of the skin cancer because tumors with noninfiltrative diagnoses can shell out easily providing firmer tactile feedback to the surgeon when tissue uninvolved by frank tumor is encountered. Benefits of curettage before the first layer of MMS include the following:

- Confirmation of the gross size and depth of a malignancy thereby avoiding unnecessary subsequent layers or allowing for a more conservative excision.
- Possible reduction in the presence of tumor floaters that may confound histologic analysis or result in false-positive interpretations.
- Tissue relaxation that may facilitate tissue processing.

Potential drawbacks include the chance of inducing skin tears or damaging adjacent epidermis, thereby rendering a Mohs layer taken through the damaged zone uninterpretable.

Scalpel-based sharp debulking may also be used. Sharp debulking is most often used to remove an exophytic tumor to facilitate taking a first Mohs stage or to debulk a tumor for histologic staging purposes. The primary pitfall of taking a debulking specimen is inadvertently taking too wide or too deep a debulk, thereby making the final Mohs excision larger than necessary. This risk can be minimized through careful technique.

Excising Mohs Tissue Specimens

The goal with each stage of MMS is to conservatively remove the malignancy in its entirety. The first stage consists of complete removal of the gross tumor as well as a narrow margin of clinically normal skin immediately around and deep to the tumor to allow for histologic processing and quality control. The specimen is removed with convex rounded contours whenever possible, and a bevel is placed around the periphery of the specimen such that the specimen is narrower at the base than it is at the surface. These actions facilitate tissue processing. If the surgeon provides a specimen that is challenging to process, then the specimen may not yield completely interpretable results even with skilled laboratory staff. This may lead to unnecessary additional stages of surgery or a greater chance of tumor recurrence for the patient.

Mohs surgeons place orienting marks on the patient's skin surrounding the specimen being excised that coordinate with marks placed on the specimen itself. This is most commonly carried out by the placement of small tissue nicks or scores with the scalpel, and the patterns of these scores can be variable based on surgeon preference. Placement of the scores in a systematized manner is important so that when the tissue is processed and interpreted, the surgeon can correlate the histologic findings with the correct location on the patient for a focused reexcision of any residual malignancy if necessary. To this end, most surgeons place tissue scores in an asymmetric manner so that the surgeon can reorient the specimen to the patient if any tissue handling error occurs during tissue processing because the specimen will only "fit" on the patient's defect one way. The most commonly deployed patterns for uncomplicated specimens include a single score in 1 location or 3 scores in a 12:00, 3:00, and 6:00 or similar asymmetric orientation (**Fig. 1**). Larger tumors are best scored with a grid or "graph paper" technique because this allows the highest possible resolution for residual tumor in the deep margin within the larger field of these tumors (see **Fig. 1**; **Fig. 2**). In this technique, scores are placed on each side of the tumor in strict 90° relation to one another such that the tissue can be divided into graph paper-like squares during tissue processing. Tissue scores, although necessary, also introduce potential error into the MMS process because each score produces an area where epidermis may be incompletely laid down into the sectioning plane. If the score results in failure to visualize focal residual tumor on a margin because of incomplete epidermal visualization, then a false negative may result.

Once the beveled incision at the periphery of the specimen is complete and scores are placed, the specimen is removed from the patient by making a flat incision across the deep margin of the specimen just below the deepest extent of the tumor. Pitfalls with incision through the deep margin of the Mohs specimen include making a jagged deep marginal incision that will create "drop out" areas on the specimen, taking an incomplete or buttonholed deep margin, grasping the tissue too firmly with toothed forceps causing triangular impressions in the deep margin that interfere with the assessment of the deep margin, and accidentally transplanting the tumor from the superficial part of the specimen to the deep part of the specimen by toothed forceps thus creating a false positive or tumor floater in the deep margin of the specimen. **Fig. 3** demonstrates proper basic technique as well as several possible pitfalls with taking of initial layers.

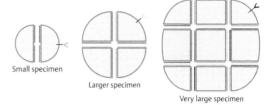

Fig. 1. Possible scoring, division, and inking patterns for various sized tissue specimens. (*From* Golda NJ, Hruza GJ. *Mohs Micrographic Surgery From Layers to Reconstruction.* 1st ed. (Harmon CB, Tolkachjov SN, eds.). © Thieme 2022.)

Taking an Initial Layer from a Recurrent or Incompletely Excised Site

Recurrent or incompletely excised sites present unique challenges because the normal anatomy has been modified by a previous closure and the tumor may now be discontiguous. This is why cure rates for tumors in these categories are lower than those for tumors treated primarily with Mohs surgery.[6–8] For incompletely excised sites, having information about whether the residual tumor is present at lateral or deep margins, or having the slides from the original excisional specimen available for review, can be helpful when planning for subsequent MMS.

Tissue Grossing

To execute the Mohs technique, the 3-dimensional tissue specimen must be converted to a 2-dimensional plane such that the epidermal, dermal, and deep margins can all be visualized in a single plane. This is accomplished during grossing by a series of relaxing cuts that allow the superficial

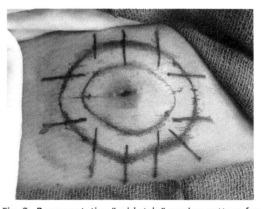

Fig. 2. Representative "grid style" scoring pattern for a larger tumor (DFSP pictured). (*From* Golda NJ, Hruza GJ. *Mohs Micrographic Surgery From Layers to Reconstruction.* 1st ed. (Harmon CB, Tolkachjov SN, eds.). © Thieme 2022.)

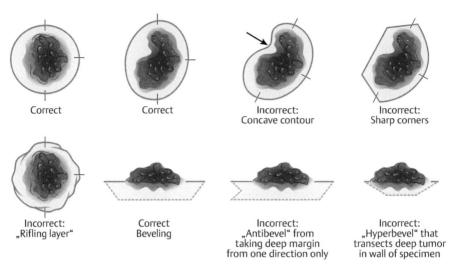

Fig. 3. Representative correct techniques and pitfalls for excision of the first layer of MMS. (*From* Golda NJ, Hruza GJ. *Mohs Micrographic Surgery From Layers to Reconstruction.* 1st ed. (Harmon CB, Tolkachjov SN, eds.). © Thieme 2022.)

part of the tissue to open like an accordion, thereby permitting the epidermal edge to lay down into the same plane as the deep margin. Tissue relaxation is facilitated as well by debulking as described previously.

Based on surgeon preference, MMS specimens can be divided before freezing and sectioning or can be processed as a single piece.[9] There are merits and drawbacks to both approaches. There may be time saved in the laboratory when a specimen is processed as a single piece but obtaining sufficient tissue relaxation to achieve full lay-down of the epidermis into the processing plane is more challenging and may result in lost time or the need for specimen recuts. A divided specimen is always required if the excised tumor is too large to fit on a microscope slide. The tissue grossing process is a source of several potential causes of false-positive findings on Mohs histologic specimens that the surgeon must be aware of:

- Dividing specimens can result in superficial tumor being pushed through to the deep margin of the specimen (**Fig. 4**).
- Following specimen division, superficial tumoral tissue in the center of the specimen may fall into continuity with the deep margin (**Fig. 5**).
- Excessive downward pressure on the specimen while freezing the tissue into the planar orientation for tangential sectioning may press tumoral tissue closer to the deep margin and predispose to false positives.
- Excessive facing into the frozen tissue block due to suboptimal epidermal relaxation and epidermal lay-down can cut into the gross

tumor when it may not have been present in the true margin if the specimen had been sectioned more conservatively.

Once the tissue is relaxed, it is marked with tissue dyes to further allow the surgeon to orient the histologic findings to the tumor site on the patient, and a map is created illustrating the tissue divisions, the tissue-inking pattern, and often the anatomic position and orientation of the tumor on the patient.

Tissue Processing

There are several techniques used to obtain a flat specimen following grossing in preparation for tissue freezing. One commonly deployed technique

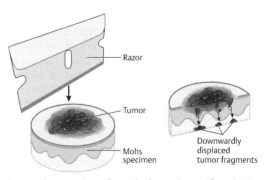

Fig. 4. The creation of "push-through" artifact during specimen division where tumor is displaced from friable tissue at the surface to create a false-positive deep margin. (*From* Golda NJ, Hruza GJ. *Mohs Micrographic Surgery From Layers to Reconstruction.* 1st ed. (Harmon CB, Tolkachjov SN, eds.). © Thieme 2022.)

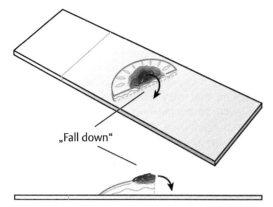

„Fall down"

Fig. 5. The mechanism for "fall over" artifact where superficial tissue from the center of a divided specimen can relax into the deep plane and create false-positive findings. (*From* Golda NJ, Hruza GJ. *Mohs Micrographic Surgery From Layers to Reconstruction.* 1st ed. (Harmon CB, Tolkachjov SN, eds.). © Thieme 2022.)

is to lay the specimen flat on a microscope slide such that the complete epidermal margin and deep margin are in full contact with the slide. The slide is then placed on a heat sink in the cryostat, covered with optimal cutting temperature medium, and a prepared cryostat chuck is placed on top of it. This is allowed to freeze, and the tissue is subsequently sectioned into thicknesses ranging from very thin 4-μm sections for immunohistochemical (IHC) staining up to 8-μm sections for traditional hematoxylin and eosin or toluidine blue staining. In certain scenarios, longer freezing times or thicker specimens may be needed to obtain excellent sections, particularly for sections with considerable fat; thus, the surgeon and laboratory staff must be able to make adjustments as necessary when certain scenarios requiring nuance arise. The tissue is then stained.

Histologic Interpretation and Mapping

A significant part of MMS fellowship training includes the proper interpretation of tangentially processed frozen section histology. Histologic interpretation requires the ability to recognize subtle changes consistent with the trailing edge of skin cancer at the margins of a Mohs excision and the ability to assess tissue specimens for quality.

An important first step in interpretation is awareness of the tumor that is being excised. Although common malignancies are easily recognized with experience, less common variants can be more challenging, and it is often helpful to review the original diagnostic biopsy slides or to take a frozen section biopsy or debulk specimen for vertical

sectioning from the center of the malignancy on the day of surgery in these cases.

Errors in slide preparation and interpretation have been shown to account for a large proportion of recurrences following MMS.[10–12] Therefore, attention to careful processes that avoid errors as well as expert interpretation of histologic specimens is important in the success of the technique.

Accuracy begins with confirming that maps and tissue specimens are correctly coordinated and identified. Next, the surgeon may inspect the specimen to confirm that there are no obvious features that indicate the specimen is incorrect such as gross size differences from what is expected, scoring patterns that do not coordinate with the map, and histologic features on the specimen that suggest an anatomic location different than that being treated. The specimen is then assessed for laboratory process and staining quality. Common issues include but are not limited to air bubbles from improper coverslipping, brown discoloration from insufficient clearing, missing stains or stain darkness issues, folded, chattered, or otherwise poorly flattened or sectioned specimens, and specimens cut too thick. A complete representation of the epidermis around the total circumference of the specimen as well as a complete deep margin with no zones of missing tissue are ideal for Mohs histologic interpretation.

Histologic Interpretation

The surgeon and pathologist being the same physician is a required element of MMS. Mohs surgeons are well-trained in the assessment and histologic mapping of frozen section tissue processed by tangential sectioning for both common and rare malignancies of the skin and are able to recognize even subtle residual malignancy in a specimen margin. A thorough description of these tumors and their features is beyond the scope of this article but common pearls and pitfalls are described herein.

Inflammation, typically manifesting as dense lymphocytic aggregates in the specimen, can occur for a variety of reasons including unrelated inflammation in the skin, inflammation related to the biopsy that was recently performed in the treatment zone, incidental chronic lymphocytic leukemia (CLL), or inflammation related to the tumor being treated. The latter cause is important to recognize because such peritumoral inflammation may alert the surgeon to small foci of invasive malignancy or may obscure tumor, thereby making it more difficult for the surgeon to diagnose.[13]

Tumoral tissue may also be artifactually present on the MMS histologic slides due to process errors during excision and tissue processing. The surgeon must be able to recognize these scenarios and work to correct the errors that underlie them. A commonly encountered artifact is a tumor floater (**Fig. 6**), which is an artifactual segment of tumor that has been dislodged and has come to rest on some portion of the margin being assessed on the histologic slide. Common causes of tumor floaters include tumor fragments that are displaced during tissue grossing, fragments transferred from the superficial to the deep margin during excision by a toothed forcep, and "fall-down artifact" that may occur in divided specimens as discussed earlier. When there is doubt, the surgeon should err on the side of excising a thin layer of additional tissue to confirm that the margins are free of tumor as oncologic cure is the most important motivating factor for performing MMS.

Proper histologic interpretation also demands that the surgeon be able to recognize benign neoplasms and normal structures in the tissue and not confuse these with malignant tissue that requires excision. Structures in the skin that may mimic malignancy include the following:

- Salivary glands can be encountered particularly on the lip or in the area immediately anterior and inferior to the ear (parotid gland)
- Hair follicles and sebaceous glands
- Goblet cells in conjunctival epithelium or urethral transitional epithelium can be confused with pagetoid cells associated with sebaceous carcinoma or extramammary Paget disease
- Follicular basaloid proliferation (benign follicular proliferation or benign follicular hamartoma)[14]

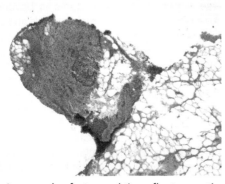

Fig. 6. An example of a tumoral tissue floater creating a false-positive deep margin. (*From* Golda NJ, Hruza GJ. *Mohs Micrographic Surgery From Layers to Reconstruction.* 1st ed. (Harmon CB, Tolkachjov SN, eds.). © Thieme 2022.)

- Benign adnexal neoplasms[14]
- Calcinosis cutis

Ideally, the Mohs surgeon will examine the tissue specimens not only for the presence or absence of malignancy but also for the presence of factors that may contribute to the patient's care such as finding and documenting features that may upstage a patient's SCC[15] and documenting the presence of lymphocytic infiltration consistent with lymphoproliferative disease, such as CLL, and initiating a workup if these features are identified.[16]

Tissue Mapping

MMS is effective because the surgeon is able to accurately pinpoint the exact location of any residual malignancy on the patient and selectively reexcise it. Histologic mapping is the tool that allows documentation of residual malignancy in relation to the patient's anatomy and the orienting marks the surgeon has placed on the patient and specimen.

Imprecise mapping may lead to selective reexcision of an incorrect site or reexcision of an inadequate breadth or depth of the correct site. Selective reexcision of the incorrect site is particularly challenging because the result will be a histologically tumor-free margin on the subsequent layer and false reassurance that the tumor was properly treated.

When mapping a tumor, the surgeon is aware that the tumor being mapped is a 3-dimensional figure with an edge, a wall, a hinge where the wall transitions to the base, and a deep margin. Often there is histologic evidence that aids the surgeon in accounting for tumor in the wall of a specimen and tumor in the hinge point or base. The most obvious form of this evidence comes from hair follicles, which are sectioned vertically in the wall and horizontally in the base. Careful attention to the precise 3-dimensional location of the residual tumor when mapping is important. Proper tumoral mapping should include the tumor type and subtype and anatomic depth. The notation of scar tissue, when observed, may aid the surgeon in resolving if the true deep or lateral margin has been reached and histologically assessed in a recurrent or incompletely excised tumor.

The surgeon may also wish to note histologic abnormalities that are not malignancies to document that these were observed and deemed to not be a positive margin. Noting actinic keratoses on the Mohs map may be helpful in that the surgeon has noted in the medical record the presence of actinic damage that did not require excision but will require subsequent superficial treatment.

The MMS map is an important part of the medical record that illustrates the observations the surgeon makes histologically and the decision-making regarding structures that will require reexcision because they were determined to be malignant and those that will be left behind because they were determined to be benign or more appropriately treated by other means such as in the case of actinic keratoses. A surgeon may wish to make written comments on the map as well to add clarity to decisions that are made based on histology and to guide selective reexcision of residual tumor.

Subsequent Layers

The rate of recurrence increases when numerous stages are required to obtain clear margins for a skin cancer being treated by MMS.[11] Tumors requiring multiple stages may be more biologically aggressive, and when multiple stages are required, there are more opportunities for a surgeon or processing error such as inaccurate mapping. Being purposeful in the planning and execution of subsequent layers is important. Although the surgeon should attempt to completely remove all residual tumor with each subsequent layer, the goal remains to also be tissue-sparing, so the surgeon should excise subsequent layers in a manner that will allow easy reorientation to the site if yet another stage is required.

The most common mechanism for indicating the extent of a subsequent layer on the patient is to place tissue scores in the skin at either side of a selective reexcision where the curvature of the edges fades back into the rounded contour of the original MMS stage although other acceptable techniques exist. The surgeon should ensure that these terminal scores on either side of a subsequent stage are discernible from those in place from earlier layers so reorientation is possible if another stage is required. Additional scores can also be placed in the span of subsequent layers to provide better resolution of the location of residual tumor if a subsequent layer persists in having tumor at the margins. Additionally, if a surgeon determines that more than one distinct tissue specimen should be excised during a single subsequent layer, these specimens can be differentiated from one another by the placement of a midpoint score in one specimen and no score in the other. Attention must be paid to inking of multiple distinct tissue specimens in one layer so they may be distinguished from one another.

At times, the surgeon may need to reexcise residual tumor that is present only in the deep margin of the specimen. Maintaining tissue orientation can be challenging when the more fragile deep tissue, consisting often of fat and possibly muscle, requires reexcision and there is no adjacent dermis, thus making orientation utilizing dermal scores or marks not possible. Below are some techniques that facilitate orientation in this scenario:

1. The necessary deep tissue can be removed as well as a nearby thin margin of dermis. The location of this dermal tag is marked by a tissue score. When tissue processing is done, the dermis is laid down as per normal Mohs tissue processing and any residual tumor in the deep margin can be mapped using this dermal tag as a reference point.
2. In large tumors where there is an extensive field of deep tissue, the surgeon uses the previously described gridding technique to accurately locate residual tumor on a deep margin. Once the appropriate zone in the grid that requires reexcision is identified, the surgeon excises the entirety of that polygon of involved tissue and inks the flat sides with different colors to correspond with the map. This allows precise location of any residual deep tumor relative to the uniquely inked margins.

Regardless of which technique is used, the critical element of deep-only layers is the same as that for all subsequent layers: complete removal of the malignancy and the ability to reorient for another selective reexcision if the margins remain involved by malignancy.

New Developments

An area of profound development in recent years is the use and acceptance of MMS for the treatment of melanoma. Although dermatologic surgeons have treated melanoma in situ as well as invasive melanoma for years using MMS,[17,18] the development of rapid protocols for melanocyte-specific IHC staining on frozen section specimens and increasing evidence supporting MMS as noninferior or superior to wide local excision, particularly on special sites,[19–21] has led to an expansion of the use of MMS for melanoma, and the most recent iteration of the Mohs AUC published by the AAD recognizes the treatment of lentigo maligna and melanoma in situ as appropriate in most scenarios.[1] An update to the AUC is expected this year that will likely further clarify the appropriateness of MMS for melanoma. The most commonly used IHC stain

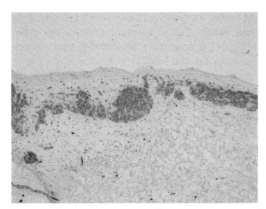

Fig. 7. Melanoma in situ MMS frozen section stained with MART-1 IHC (100×).

is the melanoma antigen recognized by T cells (MART-1) stain (**Fig. 7**), although effective protocols for SRY-related HMG-box 10 (SOX-10) and others are becoming available (**Fig. 8**). The execution of these laboratory techniques is painstaking, time-consuming, and requires well-trained laboratory staff to produce consistent results, but consensus is emerging that the use of IHC while doing Mohs surgery for melanoma is a best practice.[22,23]

The execution of the MMS procedure for melanoma is much the same as it is for conventional MMS although a few key differences exist.[24] Mohs surgeons will more commonly take sharp debulking specimens for staging purposes, which are processed with vertical sections by frozen section, permanent sections, or both. Surgeons will also start with wider margins than typically used in nonmelanoma skin cancer, often 5 mm from the visible tumor border, and will excise to a depth appropriate for melanoma treatment where anatomically appropriate.

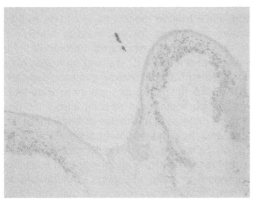

Fig. 8. Melanoma in situ MMS frozen section stained with SOX-10 IHC (40×).

SUMMARY

MMS is widely accepted as the gold standard for skin cancer care, and the surgeons who carry out this procedure are experts in the management of skin cancer. There are many potential pitfalls and challenges that a surgeon may encounter while carrying out MMS, which can increase the likelihood of tumor recurrence and increased patient morbidity. With proper training and careful processes that safeguard against errors, this procedure can provide excellent cure rates for most skin cancers, including melanoma, while maximizing tissue conservation in a low-cost outpatient clinical setting.

CLINICS CARE POINTS

- Mohs micrographic surgery (MMS) is the most effective treatment available for skin cancer but its use should be limited to only those malignancies for which it has been deemed appropriate.

- Careful processes are required at every step in the procedure (surgical, laboratory and pathologic interpretation) to achieve the dual goals of MMS: highest possible cure and maximal tissue conservation.

- Evidence and consensus support the expanding use of MMS for the treatment of melanoma, and research is underway to establish best practices.

DISCLOSURE

The authors have no relevant conflicts of interest to disclose.

REFERENCES

1. Connolly SM, Baker DR, Coldiron BM, et al. AAD/ACMS/ASDSA/ASMS 2012 appropriate use criteria for Mohs micrographic surgery: A report of the American Academy of Dermatology, American College of Mohs Surgery, American Society for Dermatologic Surgery Association, and the American Society for Mohs Surgery. J Am Acad Dermatol 2012;67(4):531–50.
2. Golda NJ, Hruza GJ. In: Harmon CB, Tolkachjov SN, editors. Mohs micrographic surgery from layers to reconstruction. 1st ed. Thieme; 2021. Available at: https://www.thieme.com/books-main/dermatology/product/6210-mohs-micrographic-surgery. Accessed December 19, 2021.

3. Tolkachjov SN, Brodland DG, Coldiron BM, et al. Understanding mohs micrographic surgery: a review and practical guide for the nondermatologist. Mayo Clin Proc 2017;92(8):1261–71.

4. Perlis CS, Campbell RM, Perlis RH, et al. Incidence of and risk factors for medical malpractice lawsuits among mohs surgeons. Dermatol Surg 2008;32(1):79–83.

5. McGinness JL, Goldstein G. The value of preoperative biopsy-site photography for identifying cutaneous lesions. Dermatol Surg 2010;36(2):194–7.

6. Rowe DE, Carroll RJ, Day CL. Mohs surgery is the treatment of choice for recurrent (previously treated) basal cell carcinoma. J Dermatol Surg Oncol 1989;15(4):424–31.

7. Rowe DE, Carroll RJ, Day CL. Prognostic factors for local recurrence, metastasis, and survival rates in squamous cell carcinoma of the skin, ear, and lip: Implications for treatment modality selection. J Am Acad Dermatol 1992;26(6):976–90.

8. Rowe DE, Carroll RJ, Day CL. Long-term recurrence rates in previously untreated (Primary) basal cell carcinoma: implications for patient follow-up. J Dermatol Surg Oncol 1989;15(3):315–28.

9. Randle HW, Zittelli J, Brodland DG, et al. Histologic preparation for mohs micrographic surgery: the single section method. J Dermatol Surg Oncol 1993;19(6):522–4.

10. Hruza GJ. Mohs micrographic surgery local recurrences. J Dermatol Surg Oncol 1994;20(9):573–7.

11.. Samie F. Surgeon error and slide quality during Mohs micrographic surgery: Is there a relationship with tumor recurrence? J Am Acad Dermatol 2021;85(2):538.

12. Zabielinski M, Leithauser L, Godsey T, et al. Laboratory errors leading to nonmelanoma skin cancer recurrence after mohs micrographic surgery. Dermatol Surg 2015;41(8):913–6.

13. Macdonald J, Sneath JR, Cowan B, et al. Tumor detection after inflammation or fibrosis on Mohs levels. Dermatol Surg 2013;39(1 Pt 1):64–6.

14. Stanoszek LM, Wang GY, Harms PW. Histologic Mimics of Basal Cell Carcinoma. Arch Pathol Lab Med 2017;141(11):1490–502.

15. Karia PS, Jambusaria-Pahlajani A, Harrington DP, et al. Evaluation of american joint committee on cancer, international union against cancer, and brigham and women's hospital tumor staging for cutaneous squamous cell carcinoma. J Clin Oncol 2014;32(4):327–34.

16. Padgett JK, Parlette HL, English JC. A diagnosis of chronic lymphocytic leukemia prompted by cutaneous lymphocytic infiltrates present in Mohs micrographic surgery frozen sections. Dermatol Surg 2003;29(7):769–71.

17. Mohs FE. Chemosurgery for melanoma. Arch Dermatol 1977;113(3):285–91.

18. Zitelli JA, Mohs FE, Larson P, et al. Mohs micrographic surgery for melanoma. Dermatol Clin 1989;7(4):833–43.

19. Rzepecki AK, Hwang CD, Etzkorn JR, et al. The rule of 10s versus the rule of 2s: High complication rates after conventional excision with postoperative margin assessment of specialty site versus trunk and proximal extremity melanomas. J Am Acad Dermatol 2021;85(2):442–52.

20. Demer AM, Hanson JL, Maher IA, et al. Association of mohs micrographic surgery vs wide local excision with overall survival outcomes for patients with melanoma of the trunk and extremities. JAMA Dermatol 2021;157(1):84–9.

21. Hanson J, Demer A, Liszewski W, et al. Improved overall survival of melanoma of the head and neck treated with Mohs micrographic surgery versus wide local excision. J Am Acad Dermatol 2020;82(1):149–55.

22. Miller CJ, Giordano CN, Higgins HW. Mohs micrographic surgery for melanoma: as use increases, so does the need for best practices. JAMA Dermatol 2019;155(11):1225–6.

23. Krausz AE, Higgins HW, Etzkorn J, et al. Systematic review of technical variations for mohs micrographic surgery for melanoma. Dermatol Surg 2021;47(12):1539–44.

24. Etzkorn JR, Sobanko JF, Elenitsas R, et al. Low recurrence rates for in situ and invasive melanomas using Mohs micrographic surgery with melanoma antigen recognized by T cells 1 (MART-1) immunostaining: Tissue processing methodology to optimize pathologic staging and margin assessment. J Am Acad Dermatol 2015;72(5):840–50.

Melanoma classification and management in the era of molecular medicine

Sarem Rashid, BS[a,b], Michael Shaughnessy, MD[c], Hensin Tsao, MD, PhD[a,c],*

KEYWORDS

- Cutaneous melanoma • Surgical treatment • Biopsy • Epidemiology • Combination therapy
- Malignant melanoma • Wide local excision

KEY POINTS

- Melanoma is the most lethal form of skin cancer caused by abnormal proliferation of pigment-producing cells called melanocytes. Most of the melanomas are believed to be caused by exposure to ultraviolet (UV) radiation
- The epidemiology of melanoma varies based on sex, race/ethnicity, geographic location, among other factors. A true biological explanation for these discrepancies has yet to be determined.
- Drug resistance is a crucial limitation of current medical treatment regimens. Combination therapy trials are currently being performed using chemotherapy, targeted therapy, and/or immunotherapy.

INTRODUCTION

Cutaneous melanoma (CM) encompasses a group of pigmented tumors that arise from skin melanocytes. Melanocytes are neural crest-derived cells that commonly migrate to the skin and hair follicles during fetal development.[1] These cells produce melanin, a UV-absorbing polymer, which provides pigment to surrounding keratinocytes.[2,3] Malignant transformation of melanocytes is most likely initiated by ultraviolet (UV) light-induced DNA mutagenesis. The stochastic nature of this process, in turn, contributes to the vast clinical heterogeneity of melanoma, which will be the focus of this review.

EPIDEMIOLOGY
General Trends

Over the past several decades, CM burden has steadily increased, comprising an estimated 106,110 cases and 7,180 deaths nationally in 2021.[4] Despite being one of the most lethal forms of skin cancer, CM has a 5-year survival rate of more than 98% if diagnosed at the localized stage (according to SEER staging), which contrasts sharply with a survival rate of 30% at the distant stage based on comprehensive data in the United States between 2011 and 2017.[4] Prognosis for patients with advanced stages of malignant melanoma (MM) is governed by the number and location of metastases.[5] For example, patients with brain metastases have a sevenfold increase in overall survival when compared with patients with lung metastases, and a twofold increase when compared with patients with digestive metastases. Wide local excision (WLE) remains the mainstay of treatment for early and localized, or Stage 0 (all stages henceforth are designated according to the AJCC 8th Edition), lesions (Table 1).[6] Surgical excision has been proven less effective for melanoma which has already metastasized,[7] although patients presenting with a limited number of metastases and metastatic sites may still be considered for WLE after clinical evaluation.

[a] Wellman Center for Photomedicine, Massachusetts General Hospital, Harvard Medical School, Boston, MA 02114, USA; [b] Boston University School of Medicine, Boston, MA 02118, USA; [c] Department of Dermatology, Massachusetts General Hospital, Boston, MA 02114, USA

* Corresponding author.
E-mail address: htsao@mgh.harvard.edu

Dermatol Clin 41 (2023) 49–63
https://doi.org/10.1016/j.det.2022.07.017

Table 1
Breakdown of pathologic staging according to the AJCC 8th Edition

Stage Group	T-Category	N-Category	M-Category
0	Tis	N0	M0
IA	T1a-T1b	N0	M0
IB	T2a	N0	M0
IIA	T2b-T3a	N0	M0
IIB	T3b-T4a	N0	M0
IIC	T4b	N0	M0
IIIA	T1a–T2a	N1a-N2a	M0
IIIB	T1a–T2a	N1b-N2b	M0
IIIC	T2a-T3a	N2c-N3c	M0
IIIC	T3b-T4a	At least N1	M0
IIIC	T4b T3b-T4a	N1a–N2c	M0
IIID	T4b	N3a-N3c	M0
IV	All T-Categories	All N-Categories	M1

The duration and pattern of ultraviolet (UV) radiation exposure is a major environmental risk factor for developing CM.[2,8] An estimated two-thirds of MM are caused by UV radiation, suggesting a critical role in early detection and sun-protective behaviors.[9] Both UVA (wavelength: 315–400 nm) and UVB (wavelength: 280–315 nm) may cause DNA damage to the skin. UVA accounts for up to 95% of solar radiation that reaches the atmosphere; the longer wavelengths penetrate deeply into the skin and dermis.[10] In contrast, UVB penetrates less deeply into the dermis, yet is more potent than UVA, more readily absorbed by the DNA in skin cells and thus more carcinogenic than UVA.[11] Ultimately, UVB-mediated cytotoxicity is highly correlated with the increased risk of sunburn and subsequently melanoma. Intermittent exposure to high-intensity radiation is associated with increased melanoma risk compared with chronic exposure to lower-intensity radiation.[12]

Race and Ethnicity

There are several noteworthy trends with regard to ethnicity and race. In the United States, CM is far more common among whites when compared with Blacks—with incidence rates of 24.9 cases per 100,000 individuals versus 1.0 case per 100,000 individuals, respectively.[4] Despite this discrepancy, overall survival is significantly better in the white population when compared with non-whites.[13] Using SEER data from 1992 to 2009, Black patients were observed to have a greater proportion of melanomas diagnosed in later stages (Stage II, III, and IV). When stratified by stage, Black patients showed significantly increased hazard ratios for Stage I (HR = 3.037;

95% CI: 2.335–3.951) and Stage III (HR = 1.864; 95% CI: 1.211–2.87) melanomas. Registry data from 2000 to 2016 report similar discrepancies in melanoma-specific survival, suggesting that racial gaps in melanoma care have persisted in recent years.[14] Although melanoma incidence is directly proportional to socioeconomic status (SES), low SES has been associated with lesions diagnosed at later stage.[15] Burden of poverty or lack of insurance disproportionately affects Blacks and Hispanics within the United States. Furthermore, these groups may be less likely to benefit from public health initiatives and clinical trials due to racial-based trends in melanoma incidence.

Another explanation may include racial-based differences in melanoma subtype prevalence. Acral lentiginous melanoma (ALM) is a rare melanoma subtype overall, but it is the most frequently diagnosed subtype with specified histology diagnosed in Blacks.[16,17] These lesions are associated with increased thickness, advanced stage upon clinical diagnosis, and poorer outcomes.[18,19] SEER analysis from 1986 to 2005 demonstrated a 5-year melanoma-specific survival rate of 80.3% in ALM compared with 91.3% for all CM[19]. While the genetic profile of ALM is distinct from more common forms of CM, a true biological explanation has yet to be established, although discrepancies in socioeconomic status, culture, sun-seeking behaviors, and the elusive clinical nature of ALMs are suspected to contribute to the discussed trends in morbidity and mortality.

Geographic Patterns

Globally speaking, white populations residing closer to the equator are predisposed to higher melanoma risk presumably due to higher UV flux. This trend has also been observed for other common skin cancer such as squamous cell carcinoma and basal cell carcinoma.[20] Australia and New Zealand report the highest melanoma incidence with age-standardized rates of 33.6 cases per 100,000 individuals and 33.3 cases per 100,000 individuals, respectively.[21] Notably, these rates are larger in men for both countries (40.4 cases per 100,000 individuals and 35.8 cases per 100,000 individuals for Australia and New Zealand, respectively).

Trends in melanoma incidence based on geographic variability have been observed even within countries. In New Zealand, the relative risk of melanoma in the southern-most location of the island (latitude 44° S; away from the equator) compared with that of the northern-most region (latitude 36° S; toward the equator) was 0.63 (95% CI: 0.60–0.67).[22] Another study compiled by the Australian Cancer Atlas showed that melanoma incidence rates are substantially lower in central and southern Australia when compared with the national average.[23]

Sex

Recent SEER analysis reports a 1.8% increase in age-adjusted rate of melanoma for men compared with 2.5% per year on average for women.[24] This gender discrepancy seems to be partially dependent on an individual's age, as women have a higher incidence up until approximately 44 years of age,[25] while men reportedly have a higher incidence from approximately 44 to 85 years.[26] Furthermore, melanoma is the most frequent cancer in women aged 15 to 24.[25,27] Until approximately 44 years of age, women show greater melanoma incidence after which melanoma incidence in men is greater until 85 years of age. Social behaviors such as the routine use of indoor tanning devices in the young female demographic have been implicated with a dose-dependent risk melanoma, as well as many other cancers.[28] While incidence has been shown to be greater in certain female subgroups, adolescent and young males are 55% more likely to die from melanoma when compared with females, even after adjusting for tumor thickness, anatomic location, and histologic subtype.[29] Differences in immune, hormonal, or other biological factors that have yet to be elucidated may explain these disparities in clinical outcomes.

Sex has also been associated with primary anatomic distribution. Men are more likely to harbor melanomas on the head and trunk,[30] whereas women are more likely to harbor melanomas on their legs.[31] These observations may be explained by differences in sun protective behavior, clothing, and hairstyle. One biological explanation is sex-based differences in childhood nevus distribution leading to site-related nevus atypia.[32] This hypothesis suggests that melanoma etiology varies with the anatomic location of the primary site, as different body sites receive different patterns of sunlight. Studies show that women are more likely to harbor banal nevi on the extremities—across all ages—when compared with men.[33,34] Six genomic loci, *IRF4, DOCK8, MTAP, 9q31.2, KITLG, and PLA2G6*, have been implicated in female nevus count location, although further mechanistic studies are required to ascertain a genetic basis for nevus distribution.[34]

PATIENT EVALUATION OVERVIEW
Clinical Picture

Although previously understood as a single disease entity, cutaneous melanoma may be further subdivided into prognostically unique subsets based on the molecular signature, sun exposure pattern, histopathological features, and treatment. Histologic subtypes for melanoma include superficial spreading (SSM), nodular (NM), lentigo maligna (LMM), and acral lentiginous (ALM) (Table 2). Of these, SSM and NM are the most frequently encountered subtypes, comprising 60% to 70% and 10% to 20% of melanoma diagnoses, respectively.[35–38] NMs are generally found to be thicker than SSM and associated with a predominant vertical growth phase (VGP). LMMs comprise 4% to 15% of diagnosed melanomas[39,40] and arise from precancerous pigmented lesions called lentigo maligna (also called Hutchinson's melanotic freckle or circumscribed precancerous melanosis of Dubreuilh).[41] ALM is the rarest melanoma subtype—comprising 2% to 5% of melanoma diagnoses—and occurs on glabrous skin (ie, palms, soles, nail units).[16,42]

Routine skin examinations are recommended for patients suspected of melanoma. During an examination, melanoma morphology is carefully examined, often with the aid of dermoscopy, to scrutinize lesion size, shape, texture, and border irregularity among other visual characteristics (Fig. 1). Patients with melanoma may report symptoms such as ongoing itch, oozing, or crusting of a pigmented lesion.[42] Other notable history may include frequent sunburns, previous tanning bed exposure, personal history of skin cancer, family history of skin cancer, and evidence of melanoma tumor syndromes such as familial atypical multiple mole melanoma (FAMMM). In the absence of such

Table 2
Clinicopathological features of each melanoma subtype with associated clinical images

Melanoma Subtype	Image	Characteristics
Superficial Spreading Melanoma		• Comprises most of the melanoma cases (60%–70%) • Usually flat, although may present with elevation in advanced stages • Ulceration, itching, and bleeding may occur • 5- and 10-y melanoma-specific survival rate is 88.43% and 79.32%, respectively[108]
Nodular Melanoma		• Comprises approximately 10%–20% of cases • Dome-shaped, firm, symmetric, "bump" above the skin surface • Presents with a single color (blue, black, red, and so forth) or multicolor pigmentation • 5- and 10-y melanoma-specific survival rate is 51.67% and 38.75%, respectively[108]
Acral Lentiginous Melanoma		• Accounts up to 5% of cases • Presents on the palms, soles, and under the nails • Amelanotic or variable pigmentation (red, black, blue, green, or brown) • Ulceration or bleeding may occur • Proportion among all melanoma subtypes greatest in blacks • 5- and 10-y melanoma-specific survival rates of 80.3% (95% CI: 77.6–83.0) and 67.5% (95% CI: 63.4–71.6)[19]
Lentigo Maligna Melanoma		• Comprises 5%–15% of cases • Arises from a precursor lesion called lentigo maligna (or Hutchinson melanotic freckle) • Presents as a smooth surface with variable pigmentation and irregular borders • 5- and 10-y melanoma-specific survival rate is 89.28% and 78.61%, respectively[108]

risk factors, there is no consensus for routine melanoma screening.[42]

Lesions may present as nevus-associated melanomas or may arise spontaneously (without a pre-existing nevus) as *de novo* melanomas. Nevus-associated melanomas comprise approximately one-third of all melanoma diagnoses and commonly arise in younger patients—particularly those with a history of frequent sunburns and high baseline nevus count.[43,44] It has been estimated that, for a 20 years old, the risk of any mole transforming into melanoma by age 80 years is approximately 1 in 3,164 for men and 1 in 10,800 for women.[45] Lesions are preferentially located in the truncal areas. Prognostically, nevus-associated melanomas demonstrate better outcomes because lesions are generally thinner and detected earlier.[43] Contrarily, *de novo* melanoma is less frequently

encountered but considered more aggressive to its counterpart.[46] These lesions are more likely to resemble ALMs or LMMs histologically, although it is important to note that all subtypes may be encountered in both subgroups.[46]

Characterizing Atypical Lesions

For lesions suspected to be skin cancer, visual recognition tools such as the "ABCDE criteria" and "ugly duckling sign" may be used to usher a diagnosis. The ABCDE criteria describe the following set of atypical characteristics: A is for asymmetry, B is for border irregularity, C is for color heterogeneity, D is for diameter larger than 6 mm, and E is for evolution with regards to shape, size, or elevation. Secondly, the ugly duckling sign approach relies on the understanding that banal nevi on the body should closely resemble one

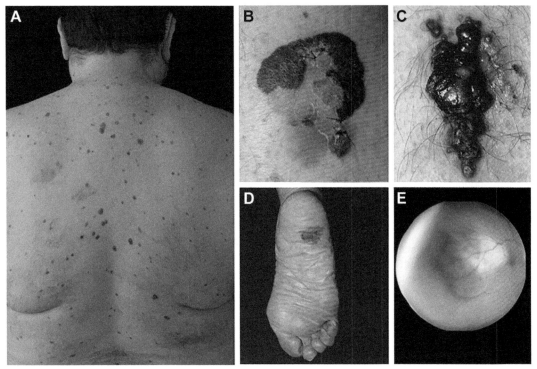

Fig. 1. Clinical presentation of cutaneous melanoma. (A) Approximately 20% to 30% of melanomas arise from pre-existing nevi of the skin, which predominantly harbor the superficial spreading subtype and BRAFV600 E mutation. Such nevi commonly present on the trunk and extremities in younger patients. Of the histologic subtypes, (B) superficial spreading melanomas are most common, followed by (C) nodular melanomas and (D) acral lentiginous melanomas. (E) Uveal melanomas arise from melanocytes in the pigmented tissues of the iris, ciliary body, and iris. These tumors may be asymptomatic and present during the routine eye examination. Image reprinted with permission.[116]

another. Nevi that are atypical from other nevi on the body may require further inspection with dermatoscopy. Once a suspicious skin lesion is detected, a biopsy may be performed to further establish diagnosis and staging.

Staging

Published in 2016, the 8th edition American Joint Commission for Cancer (AJCC) Cancer Staging Manual is a tumor-node-metastasis (TNM)-based classification scheme that classifies the size and ulceration of the primary tumor (T), spread to nearby lymph nodes (N), and spread to distant body sites (M).[47] Adequate sampling should include a primary tumor biopsy with controlled margins followed by pathologic assessment. Sentinel lymph node biopsy (SLNB) may be indicated for lesions suspected to be advanced melanoma. For biopsies containing multiple samples, the summative worst features should be incorporated into staging results.[48] In patients with multiple primary CM, the single highest stage group should be included.

T category

Current T-category features include thickness and ulceration. Thickness is measured using Breslow depth, or primary tumor depth of invasion from the granular layer of the epidermis to the deepest point of the tumor. This measurement should be calculated to the nearest tenth of a millimeter, as the measurement to the nearest 0.01 mm offers little prognostic advantage.[49] Current thresholds for melanoma thickness are defined as follows: no reported thickness for T0 (or melanoma in situ), $\leq$1.0 mm for T1, >1.0 to 2.0 mm for T2, >2.0 to 4.0 mm for T3, and >4.0 mm for T4.

The presence of ulceration in the primary tumors is indicated by the "b" subcategory for stage T1–T4 melanomas. Ulcerated tumors should be measured starting from the base of the ulceration.[50] Similar to Breslow thickness, ulceration is considered a strong independent prognostic factor in CM.[51,52] Epidermal disruption due to previous surgery, biopsy, or excoriation is not considered for prognosis and should not be mistaken for ulceration during the assessment.

Previously, the mitotic rate was included as a T-category feature but was removed following the 7th Edition AJCC guidelines. This recent removal is due to conflicting reports regarding the prognostic ability of mitotic rate. For example, multivariate analysis of the International Melanoma Database and Discovery Platform (IMDDP) showed that melanomas with a mitotic rate ≥ 1 mitosis/mm^2 squared had decreased survival compared with melanomas with a mitotic rate <1 mitosis/mm^2, although this finding was not found to be significant.[49] Other studies regard mitotic rate to be an important independent prognosticator for melanoma, similar to Breslow thickness.[53,54]

N category

The N-category in AJCC staging refers to metastatic spread to regional lymph nodes (LN). "Clinically occult" metastases refer to tumor-involved regional nodal metastases which are detected by SLNB but not detected through clinical or radiographical examination.[55] If regional nodal metastases can be detected either clinically or radiographically, then patients are defined as having "clinically detected" (N1a, N2a, N3a) metastases. Clinically occult (N1b, N2b, N2c) regional nodal metastases comprise most of the regional metastases during AJCC staging and have better outcomes.[49]

Microsatellite and intralymphatic metastases (N1c, N2c, N3c), such as satellites or in-transit metastases, are also included as an N-subcategory. The term microsatellite is defined by the AJCC 8th edition as "microscopic cutaneous and/or subcutaneous metastasis adjacent to or deep to and completely discontinuous from a primary melanoma with unaffected stroma occupying the space between."[47,56] Satellites include any skin or subcutaneous metastasis >2 cm from the primary lesion (although not surpassing the regional nodal basin).[47] In contrast, in-transit metastases occur ≤ 2 cm from the primary tumor and may develop in up to 5% to 10% of patients.[57] All 3 lesions (microsatellites, satellites, and in-transit metastases) demonstrate similar survival outcomes according to the recent analysis of the AJCC database and are therefore not distinguished from one another during staging.[49]

M category

M-category features incorporate the anatomic site of metastasis and serum lactate dehydrogenase (LDH) at the time of Stage IV diagnosis.[47] Serum LDH catalyzes the conversion of pyruvate to lactate in low oxygen states and has been found to be an important prognosticator in advanced melanoma.[58]

Overall, median survival for patients with distant metastases is approximately 6 to 8 months.[59] Although patients with distant metastases to the skin, subcutaneous tissue, muscle, or distant LN (M1a) fare better outcomes compared with patients with metastases to all other sites included in AJCC staging (M1b-M1d).[49,59,60]

SURGICAL TREATMENT OPTIONS
Excision

Surgical excision is the primary treatment of localized melanomas. WLE is performed with extended margins, determined based on tumor thickness, to ensure complete removal of the lesion, and adequate sampling for biopsy. For melanoma in situ and primary melanomas with thickness ≤ 1.0, 1.01 to 2, 2.01 to 4, and >4 mm, the NCCN recommends margins of 0.5 to 1, 1, 1 to 2, 2, and 2 cm, respectively (**Table 3**).[61–63]

Margins for invasive melanomas should be ≥ 1 cm and ≤ 2 cm around the primary lesion. Of the different biopsy techniques (shave, incisional, excisional, and punch), the AJCC and NCCN both recommend excisional biopsy due to the mitigation of potential sampling error.[47,64] Punch and incisional biopsies may be indicated for focally suspicious samples in larger lesions. Mohs micrographic surgery, commonly used for excision of keratinocyte carcinomas, is not currently recommended for routine melanoma removal unless the lesion resides in cosmetically sensitive areas (such as the face or hands).[65] For each procedure, careful evaluation of benefits and risks should be performed on an individual patient basis with guidance from clinical experts.

Sentinel Lymph Node Biopsy

Lymphatic mapping (LM) and SLN status are important for the accurate detection of nodal

Table 3	
NCCN guidelines for surgical margins during wide local excision of melanoma	
Thickness (mm)	Margin (cm)
Melanoma in situ	0.5–1.0
≤ 1.0	1.0
1.01–2.00	1.0–2.0
2.01–4.00	2.0
>4.00	2.0

During this procedure, all tissue up until the fascia should be removed. Resection margins may be further modified on a per-patient basis to accommodate anatomic or functional factors, although smaller margins may pose an increased risk for local recurrence groups at risk for metastases. During LM (or lymphoscintigraphy), vital blue dye is injected around the primary tumor site and nodal groups are visualized using technetium-99 sulfur colloid.[62] It is recommended that both procedures should be performed preoperatively before excision of the primary tumor.[66] SLNB is not routinely recommended for T1a lesions <0.8 cm (without ulceration) unless high-risk features are present. These features include but are not limited to young patient age, presence of lymphovascular invasion, and high mitotic rate. For lesions staged T2a and above, SLNB may be indicated after the acknowledgment of procedure benefits and risks.

Complete removal of all LN within the affected lymphatic basin (ie, completion lymph node dissection (CLND))[67] is rarely performed now. A Phase III trial of 483 patients with melanoma demonstrated no improvement in overall survival for patients who received a CLND following positive SLNB compared with those who did not, even when controlling for thickness, ulceration, and tumor burden.[68] Thus, organizations such as the NCCN recommend careful evaluation of CLND versus active nodal basin surveillance with ultrasound following a positive SLNB result.[64]

MEDICAL TREATMENT
Targeted Therapies

Melanoma is one of the few tumors in which molecular classification has successfully guided the development of individualized therapies with improved clinical outcomes. Melanoma targeted therapy was first founded on the observation that 66% of MM were found to harbor protein kinase B-raf (*BRAF*) somatic missense mutations.[69] *BRAF* mutations result in elevated serine/threonine kinase activity and mediate cell proliferation through the regulation of the mitogen-activated protein kinase (MAPK) signaling pathway. The most common variant is a val-to-glu point mutation at codon 600 (V600 E), although more than 60 variants have been identified in the BRAF gene including other V600 changes (eg, p.V600D (GTG > GAT), p.V600 K (GTG > AAG), and p.V600 R (GTG > AGG/CGG).[69–71] Clinically, these mutations have been associated with tumors exhibiting superficial spreading and nodular subtypes, earlier onset of disease, and increased presence of mitotic figures[72,73]

BRAF(V600 E/K) inhibitors—such as dabrafenib, encorafenib, and vemurafenib—target the MAPK signaling pathway in melanocytes which regulates cell proliferation and survival in melanocytes. A Phase III study (BRIM-3) conducted by McArthur and colleagues showed median overall survival and progression-free survival of 13.6 and 6.9 months in the vemurafenib group compared with 9.7 and 1.6 months in the dacarbazine group for *BRAF(V600 E)*-mutant melanomas.[74] Dacarbazine (DTIC), or imidazole carboxamide, is the first monotherapy agent approved by the FDA to show improved clinical benefit in patients with metastatic melanoma.[75] Vemurafenib was observed to have a 63% relative reduction in the risk of death and 70% reduction in the risk of tumor progression compared with dacarbazine.[76] However, BRAF(V600 E) inhibitor treatment is rarely curative due to the almost-certain development of acquired resistance, which can be due to target site neutralization through a resistance-associated BRAF splice variant,[77] MAPK pathway re-engagement (such as *NRAS* or *MAP2K1/MAP2K2* mutagenesis)[78] or secondary activation of various receptor tyrosine kinases (RTK).[79]

Given the high likelihood of tumor escape and resistance during medical treatment, combination therapy offers the potential for increased therapeutic efficacy and response durability. The current recommended use of these agents is outlined in a later section. Since 2014, the FDA has approved the following combination regimens for melanoma: atezolizumab, vemurafenib and cobimetinib[80]; encorafenib and binimetinib[81]; dabrafenib and trametinib[82]; nivolumab and ipilimumab[83]; and vemurafenib and cobimetinib.[84]

MEK is a kinase enzyme downstream to RAF that may be constitutively active in up to 8% of melanomas.[85] When used in combination therapy, trametinib was found to improve response rate, progression-free survival, and overall survival in melanomas harboring BRAF V600 E and V600 K mutations when compared with dabrafenib or vemurafenib alone. The addition of a MEK inhibitor to this regimen was also found to influence adverse side effect profiles. For example, patients in the study became less susceptible to squamous cell carcinoma and hyperkeratosis following treatment; however, they also became more susceptible to nonspecific fever and nausea.[86] Notably, 3-year survival overall survival with this dabrafenib and trametinib regimen is 62% in patient subgroups with normal serum LDH and <3 organ sites with metastases; however, only 25% in subgroups with elevated serum LDH.[87] Other BRAF/MEK inhibitor regimens (encorafenib plus binimetinib and vemurafenib plus cobimetinib) were found to have similar improvements in response rate and overall survival but adverse side effect profiles were reported to be variable.

NRAS is the second most common driver mutation in CM and may occur in up to 30% of cases.[88] These mutations most frequently occur at position 61 thereby impairing GTPase binding and activity.[89] Studies using small interfering RNA (siRNA)-mediated knockdown of *NRAS* show growth inhibition of melanocytes with decreased expression of cyclins D1 and E2.[90] Unlike for *BRAF*-mutant melanomas, the development of *NRAS* inhibitors has proved challenging due to many factors including the inaccessibility of targetable hydrophobic pockets within the protein structure.

Immune Checkpoint Inhibitors

Immune checkpoint inhibitors were among the first agents to show improved survival in patients with advanced melanoma (**Fig. 2**).[91] James Allison first suggested that CTLA-4 blockade could potentiate tumor regression in mice in 1996.[92] CTLA-4, a constitutively expressed T-cell surface protein, binds to B7 (CD80/CD86) on antigen-presenting cells in the early stages of immune engagement. In the presence of CD80/CD86 on antigen-presenting cells, CTLA-4 binding propagates an inhibitory immune response and prevents binding to the costimulatory receptor, CD28. Thus, CTLA-4 acts as a molecular "off switch" that decreases physiologic T-cell response[93(p28)]. Ipilimumab was the first CTLA-4 antibody approved for melanoma use by the FDA in 2011. Tremelimumab is an IgG2 antibody that has been shown to demonstrate inferior antibody-dependent cellular cytotoxicity when compared with ipilimumab, an IgG1 antibody. In a Phase III study, the 5-year survival rate of patients with advanced melanoma receiving ipilimumab plus dacarbazine was 18.2% (95% CI: 13.6%-23.4%) compared with 8.8% (95% CI: 5.7%-12.8%) for dacarbazine alone.[94]

During antigen recognition, the host immune system relies on several "checkpoints" during which tumorigenic cells can be distinguished from normal cells. The PD-1 checkpoint on T-cells—and subsequently its interaction with PD-L1 on tumor cells—is of particular interest in melanoma therapeutics. This binding interaction acts via phosphatase SHP2 to This binding interaction acts via phosphatase SHP2 to induce T-cell apoptosis while inhibiting proliferation and the release of cytokines.[95] Inhibition of PD-1/PD-L1 binding thus decreases PD-1 mediated signaling and promotes T-cell proliferation and function.[96] Nivolumab is a IgG4 human monoclonal human antibody that functions to block the PD-1/PD-L1 interaction. A Phase I study of patients with advanced melanoma, nonsmall-cell lung cancer, castration-resistant prostate cancer,

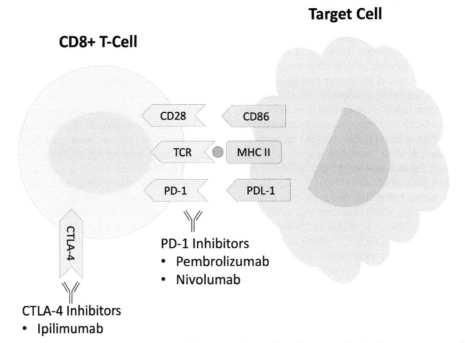

Fig. 2. The interaction of immune checkpoint inhibitors with T-cells and target cells (malignant or nonmalignant). Immune checkpoint blockade is achieved by blocking the interaction of receptors which attenuate T-cell activation and immune response. Current clinical trials are exploring the use of these agents in combination with targeted therapies.

renal-cell, and colorectal cancer showed an objective response rate (ORR) of 28% and median duration of response of 2 years.[97] Response rate was found to be slightly increase with dose escalation (ORR = 31%) and treatment was generally well tolerated. Another Phase III double-blind, randomized controlled trial (Checkmate 066) of untreated patients with advanced melanoma further showed an ORR of 40% for patients treated with nivolumab compared with 13.9% for those treated with dacarbazine.[98] Taken together, the durable response and low toxicity profile observed with these immunotherapy agents has yielded promising results for late-stage and adjuvant treatment.

Combination immune checkpoint therapy has extended 5-year survival to approximately 50% in recent studies.[99] According to the Checkmate 067 study, treatment with nivolumab plus ipilimumab resulted in significantly higher overall survival, progression-free survival, and response durability when compared with ipilimumab alone.[83] Combined targeted and immune checkpoint therapy (atezolizumab, vemurafenib, and cobimetinib) has also been shown to improve the duration of response when compared with vemurafenib or cobimetinib alone, suggesting triple combination therapy to be a viable treatment option in future trial studies. Results from the IMspire150 trial show a significant improvement in progression-free survival (PFS = 15.1 months; response duration = 21.0 months) in the vemurafenib, cobimetinib, and atezolizumab arm when compared with the vemurafenib, cobimetinib and placebo arm (PFS = 10.1 months; response duration = 12.6 months).[100]

Combined CTLA-4 and PD-1 inhibition has drastically improved the therapeutic landscape for advanced melanoma, although early clinical trials are limited by their low response rates and high toxicity profiles. Emerging studies have thus explored the inhibition of other immunomodulatory targets in an effort to prolong antitumor control. Lymphocyte activation gene-3 (LAG-3), or CD223, is another promising T-cell marker that serves to maintain immune homeostasis, cytokine production, and T-cell activation (Fig. 3).[101,102] Continuous antigen stimulation, such as in cancer, is associated with chronically elevated levels of LAG-3 subsequent T-cell exhaustion.[102] In a recent Phase II-III trial, fixed combination of relatlimab (a LAG-3 inhibitor) and nivolumab was associated with improved progression-free survival (10.1 months; 95% CI: 6.4–15.7) when compared with nivolumab (4.6 months; 95% CI: 3.4–5.6) alone.[103] Approximately 18.9% of participants experienced grade 3 or 4 immune-related adverse events, compared with 9.7% for nivolumab alone.

While the response and safety profile of combination LAG-3 inhibitor therapy is promising in early studies, data from additional Phase III trials will be required to ascertain the efficacy of this regimen in routine clinical care.

Treatment Guidelines

According to clinical practice guidelines from the National Comprehensive Cancer Network (NCCN) and European Society for Medical Oncology (ESMO), systemic therapy is recommended for Stage III and IV BRAF wild-type tumors following WLE with or without SLNB (Table 4).[64,104] High dose IFN-alpha was previously used for adjuvant treatment, but it has since been replaced by targeted and immune checkpoint therapies. Current first-line treatment may include CTLA-4 inhibitors (ipilimumab) and PD-1 inhibitors (nivolumab, pembrolizumab), in addition to targeted therapy (BRAF and MEK inhibitors). Certain high-risk features (thickness >4 mm, head/neck location, peri-neural invasion, and so forth) may also indicate the administration of adjuvant radiation therapy following primary excision. Melanomas refractory to combined BRAF and MEK inhibitor treatment, anti–PD-1 therapy, and ipilimumab, may consider other treatment options such as T-VEC, high-dose IL-2, cytotoxic chemotherapy, or other clinical trials.[105]

According to the American Society of Clinical Oncology (ASCO) Expert Panel,[106] patients with resected stage IIIA, IIB, IIIC, or IIID BRAF wild-type CM should be treated first-line with nivolumab or pembrolizumab. For BRAF-mutant melanoma, nivolumab, pembrolizumab, or a combination of dabrafenib and trametinib is recommended. Late-stage or unresectable melanomas that are BRAF wild-type should be treated with either ipilimumab plus nivolumab, nivolumab alone, or pembrolizumab alone. These same regimens, or combination BRAF/MEK inhibitor therapy, should be used for BRAF-mutant unresectable melanomas.

TREATMENT RESISTANCE

A significant barrier to targeted therapy remains to be the rapid development of resistance after the initial response. Of particular interest is the set of genetic or epigenetic changes responsible for MAPK pathway reactivation (or PI3K–Akt activation) and BRAF dimerization. Genetic alterations causing resistance may occur in NRAS, MAP2K1, MAP2K2, MITF, and HOXD8. Nongenetic alterations are far less common and may include receptor tyrosine kinase (RTK) dysregulation, EGFR activation, stromal growth factor

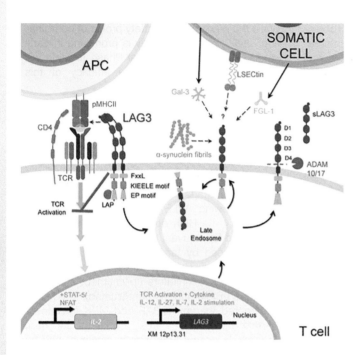

Fig. 3. Mechanisms for LAG-3 activation in T-cells. (*From* Graydon CG, Mohideen S, Fowke KR. LAG3's Enigmatic Mechanism of Action. Front Immunol. 2021 Jan 8;11:615317; with permission.)[117]

T cell

secretion, and alternative BRAF splicing. In *BRAF(V600 E)*-mutant melanomas, dimerization of aberrantly spliced p61BRAF(V600 E) lacking a RAS-binding domain has been associated with ERK signaling that is resistant to vemurafenib treatment.[77] Therefore, compensatory ERK signaling in certain isoforms may be dimerized in a RAS-independent fashion. Constitutively active RAS-GTP observed in *RAS* activating mutations may cause an increase in BRAF dimerization and resistance.[78] Taken together, our collective understanding of the mechanisms underlying resistance in *BRAF*-mutant melanomas is far from complete, but screening for "resistance genes" may provide important insight for therapeutic selection.

Table 4
Summary of targeted therapies used for metastatic melanoma

	Treatment	Class	Indication
Combination Therapy	Dabrafenib/Trametinib[109]	BRAF inhibitor/MEK inhibitor	*BRAFV600*-mutant melanoma
	Vemurafenib/Cobimetinib[84]	BRAF inhibitor/MEK inhibitor	*BRAFV600*-mutant melanoma
	Vemurafenib/Cobimetinib + Atezolizumab[80]	BRAF inhibitor/MEK inhibitor + Checkpoint Inhibitor	*BRAFV600*-mutant melanoma
	Encorafenib/Binimetinib[81]	BRAF Inhibitor/MEK Inhibitor	*BRAFV600*-mutant melanoma
Monotherapy	Vemurafenib[110]	BRAF Inhibitor	*BRAFV600*-mutant melanoma
	Dabrafenib[111]	BRAF Inhibitor	*BRAF*-mutant melanoma
	Imatinib[112]	Tyrosine Kinase Inhibitor	Activating *KIT* mutations
	Larotrectinib[113]	Tyrosine Kinase Inhibitor	*NTRK* gene fusion-positive tumors
	Entrectinib[114]	Tyrosine Kinase Inhibitor	*NTRK* gene fusion-positive tumors
	Binimetinib[115]	MEK Inhibitor	*NRAS*-mutant melanoma

FOLLOW-UP RECOMMENDATIONS

Routine skin examinations are recommended for patients with melanoma regardless of stage and symptoms. The frequency of these examinations should take into consideration the patient history of skin cancer (or other cancers), presence of atypical nevi, family history of skin cancer, tumor phenotype, and associated symptoms. Furthermore, patients should be instructed on how to perform at-home self-exams for skin and LN surveillance. Per NCCN guidelines, Stage IA–IIA melanomas should be monitored every 3 to 12 months. Stage IIB–V melanomas should be monitored for 3 to 6 months for 2 years, then every 3 to 12 months for 3 years, and annually for periods extending three years.[64,107]

Additional imaging such as computed tomography (CT), positron emission tomography (PET), and magnetic resonance imaging (MRI) may be performed at least annually to monitor spread and recurrence. The NCCN makes no recommendations for routine blood testing in melanoma surveillance. Should blood testing be performed, the ESMO considers serum S100 levels to have higher specificity for disease progression when compared with LDH.[104]

SUMMARY

Melanoma is the most severe and lethal form of skin cancer. Recent classification efforts have determined that melanoma is not one single disease but rather a grouping of disease entities with distinct genetics, histopathology, and clinical outcomes. A better understanding of these distinctions may translate into improvements in preventative care and precision medicine. The burgeoning success of combined therapy regimens continues to blossom with immunotherapy and the development of novel druggable targets. These early victories underscore how interdisciplinary approaches rooted in basic science research and clinical context are crucial in the fight against melanoma.

CLINICS CARE POINTS

- The 4 main histologic subtypes for melanoma include superficial spreading melanoma, nodular melanoma, acral lentiginous melanoma, and lentigo maligna melanoma
- Molecular classification is emerging with new advances in next-generation sequencing. Common gene mutations may provide novel druggable targets in future treatments
- Important risk factors for melanoma include exposure to ultraviolet (UV) radiation, family/personal history of skin cancer, fair skin, tanning bed exposure, increased numbers of atypical nevi, and more
- Treatment of melanoma is primarily wide local excision; margin width for this procedure varies based on the thickness of the primary lesion

DISCLOSURE

The authors have nothing to disclose.

REFERENCES

1. Mort RL, Jackson IJ, Patton EE. The melanocyte lineage in development and disease. Development 2015;142(4):620–32.
2. Lin JY, Fisher DE. Melanocyte biology and skin pigmentation. Nature 2007;445(7130):843–50.
3. Vergara IA, Mintoff CP, Sandhu S, et al. Evolution of late-stage metastatic melanoma is dominated by aneuploidy and whole genome doubling. Nat Commun 2021;12(1):1434.
4. Melanoma of the Skin - Cancer Stat Facts. SEER. Available at: https://seer.cancer.gov/statfacts/html/melan.html. Accessed March 8, 2021.
5. Sandru A, Voinea S, Panaitescu E, et al. Survival rates of patients with metastatic malignant melanoma. J Med Life 2014;7(4):572–6.
6. Joyce KM. Surgical Management of Melanoma. In: Ward WH, Farma JM, editors. Cutaneous melanoma: etiology and therapy. Codon Publications; 2017. Available at: http://www.ncbi.nlm.nih.gov/books/NBK481850/. Accessed February 28, 2022.
7. Essner R, Lee JH, Wanek LA, et al. Contemporary surgical treatment of advanced-stage melanoma. Arch Surg 2004;139(9):961–6. ; discussion 966-967.
8. Erdei E, Torres SM. A new understanding in the epidemiology of melanoma. Expert Rev Anticancer Ther 2010;10(11):1811–23.
9. Koh HK, Geller AC, Miller DR, et al. Prevention and early detection strategies for melanoma and skin cancer. Current status. Arch Dermatol 1996;132(4):436–43.
10. Brem R, Guven M, Karran P. Oxidatively-generated damage to DNA and proteins mediated by photosensitized UVA. Free Radic Biol Med 2017;107:101–9.
11. Bruls WA, Slaper H, van der Leun JC, et al. Transmission of human epidermis and stratum corneum as a function of thickness in the ultraviolet and visible wavelengths. Photochem Photobiol 1984;40(4):485–94.

12. Leonardi GC, Falzone L, Salemi R, et al. Cutaneous melanoma: From pathogenesis to therapy (Review). Int J Oncol 2018;52(4):1071–80.

13. Dawes SM, Tsai S, Gittleman H, et al. Racial disparities in melanoma survival. J Am Acad Dermatol 2016;75(5):983–91.

14. Brady J, Kashlan R, Ruterbusch J, et al. Racial Disparities in Patients with Melanoma: A Multivariate Survival Analysis. Clin Cosmet Investig Dermatol 2021;14:547–50.

15. Zell JA, Cinar P, Mobasher M, et al. Survival for patients with invasive cutaneous melanoma among ethnic groups: the effects of socioeconomic status and treatment. J Clin Oncol 2008;26(1):66–75.

16. Hall KH, Rapini RP. Acral Lentiginous Melanoma. In: StatPearls. StatPearls Publishing; 2022. Available at: http://www.ncbi.nlm.nih.gov/books/NBK559113/. Accessed February 26, 2022.

17. Wang Y, Zhao Y, Ma S. Racial differences in six major subtypes of melanoma: descriptive epidemiology. BMC Cancer 2016;16(1):691.

18. Basurto-Lozada P, Molina-Aguilar C, Castaneda-Garcia C, et al. Acral lentiginous melanoma: Basic facts, biological characteristics and research perspectives of an understudied disease. Pigment Cell Melanoma Res 2021;34(1):59–71.

19. Bradford PT, Goldstein AM, McMaster ML, et al. Acral Lentiginous Melanoma: Incidence and Survival Patterns in the United States, 1986-2005. Arch Dermatol 2009;145(4).

20. Suzuki T, Ueda M, Ogata K, et al. Doses of solar ultraviolet radiation correlate with skin cancer rates in Japan. Kobe J Med Sci 1996;42(6):375–88.

21. Sung H, Ferlay J, Siegel RL, et al. Global Cancer Statistics 2020: GLOBOCAN Estimates of Incidence and Mortality Worldwide for 36 Cancers in 185 Countries. CA: A Cancer J Clinicians 2021; 71(3):209–49.

22. Bulliard JL, Cox B, Elwood JM. Latitude gradients in melanoma incidence and mortality in the non-Maori population of New Zealand. Cancer Causes Control 1994;5(3):234–40.

23. Duncan EW, Cramb SM, Aitken JF, et al. Development of the Australian Cancer Atlas: spatial modelling, visualisation, and reporting of estimates. Int J Health Geogr 2019;18(1):21.

24. Melanoma Incidence and Mortality, United States–2012–2016 | CDC. Available at: https://www.cdc.gov/cancer/uscs/about/data-briefs/no9-melanoma-incidence-mortality-UnitedStates-2012-2016.htm. Accessed November 30, 2020.

25. Nikolaou V, Stratigos AJ. Emerging trends in the epidemiology of melanoma. Br J Dermatol 2014; 170(1):11–9.

26. Urban K, Mehrmal S, Uppal P, et al. The global burden of skin cancer: A longitudinal analysis from the Global Burden of Disease Study, 1990-2017. JAAD Int 2021;2:98–108.

27. Purdue MP, Freeman LB, Anderson WF, et al. Recent trends in incidence of cutaneous melanoma among U.S. Caucasian young adults. J Invest Dermatol 2008;128(12):2905–8.

28. Zhang M, Qureshi AA, Geller AC, et al. Use of Tanning Beds and Incidence of Skin Cancer. J Clin Oncol 2012;30(14):1588–93.

29. Gamba CS, Clarke CA, Keegan THM, et al. Melanoma Survival Disadvantage in Young, Non-Hispanic White Males Compared With Females. JAMA Dermatol 2013;149(8):912–20.

30. Cho E, Rosner BA, Colditz GA. Risk factors for melanoma by body site. Cancer Epidemiol Biomarkers Prev 2005;14(5):1241–4.

31. Stanienda-Sokół K, Salwowska N, Sławińska M, et al. Primary Locations of Malignant Melanoma Lesions Depending on Patients' Gender and Age. Asian Pac J Cancer Prev 2017;18(11):3081–6.

32. Juhl AL, Byers TE, Robinson WA, et al. The anatomic distribution of melanoma and relationships with childhood nevus distribution in Colorado. Melanoma Res 2009;19(4):252–9.

33. Kwan TY, Belke TW, Enta T. Sex differences in the anatomical distribution of melanocytic nevi in Canadian Hutterite children. J Cutan Med Surg 2000;4(2):58–62.

34. Visconti A, Ribero S, Sanna M, et al. Body site-specific genetic effects influence naevus count distribution in women. Pigment Cell Melanoma Res 2020;33(2):326–33.

35. Greenwald HS, Friedman EB, Osman I. Superficial spreading and nodular melanoma are distinct biological entities: a challenge to the linear progression model. Melanoma Res 2012; 22(1):1–8.

36. Morton DL, Wen DR, Wong JH, et al. Technical details of intraoperative lymphatic mapping for early stage melanoma. Arch Surg 1992;127(4):392–9.

37. Kelly JW, Chamberlain AJ, Staples MP, et al. Nodular melanoma. No longer as simple as ABC. Aust Fam Physician 2003;32(9):706–9.

38. Shaikh WR, Xiong M, Weinstock MA. The contribution of nodular subtype to melanoma mortality in the United States, 1978 to 2007. Arch Dermatol 2012;148(1):30–6.

39. Collgros H, Rodriguez-Lomba E, Regio Pereira A, et al. Lentiginous melanoma (lentigo maligna and lentigo maligna melanoma) in Australia: clinico-pathological characteristics, management and recurrence rates after 10-year follow-up at a tertiary centre. J Eur Acad Dermatol Venereol 2021;35(6): 1315–22.

40. Morton DL, Essner R, Kirkwood JM, et al. Clinical characteristics. 6th edition. Holland-Frei Cancer Medicine; 2003. Available at: https://www.ncbi.nlm.

nih.gov/books/NBK13375/. Accessed January 17, 2021.

41. Wayte DM, Helwig EB. Melanotic freckle of Hutchinson. Cancer 1968;21(5):893–911.

42. Ward WH, Lambreton F, Goel N, et al. Clinical Presentation and Staging of Melanoma. In: Ward WH, Farma JM, editors. Cutaneous melanoma: etiology and therapy. Codon Publications; 2017. Available at: http://www.ncbi.nlm.nih.gov/books/NBK481857/. Accessed January 17, 2021.

43. Pampena R, Lai M, Piana S, et al. Nevus-associated melanoma: facts and controversies. G Ital Dermatol Venereol 2020;155(1):65–75.

44. Lin WM, Luo S, Muzikansky A, et al. Outcome of patients with de novo versus nevus-associated melanoma. J Am Acad Dermatol 2015;72(1):54–8.

45. Tsao H, Bevona C, Goggins W, et al. The transformation rate of moles (melanocytic nevi) into cutaneous melanoma: a population-based estimate. Arch Dermatol 2003;139(3):282–8.

46. Cymerman RM, Shao Y, Wang K, et al. De Novo vs Nevus-Associated Melanomas: Differences in Associations With Prognostic Indicators and Survival. J Natl Cancer Inst 2016;108(10). https://doi.org/10.1093/jnci/djw121.

47. AJCC cancer staging manual. 8th ed. New York: Springer International Publishing; 2017.

48. Scolyer RA, Rawson RV, Gershenwald JE, et al. Melanoma pathology reporting and staging. Mod Pathol 2020;33(1):15–24.

49. Gershenwald JE, Scolyer RA, Hess KR, et al. Melanoma Staging: Evidence-Based Changes in the American Joint Committee on Cancer Eighth Edition Cancer Staging Manual. CA Cancer J Clin 2017;67(6):472–92.

50. Trinidad CM, Torres-Cabala CA, Curry JL, et al. Update on eighth edition American Joint Committee on Cancer classification for cutaneous melanoma and overview of potential pitfalls in histological examination of staging parameters. J Clin Pathol 2019;72(4):265–70.

51. Balch CM, Wilkerson JA, Murad TM, et al. The prognostic significance of ulceration of cutaneous melanoma. Cancer 1980;45(12):3012–7.

52. Eigentler TK, Buettner PG, Leiter U, et al. Impact of Ulceration in Stages I to III Cutaneous Melanoma As Staged by the American Joint Committee on Cancer Staging System: An Analysis of the German Central Malignant Melanoma Registry. JCO 2004;22(21):4376–83.

53. Donizy P, Kaczorowski M, Leskiewicz M, et al. Mitotic rate is a more reliable unfavorable prognosticator than ulceration for early cutaneous melanoma: A 5-year survival analysis. Oncol Rep 2014;32(6):2735–43.

54. Thompson JF, Soong SJ, Balch CM, et al. Prognostic significance of mitotic rate in localized primary cutaneous melanoma: an analysis of patients in the multi-institutional American Joint Committee on Cancer melanoma staging database. J Clin Oncol 2011;29(16):2199–205.

55. Hawes D, Neville AM, Cote RJ. Occult metastasis. Biomed Pharmacother 2001;55(4):229–42.

56. Niebling MG, Haydu LE, Lo SN, et al. The prognostic significance of microsatellites in cutaneous melanoma. Mod Pathol 2020;33(7):1369–79.

57. Read RL, Haydu L, Saw RPM, et al. In-transit melanoma metastases: incidence, prognosis, and the role of lymphadenectomy. Ann Surg Oncol 2015; 22(2):475–81.

58. Palmer SR, Erickson LA, Ichetovkin I, et al. Circulating Serologic and Molecular Biomarkers in Malignant Melanoma. Mayo Clin Proc 2011;86(10): 981–90.

59. Brand CU, Ellwanger U, Stroebel W, et al. Prolonged survival of 2 years or longer for patients with disseminated melanoma. An analysis of related prognostic factors. Cancer 1997;79(12): 2345–53.

60. Barth A, Wanek LA, Morton DL. Prognostic factors in 1,521 melanoma patients with distant metastases. J Am Coll Surg 1995;181(3):193–201.

61. Gupta S, Tsao H. Epidemiology of Melanoma. In: ; 2017. doi:10.1007/978-3-319-35153-7_31.

62. Swetter SM, Tsao H, Bichakjian CK, et al. Guidelines of care for the management of primary cutaneous melanoma. J Am Acad Dermatol 2019; 80(1):208–50.

63. Niknam Leilabadi S, Chen A, Tsai S, et al. Update and Review on the Surgical Management of Primary Cutaneous Melanoma. Healthcare (Basel) 2014;2(2):234–49.

64. Coit DG, Thompson JA, Albertini MR, et al. Cutaneous Melanoma, Version 2.2019, NCCN Clinical Practice Guidelines in Oncology. J Natl Compr Canc Netw 2019;17(4):367–402.

65. Pathak S, Zito PM. Clinical Guidelines For The Staging, Diagnosis, and Management Of Cutaneous Malignant Melanoma. In: StatPearls. StatPearls Publishing; 2022. Available at: http://www.ncbi.nlm.nih.gov/books/NBK572149/. Accessed March 7, 2022.

66. Gannon CJ, Rousseau DL Jr, Ross MI, et al. Accuracy of lymphatic mapping and sentinel lymph node biopsy after previous wide local excision in patients with primary melanoma. Cancer 2006; 107(11):2647–52.

67. Dzwierzynski WW. Complete lymph node dissection for regional nodal metastasis. Clin Plast Surg 2010;37(1):113–25.

68. Leiter U, Stadler R, Mauch C, et al. Complete lymph node dissection versus no dissection in patients with sentinel lymph node biopsy positive

melanoma (DeCOG-SLT): a multicentre, randomised, phase 3 trial. Lancet Oncol 2016;17(6):757–67.

69. Davies H, Bignell GR, Cox C, et al. Mutations of the BRAF gene in human cancer. Nature 2002;417(6892):949–54.

70. Cheng S, Chu P, Hinshaw M, et al. Frequency of mutations associated with targeted therapy in malignant melanoma patients. JCO 2011;29(15_suppl):8597.

71. Alqathama A. BRAF in malignant melanoma progression and metastasis: potentials and challenges. Am J Cancer Res 2020;10(4):1103–14.

72. Hugdahl E, Kalvenes MB, Puntervoll HE, et al. BRAF-V600E expression in primary nodular melanoma is associated with aggressive tumour features and reduced survival. Br J Cancer 2016;114(7):801–8.

73. Eigentler T, Assi Z, Hassel JC, et al. Which melanoma patient carries a BRAF-mutation? A comparison of predictive models. Oncotarget 2016;7(24):36130–7.

74. McArthur GA, Chapman PB, Robert C, et al. Safety and efficacy of vemurafenib in BRAFV600E and BRAFV600K mutation-positive melanoma (BRIM-3): extended follow-up of a phase 3, randomised, open-label study. Lancet Oncol 2014;15(3):323–32.

75. Serrone L, Zeuli M, Sega FM, et al. Dacarbazine-based chemotherapy for metastatic melanoma: thirty-year experience overview. J Exp Clin Cancer Res 2000;19(1):21–34.

76. Chapman PB, Hauschild A, Robert C, et al. Improved Survival with Vemurafenib in Melanoma with BRAF V600E Mutation. New Engl J Med 2011;364(26):2507–16.

77. Poulikakos PI, Persaud Y, Janakiraman M, et al. RAF inhibitor resistance is mediated by dimerization of aberrantly spliced BRAF(V600E). Nature 2011;480(7377):387–90.

78. Kakadia S, Yarlagadda N, Awad R, et al. Mechanisms of resistance to BRAF and MEK inhibitors and clinical update of US Food and Drug Administration-approved targeted therapy in advanced melanoma. Onco Targets Ther 2018;11:7095–107.

79. Nazarian R, Shi H, Wang Q, et al. Melanomas acquire resistance to B-RAF(V600E) inhibition by RTK or N-RAS upregulation. Nature 2010;468(7326):973–7.

80. Gutzmer R, Stroyakovskiy D, Gogas H, et al. Atezolizumab, vemurafenib, and cobimetinib as first-line treatment for unresectable advanced BRAFV600 mutation-positive melanoma (IMspire150): primary analysis of the randomised, double-blind, placebo-controlled, phase 3 trial. Lancet 2020;395(10240):1835–44.

81. Dummer R, Ascierto PA, Gogas HJ, et al. Encorafenib plus binimetinib versus vemurafenib or encorafenib in patients with BRAF-mutant melanoma (COLUMBUS): a multicentre, open-label, randomised phase 3 trial. Lancet Oncol 2018;19(5):603–15.

82. Robert C, Karaszewska B, Schachter J, et al. Improved overall survival in melanoma with combined dabrafenib and trametinib. N Engl J Med 2015;372(1):30–9.

83. Wolchok JD, Chiarion-Sileni V, Gonzalez R, et al. Overall Survival with Combined Nivolumab and Ipilimumab in Advanced Melanoma. N Engl J Med 2017;377(14):1345–56.

84. Larkin J, Ascierto PA, Dréno B, et al. Combined Vemurafenib and Cobimetinib in BRAF-Mutated Melanoma. New Engl J Med 2014;371(20):1867–76.

85. Kunz M, Dannemann M, Kelso J. High-throughput sequencing of the melanoma genome. Exp Dermatol 2013;22(1):10–7.

86. Spain L, Julve M, Larkin J. Combination dabrafenib and trametinib in the management of advanced melanoma with BRAFV600 mutations. Expert Opin Pharmacother 2016;17(7):1031–8.

87. Ribas A, Flaherty KT. BRAF targeted therapy changes the treatment paradigm in melanoma. Nat Rev Clin Oncol 2011;8(7):426–33.

88. Hayward NK, Wilmott JS, Waddell N, et al. Whole-genome landscapes of major melanoma subtypes. Nature 2017;545(7653):175–80.

89. Fedorenko IV, Gibney GT, Smalley KSM. NRAS mutant melanoma: biological behavior and future strategies for therapeutic management. Oncogene 2013;32(25):3009–18.

90. Eskandarpour M, Hashemi J, Kanter L, et al. Frequency of UV-Inducible NRAS Mutations in Melanomas of Patients With Germline CDKN2A Mutations. JNCI: J Natl Cancer Inst 2003;95(11):790–8.

91. Callahan MK, Postow MA, Wolchok JD. Targeting T Cell Co-receptors for Cancer Therapy. Immunity 2016;44(5):1069–78.

92. Leach DR, Krummel MF, Allison JP. Enhancement of antitumor immunity by CTLA-4 blockade. Science 1996;271(5256):1734–6.

93. Alegre ML, Frauwirth KA, Thompson CB. T-cell regulation by CD28 and CTLA-4. Nat Rev Immunol 2001;1(3):220–8.

94. Maio M, Grob JJ, Aamdal S, et al. Five-year survival rates for treatment-naive patients with advanced melanoma who received ipilimumab plus dacarbazine in a phase III trial. J Clin Oncol 2015;33(10):1191–6.

95. Pardoll DM. The blockade of immune checkpoints in cancer immunotherapy. Nat Rev Cancer 2012;12(4):252–64.

96. Tang F, Zheng P. Tumor cells versus host immune cells: whose PD-L1 contributes to PD-1/PD-L1

blockade mediated cancer immunotherapy? Cell Biosci 2018;8:34.

97. Topalian SL, Hodi FS, Brahmer JR, et al. Safety, activity, and immune correlates of anti-PD-1 antibody in cancer. N Engl J Med 2012;366(26):2443–54.

98. Robert C, Long GV, Brady B, et al. Nivolumab in previously untreated melanoma without BRAF mutation. N Engl J Med 2015;372(4):320–30.

99. Frampton AE, Sivakumar S. A New Combination Immunotherapy in Advanced Melanoma. New Engl J Med 2022;386(1):91–2.

100. Czarnecka AM, Bartnik E, Fiedorowicz M, et al. Targeted Therapy in Melanoma and Mechanisms of Resistance. Int J Mol Sci 2020;21(13):4576.

101. Goldberg MV, Drake CG. LAG-3 in Cancer Immunotherapy. Curr Top Microbiol Immunol 2011;344: 269–78.

102. Ruffo E, Wu R, Bruno TC, et al. Lymphocyte-Activation Gene 3 (LAG3): the Next Immune Checkpoint Receptor. Semin Immunol 2019;42:101305.

103. Tawbi HA, Schadendorf D, Lipson EJ, et al. Relatlimab and Nivolumab versus Nivolumab in Untreated Advanced Melanoma. N Engl J Med 2022;386(1):24–34.

104. Michielin O, van Akkooi ACJ, Ascierto PA, et al, ESMO Guidelines Committee. Electronic address: clinicalguidelines@esmo.org. Cutaneous melanoma: ESMO Clinical Practice Guidelines for diagnosis, treatment and follow-up. Ann Oncol 2019; 30(12):1884–901.

105. Swetter S, Thompson JA. NCCN Clinical Practice Guidelines in Oncology, Melanoma: Cutaneous. NCCN.org. 2022;2:2022.

106. Seth R, Messersmith H, Kaur V, et al. Systemic Therapy for Melanoma: ASCO Guideline. JCO 2020;38(33):3947–70.

107. Trotter SC, Sroa N, Winkelmann RR, et al. A Global Review of Melanoma Follow-up Guidelines. J Clin Aesthet Dermatol 2013;6(9):18–26.

108. Lideikaitė A, Mozūraitienė J, Letautienė S. Analysis of prognostic factors for melanoma patients. Acta Med Litu 2017;24(1):25–34.

109. Long GV, Stroyakovskiy D, Gogas H, et al. Dabrafenib and trametinib versus dabrafenib and placebo for Val600 BRAF-mutant melanoma: a multicentre, double-blind, phase 3 randomised controlled trial. Lancet 2015;386(9992):444–51.

110. Sosman JA, Kim KB, Schuchter L, et al. Survival in BRAF V600-mutant advanced melanoma treated with vemurafenib. N Engl J Med 2012;366(8): 707–14.

111. Long GV, Trefzer U, Davies MA, et al. Dabrafenib in patients with Val600Glu or Val600Lys BRAF-mutant melanoma metastatic to the brain (BREAK-MB): a multicentre, open-label, phase 2 trial. Lancet Oncol 2012;13(11):1087–95.

112. Hodi FS, O'Day SJ, McDermott DF, et al. Improved Survival with Ipilimumab in Patients with Metastatic Melanoma. N Engl J Med 2010;363(8):711–23.

113. Drilon A, Laetsch TW, Kummar S, et al. Efficacy of Larotrectinib in TRK Fusion–Positive Cancers in Adults and Children. New Engl J Med 2018; 378(8):731–9.

114. Doebele RC, Drilon A, Paz-Ares L, et al. Entrectinib in patients with advanced or metastatic NTRK fusion-positive solid tumours: integrated analysis of three phase 1-2 trials. Lancet Oncol 2020; 21(2):271–82.

115. Dummer R, Schadendorf D, Ascierto PA, et al. Binimetinib versus dacarbazine in patients with advanced NRAS-mutant melanoma (NEMO): a multicentre, open-label, randomised, phase 3 trial. Lancet Oncol 2017;18(4):435–45.

116. Tsao H, Chin L, Garraway LA, et al. Melanoma: from mutations to medicine. Genes Dev 2012; 26(11):1131–55.

117. Graydon CG, Mohideen S, Fowke KR. LAG3's Enigmatic Mechanism of Action. Front Immunol 2020;11:615317.

Targeted Therapy and Immunotherapy in Melanoma

Jake Lazaroff, MD*, Diana Bolotin, MD, PhD

KEYWORDS

• Melanoma • Targeted • Therapy • Immunotherapy

KEY POINTS

- Targeted therapy and immunotherapy have improved outcomes in metastatic melanoma.
- BRAF and MEK inhibitors exert their effects on the MAPK pathway and can be effective as monotherapies, but are more effective in combination for advanced melanoma.
- Immunotherapy downregulates inhibitory immune signals expressed by malignancies and has demonstrated improved progression-free and overall survival (OS) in the treatment of melanoma.
- Current NCCN guidelines recommend treatment with targeted BRAF/MEK therapy or immunotherapy, depending on BRAF status, for unresectable stage III or stage IV melanoma 3.
- Immunotherapy may lead to improved long-term outcomes but generally has a slower onset, with some patients having late responses up to a year after initiating treatment, while BRAF and MEK inhibition can lead to quick symptom control and higher early response rates but often leads to resistance and progression [3, 61, 69, 116].

INTRODUCTION

Incidence of melanoma has grown by 320% between 1975 and 2018.[1] Risk factors include sun exposure, indoor tanning, family history, and number of nevi.[1] Definitive diagnosis is made via biopsy for histopathologic staging and to guide management decisions.[2]

Early stage I–II melanoma is treated with complete surgical excision and has an excellent 5-year survival rate at 99.4%.[1–3] However, advanced stages carry a worse prognosis with 5-year survival rates of stage III and IV melanoma of 68% and 29.8%, respectively.[1,3]

Emergence of targeted and immunotherapy agents has transformed the treatment of advanced melanoma in recent years. Prior to these treatments, dacarbazine was the only FDA-approved chemotherapeutic for metastatic melanoma and carried a modest response rate of 7% to 12% that increased median overall survival (OS) from 5.6 to 7.8 months.[4] The 1-year survival rate of melanoma between 2008 and 2010 was 42%.[5] This subsequently improved significantly to 55% between 2013 and 2015, which coincided with the introduction and approval of targeted therapy and immunotherapy.[5]

TARGETED THERAPIES IN MELANOMA
BRAF and MAPK pathways in melanoma

Tumorigenesis is the result of genetic mutations that allow for dysregulated and uncontrolled growth. In melanoma, the mitogen-activated protein kinase (MAPK) pathway, which regulates cellular proliferation, is frequently altered and considered a driver mutation.[6]

The MAPK pathway consists of RAS, RAF, ERK, and mitogen-activated extracellular signal-regulated kinase (MEK) which relay proliferative signals. Under normal circumstances, this cascade is initiated by the stimulation of a receptor tyrosine kinase, leading to the activation of RAS that recruits downstream RAF, MEK, and ERK to

Department of Medicine, Section of Dermatology, University of Chicago, The University of Chicago Medicine, 5841 S Maryland Avenue MC 5067, Chicago, IL 60637, USA
* Corresponding author.
E-mail address: Jake.Lazaroff@uchospitals.edu

Dermatol Clin 41 (2023) 65–77
https://doi.org/10.1016/j.det.2022.07.007
0733-8635/23/© 2022 Elsevier Inc. All rights reserved.

positively regulate proliferation and modify apoptotic pathways (**Fig. 1**).[6]

Approximately 40% to 60% of melanomas carry a mutation in v-raf murine sarcoma viral oncogene homolog B1 (BRAF) resulting in hyperactive MAPK signaling leading to uncontrolled cell proliferation.[4] The most common BRAF mutation is the substitution of glutamic acid (E) for valine (V), BRAF-V600 E, which accounts for 70% to 90% of mutations.[6,7] The BRAF-V600 K mutation substitutes a lysine (K) for valine (V) and accounts for an additional 10% to 20% of mutations.[6,7]

BRAF inhibitors

Agents targeting BRAF mutant tumors were some of the first successful targeted treatments for advanced and metastatic melanoma. Vemurafenib and dabrafenib competitively inhibit BRAF-V600 E with minimal effect on wild-type (WT) BRAF. Testing for BRAF-mutation status is recommended for high-risk melanomas as it can help guide treatment decisions.[2]

Vemurafenib was FDA-approved in 2011 for the treatment of metastatic melanoma with BRAF-V600 E mutations. A phase III (BRIM-3) trial demonstrated an increased OS of 13.6 months with vemurafenib vs. 9.7 months with dacarbazine (**Table 1**).[4,8–10] Progression-free survival (PFS) with vemurafenib was shown to be 5.3 months compared with 2.7 months in the dacarbazine group.[4] Vemurafenib was associated with a relative risk reduction of death of 63% and reduction in tumor progression of 74%.[4,10]

Dabrafenib was approved in 2013 for unresectable or metastatic melanoma with BRAF-V600 E mutations. Phase III data from the BREAK-3 trial demonstrated an overall response rate (ORR) of 59% and a similar OS and PFS to vemurafenib (see **Table 1**).[11]

Encorafenib is the newest BRAF-inhibitor that gained FDA approval for use with binimetinib in unresectable or metastatic melanoma with V600 E or V600 K mutations.[12] In clinical trials encorafenib as a monotherapy exhibited an OS rate of 60% and median PFS of 12.4 months in BRAF-inhibitor naïve patients.[12]

Common adverse events (AEs) of BRAF-inhibitors include arthralgias, headaches, fevers, and fatigue with the majority of these being mild and not necessitating the discontinuation of treatment.[4] Additionally, cutaneous eruptions and photosensitivity can occur, rarely resulting in blistering.[4]

Approximately 14% to 26% of patients on BRAF-inhibitor monotherapy develop cutaneous squamous cell carcinomas (cSCCs) and keratoacanthomas (KAs) as a result of BRAF inhibition causing a paradoxic activation of the downstream MAPK pathway.[13] Rates of keratinocyte carcinomas vary depending on the agent used with vemurafenib, dabrafenib, and encorafenib having rates of 22%, 6% and 2.7%, respectively.[14]

One of the greatest limitations of BRAF-inhibitor monotherapy is that approximately half of the treated patients develop resistance within 6 to 10 months.[15] Resistance with BRAF-inhibitor monotherapy is thought to be mediated by selective pressure on tumor microenvironment. Several mechanisms of resistance have been identified including downstream mutations or MAPK activation independent of BRAF, BRAF gene amplification, alternative splicing of BRAF, or loss of other tumor suppressors.[15]

MEK inhibitors

MEK is downstream of BRAF in the MAPK signaling pathway making it an attractive target for melanoma treatment (see **Fig. 1**).[16] Unlike BRAF-inhibitor therapies that target tumor cells with mutant BRAF, MEK-inhibitors suppress function in tumor and normal cells which limits dosage, tolerance and leads to potential for more toxicities.[16]

Trametinib was approved for use as a single agent therapy in 2013 for patients with metastatic melanoma harboring BRAF mutations.[17] In METRIC, a phase III study, trametinib increased PFS resulting in a hazard ratio (HR) of disease progression or death of 0.45 (see **Table 1**).[17–19] Additionally, the 6-month OS was 81% versus 67% in the dacarbazine or paclitaxel groups.[17]

Common AEs of trametinib include rash, diarrhea, edema, and fatigue.[17] Only 8% of cutaneous AEs in the treatment group were severe (grade 3 or 4).[17] Other AEs included decreased ejection fraction/ventricular dysfunction and ocular toxicities.[17] AEs necessitated dose interruptions in 35% and dose reductions in 27% of patients.[16,17]

Cobimetinib and binimetinib are other MEK-inhibitors approved for use in melanoma in

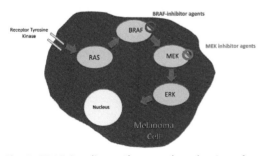

Fig. 1. BRAF signaling pathway and mechanism of action of targeted agents in melanoma.

Table 1
Phase III trial data for targeted therapy and immunotherapy

Trial	Name/Reference	Treatment	PFS (Months)	OS (Months)
BRIM-3	McArthur et al[8] 2014	Vemurafenib	6.9	13.6
		Dacarbazine	1.6	9.7
	Chapman et al[9] 2017	Vemurafenib	–	13.6
		Dacarbazine	–	9.7
BREAK-3	Hauschild et al[11] 2012	Dabrafenib	5.1	–
		Dacarbazine	2.7	–
METRIC	Flaherty et al[17] 2012	Trametinib	4.8	–
		Dacarbazine or paclitaxel	1.5	–
	Schadendorf et al[18] 2013	Trametinib	–	15.6
		Dacarbazine or paclitaxel	–	11.3
	Robert et al[19] 2019	Trametinib	4.9	15.6
		Dacarbazine or paclitaxel	1.5	11.3
coBRIM	Larkin et al[21] 2014	Vemurafenib + cobimetinib	9.9	–
		Vemurafenib + placebo	6.2	–
	Ascierto et al[22] 2016	Cobimetinib + vemurafenib	12.3	22.3
		Vemurafenib + placebo	7.2	17.4
	Dréno et al[23] 2018	Cobimetinib + vemurafenib	–	22.5
		Vemurafenib + placebo	–	17.4
COMBI-d	Long et al[24] 2014	Dabrafenib + trametinib	9.3	–
		Dabrafenib + placebo	8.8	–
	Long et al[25] 2015	Dabrafenib + trametinib	11	25.1
		Dabrafenib + placebo	8.8	18.7
COMBI-v	Robert et al[27] 2015	Dabrafenib + trametinib	11.4	–
		Vemurafenib	7.3	17.2
	Robert et al[28] 2016	Dabrafenib + trametinib	12.1	26.1
		Vemurafenib	7.3	17.8
COLUMBUS Part 1	Dummer et al[29] 2016	Encorafenib + binimetinib	14.9	–
		Encorafenib	9.6	–
		Vemurafenib	7.3	–
	Dummer et al[12] 2018, Dummer et al[30] 2018	Encorafenib + binimetinib	14.9	33.6
		Encorafenib	9.6	23.5
		Vemurafenib	7.3	16.9
COLUMBUS Part 2	Dummer et al[31] 2017	Encorafenib + binimetinib	12.9	–
		Encorafenib	9.2	–
		Encorafenib	7.4	–
NCT00094653	Hodi et al[36] 2010	Ipilimumab	–	10.1
		Ipilimumab + gp100	–	10
		gp100	–	6.4
MDX010	Robert et al[37] 2011	Ipilimumab + dacarbazine	–	11.2
		Dacarbazine + placebo	–	9.1
CheckMate 066	Robert et al[38] 2015	Nivolumab + Placebo	5.1	–
		Dacarbazine + Placebo	2.2	10.8
CheckMate 037	Weber et al[39] 2015	Nivolumab	4.7	–
		Dacarbazine or carboplatin + paclitaxel	4.2	–
	Weber et al[40] 2016	Nivolumab	3.1	15.7
		Dacarbazine or carboplatin + paclitaxel	3.7	14.4

(continued on next page)

Table 1
(continued)

Trial	Name/Reference	Treatment	PFS (Months)	OS (Months)
KEYNOTE-006	Robert et al[41] 2015	Pembrolizumab q2 weeks	5.5	–
		Pembrolizumab q3 weeks	4.1	–
		Ipilimumab	2.8	–
	Schachter et al[42] 2017	Pembrolizumab q2 weeks	5.6	–
		Pembrolizumab q3 weeks	4.1	–
		Ipilimumab	2.8	16
	Long et al[43] 2018	Pembrolizumab q2 or q3 weeks	8.3	32.7
		Ipilimumab	3.3	15.9
CheckMate 067	Larkin et al[48] 2015	Nivolumab + ipilimumab	11.5	–
		Nivolumab	6.9	–
		Ipilimumab	2.9	–
	Wolchok et al[49] 2016	Nivolumab + ipilimumab	11.5	–
		Nivolumab	6.9	–
		Ipilimumab	2.9	–
	Wolchok et al[50] 2017	Nivolumab + ipilimumab	11.5	–
		Nivolumab	6.9	37.6
		Ipilimumab	2.9	19.9
	Hodi et al[51] 2018	Nivolumab + ipilimumab	11.5	–
		Nivolumab	6.9	36.9
		Ipilimumab	2.9	19.9
	Larkin et al[52] 2019	Nivolumab + ipilimumab	11.5	–
		Nivolumab	6.9	36.9
		Ipilimumab	2.9	19.9

combination with BRAF-inhibitors as will be discussed subsequently.[20]

BRAF-MEK combination therapy

Combination approaches to targeted therapy were borne of the observation that resistance to BRAF-inhibitor monotherapy typically occurs within 6 to 7 months.[11] Use of combination therapy of BRAF and MEK-inhibitors is aimed to block multiple points in the MAPK pathway reducing the risk of resistance.

Combination of vemurafenib and cobimetinib was studied in the coBRIM trial which demonstrated an increased PFS of 9.9 months compared with 6.2 months with vemurafenib monotherapy (see **Table 1**).[21–23] Additionally, with combination therapy, the ORR was 68% compared with 45% with vemurafenib monotherapy.[21] Patients in the combination therapy arm had higher rates of central serous retinopathy, gastrointestinal events, photosensitivity, transaminitis, and increased creatine kinase levels but the majority of these were low grade.[21]

Subsequent studies evaluated the efficacy of combining dabrafenib and trametinib.[24–29] COMBI-d compared dabrafenib and trametinib to dabrafenib monotherapy; combination therapy provided an improved ORR (67% vs 51%) (see **Table 1**).[24] Use of this combination also significantly decreased the rates of cSCCs to 2%, but did result in an increased number of patients experiencing pyrexia, at nearly 50%.[24] The COMBI-v trial went on to compare dabrafenib and trametinib to vemurafenib monotherapy (see **Table 1**).[27,28] This study demonstrated improved efficacy for combination therapy and a 72% OS at 12 months, compared with 65% with vemurafenib alone.[27]

COLUMBUS trials have demonstrated a similar benefit with the combination of encorafenib and binimetinib showing an ORR of 63% and a the median duration of response of 18.6 months compared with 40% and 12.3 months with vemurafenib (see **Table 1**).[12,29–31] The most common AEs of encorafenib plus binimetinib were increased serum γ-glutamyl transferase and creatine phosphokinase levels, and hypertension.[12]

The rates of cSCCs were significantly lower with the use of any of the combination BRAF/MEK therapies.[32] A meta-analysis showed rates of cSCCs around 3% with BRAF/MEK dual therapy compared with 12.5% with BRAF-inhibitor monotherapy.[33] The reduced risk of cSCCs with combination therapy makes sense mechanistically as the MEK inhibitor blocks the reactivation of downstream MAPK pathway observed with BRAF monotherapy.

Even though combination BRAF and MEK therapy is utilized in part to help reduce resistance with monotherapy, resistance to combinatorial treatments still occurs. Nonetheless, the time until resistance with combination therapy is 11 to 15 months which is significantly longer than with monotherapy.[7] Current NCCN guidelines consider combination BRAF and MEK therapy a first-line option for the treatment of metastatic or unresectable melanoma if BRAF-V600 activating mutations are confirmed.[2]

Immunotherapy

Over the last decade, the field of immunotherapy has revolutionized the treatment of many tumors, with melanoma being one of the earliest malignancies treated with this approach. One of the immune system's functions is to monitor and destroy aberrantly proliferating cells. Under normal circumstances, there are checks and balances in place to ensure proper activation and inhibition of the immune system to avoid autoimmune consequences. Tumors can take advantage of these inhibitory mechanisms to escape immune surveillance. Several inhibitory signaling pathways have been elucidated. One pathway is the interaction of PD-1 with its ligand PD-L1, which induces T-lymphocyte apoptosis and downregulates the T-cell immunologic response (**Fig. 2**). Another relevant pathway includes CD28 binding to B7 to act as a costimulatory signal to upregulate T-cell activation. Cytotoxic T-lymphocyte antigen-4 (CTLA-4) acts as a break in this pathway by competitively binding to B7, thus removing the activating signals and down-regulating immune response (see **Fig. 2**).

Melanoma is known to be a highly immunogenic malignancy.[34] The complex and multifactorial process in which melanoma develops the ability to evade the immune system is termed "immune editing."[34] Several key features of this process include defective immune recognition, increased resistance to apoptosis, and alterations in the cellular microenvironment to promote immunosuppression.[34] In addition, the continuous antigenic stimulation leads to T-cell exhaustion and immune escape.[34]

However, owing to its high immunogenicity, melanoma is a great target for immunotherapy which works by blocking the cellular interactions that dampen host immune response and allow for uncontrolled tumor growth.[34] Currently two classes of immunotherapy target these immune-inhibitory pathways: anti-CTLA4 antibody, which acts at the level of the lymph nodes and agents that target the PD-1 and PDL-1 interaction in lymphoid, peripheral and tumoral tissues.[35] Use of these medications has proven to be an effective and often durable therapy for advanced and metastatic melanoma.

Anti-CTLA4 therapy

Ipilimumab is a fully humanized monoclonal antibody that was approved by the FDA in 2011 for use in metastatic melanoma.[36] Ipilimumab augments T-cell activity by blocking the immunosuppressive interaction of CTLA-4 with B7.[36]

In a landmark trial evaluating its efficacy, ipilimumab was used in conjunction with standard of care dacarbazine (see **Table 1**).[37] OS in patients receiving ipilimumab and dacarbazine was 11.2 months compared with 9.1 months with dacarbazine and the estimated survival at 1 year with ipilimumab was increased to 47.3% from 36.3% with dacarbazine.[37] The average response duration was 19.3 months for the ipilimumab group compared with 8.1 months for dacarbazine.[37]

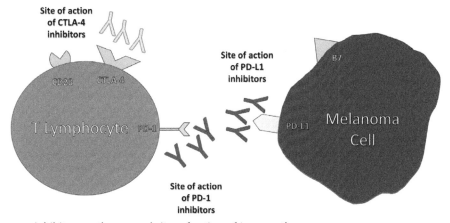

Fig. 2. Immune inhibitory pathways and sites of action of immunotherapy.

Anti-PD-1 and anti-PDL-1 therapy

Several agents targeting the PD-1/PD-L1 pathway have now been approved for use in melanoma—nivolumab, pembrolizumab, and atezolizumab. Pivotal phase III trials of nivolumab include Check-Mate 066 and CheckMate 037 (see **Table 1**).[38–40] In the CheckMate 066 trial, which evaluated previously untreated metastatic melanomas, patients treated with nivolumab had a 1-year OS of 72.9% compared with only 42.1% in the control group treated with dacarbazine.[38] Furthermore, the median PFS of patients treated with nivolumab was 5.1 months versus 2.2 months with standard chemotherapy.[38]

Weber and colleagues, (CheckMate 037), went on to evaluate the efficacy of nivolumab in patients whose melanoma progressed after ipilimumab and/or the use of a BRAF-inhibitor. This study demonstrated nivolumab to have an ORR of 31.7% compared with 10.6% with chemotherapy (dacarbazine or paclitaxel).[39]

Pembrolizumab is an anti-PD-1 monoclonal antibody that has been approved for use in unresectable or metastatic melanoma.[41] KEYNOTE-006 was a phase III study that directly compared the efficacy of pembrolizumab at various dosing regimens to ipilimumab (see **Table 1**).[41–43] The RR was 33.7% with pembrolizumab every 2 weeks, 32.9% every 3 weeks, and 11.9% with ipilimumab. Additionally, the estimated 12-month survival rates for pembrolizumab dosed every 2 and every 3 weeks were 74.1% and 68.4%, respectively, compared with 58.2% with ipilimumab.[41]

Regarding treatment endpoints with the use of anti-PD1 immunotherapy, The European Society for Medical Oncology (ESMO), has recommended that patients with a complete response (CR) evaluated radiologically and having received at least 6 months of therapy can be considered for treatment discontinuation.[44] Studies demonstrated that at 2 years following the discontinuation of pembrolizumab in this manner, over 85% of responders did not have evidence of relapse.[45] This result was substantiated in patients who electively discontinued treatment with either pembrolizumab or nivolumab. However, it was observed that relapse was more likely after less than 6 months of therapy.[46] NCCN recommends immunotherapy with PD-1 inhibitors as another first-line option for advanced and metastatic melanoma; however, no optimal duration of treatment is suggested as there is limited prospective data.[2]

Combination immunotherapy

Given potential for synergy between the two classes of immunotherapy to stimulate different parts of the immune cascade, the next evolution in treatment led to trials of combination therapies. Phase II study CheckMate-069 administered ipilimumab combined with nivolumab to patients with BRAF-V600 WT melanoma.[47] This trial went on to demonstrate an ORR of 61% for combination therapy compared with 11% in patients treated with ipilimumab and placebo.[47] Of that, CRs were observed in 22% of the combination therapy group versus 0% of the ipilimumab cohort.[47]

The phase III trial CheckMate-067 subsequently assessed efficacy in BRAF-mutant and WT melanoma (see **Table 1**).[48–52] Results showed a median PFS with ipilimumab and nivolumab of 11.5 months, 6.9 months with nivolumab monotherapy, and 2.9 months with ipilimumab monotherapy.[48–52] Differences between patients with BRAF-mutant and WT did not reach statistical significance.[48]

Currently, NCCN recommends nivolumab/ipilimumab or pembrolizumab/ipilimumab combination therapy as options for metastatic and unresectable disease. Relative indications for combination as opposed to PD-1 agent monotherapy include patient willingness to risk immune-related adverse events (irAEs), lack of comorbidities that increase the risk of irAEs, social support, and expected compliance with the management of toxicities.[2]

Immune-related adverse events

Upregulation of host immune response by immunotherapy is not limited to the tumor and can have off-target effects. This creates a unique subset of adverse events referred to as irAEs that may be severe and continue to evolve in the literature.[53] Rates of irAEs vary widely based on the agent used but have been reported to be between 15% and 90% and severe (grade 3/4) irAEs between 0.5% and 13% with the use of immune checkpoint monotherapy.[53] Combined therapy is associated with increased toxicity and high rate of irAEs occurring in 55% to 60% cases.[53]

Skin manifestations are the most common irAEs and include but are not limited to psoriasis, bullous pemphigoid, lichenoid reactions, lupus erythematosus, and vitiligo.[54] The time course for developing irAEs varies but skin manifestations can begin as early as 2 to 3 weeks after initiation or as late as after discontinuation.[55]

Systemic irAEs include enterocolitis, hepatitis, pneumonitis, and endocrinopathies.[53] Severe irAEs have been described and result in death in up to 2% of patients.[55] Prompt recognition is critical for management.[56] Steroids and holding/discontinuing immunotherapy are the backbone of management of severe irAEs but some refractory cases require long-term alternate immunosuppressive regimens.[53,56]

A systematic review demonstrated a positive association between the development of irAEs and ORR, PFS, and OS.[57] Patients with stage IV or locally advanced melanoma treated with immunotherapy who developed irAEs had an improved RR compared with patients without irAEs.[57] OS was 15.24 months in patients with any grade irAE compared with 8.94 months in patients with none.[57]

Intralesional and topical immunotherapies

Talimogene Laherparepvec (T-VEC) is an oncolytic virus that is FDA-approved for use in melanoma and is administered intralesionally.[58] It is a genetically modified herpes-simplex-1 virus (HSV-1) that lacks genes necessary for neurotropism and includes granulocyte-macrophage colony-stimulating factor (GM-CSF) to stimulate immunogenicity.[58] This modification allows T-VEC to preferentially multiply within tumor cells, cause tumor lysis, and promote an immune response targeting tumoral cells without the latency seen with wild-type HSV1.[58] Several trials have demonstrated both improvements in ORR and decreases in sizes of injected and uninjected lesions treated with T-VEC (**Table 2**).[59,60] Trials combining T-VEC with ipilimumab have also shown promising results and other combinations are under investigation.[61,62] In addition, other intralesional agents such as interleukin-2 and topical agents such as imiquimod and diphencyprone have been utilized with varying degrees of success; their role in the management of melanoma remains unclear (see **Table 2**).[63–66]

Novel Approaches

Even though immunotherapy and targeted therapy have shown significant benefits in the treatment of melanoma, a number of tumors either fail to respond or eventually progress despite these treatments. While a significant improvement in chemotherapy, response rates, and irAEs to these treatments leave room for improvement. Novel approaches to optimize the use of systemic agents, reduce irAEs and predict response are actively being investigated.[7,10]

BRAF/MEK-inhibitors plus immunotherapy

One such approach is the so-called "triplet" therapy in which patients receive BRAF-inhibitors, MEK-inhibitors, and immunotherapy. The Keynote-022 trial and NCT02130466 trial, were both phase II studies comparing dabrafenib, trametinib, and pembrolizumab to dabrafenib, trametinib, and placebo (**Table 3**).[67,68] Results were comparable and Keynote-022 showed PFS with triplet therapy for 16.9 months compared with 10.7 months in the control arm. Additionally, median duration of response was 25.1 months with triplet therapy versus 12.1 months with dabrafenib and trametinib.

IMspire150, a phase III trial, compared combination atezolizumab, vemurafenib, and cobimetinib to vemurafenib, cobimetinib, and placebo (see **Table 3**).[69] Triplet therapy resulted in a PFS increase from 10.6 to 15.1 months leading to approval of the combination of atezolizumab, cobimetinib and vemurafenib for patients with unresectable or metastatic melanoma harboring BRAF-V600 mutations [91]. In all trials of triple therapy, patients in the triple therapy arm were more likely to experience grade 3/4 AEs; however, the percentage of patients that stopped treatment as a result of AEs was similar to the control groups.[67–69]

Adjuvant and neoadjuvant uses

Adjuvant and neoadjuvant approaches using immunotherapy and targeted therapy in combination with surgery have also shown promising results in early studies. EORTC-18071 was a phase III trial comparing THE use of adjuvant ipilimumab to placebo following complete resection of stage III melanoma (**Table 4**).[70] Results demonstrated improved 5-year recurrence-free survival (RFS) and OS.[70]

Use of PD-1 inhibitor, nivolumab showed even more promising results in the CheckMate-238 trial (see **Table 4**).[71] This trial demonstrated RFS of 70.5% with the use of adjuvant nivolumab and 60.8% with adjuvant ipilimumab at 12 months.[71] Furthermore, grade 3/4 irAEs were seen in 14.4% of patients receiving nivolumab as opposed to 45.9% in the ipilimumab group.[71]

Adjuvant pembrolizumab in patients with resected stage III melanoma in phase III Keynote-054 trial showed similar results (see **Table 4**).[72] At the 3.5-year mark, metastasis-free survival increased to 65.3% with the use of pembrolizumab compared with 49.4% in the control group.[72] Current NCCN guidelines recommend nivolumab or pembrolizumab as the preferred immunotherapy adjuvant treatment.[2]

The NCCN also recommends dabrafenib/trametinib as an option for adjuvant therapy in resected stage III melanomas harboring BRAF-V600 mutations based on the COMBI-AD trial (see **Table 4**).[2,73] This phase III trial demonstrated improved 3-year RFS and OS compared with placebo.[73]

BRIM8 trial evaluated adjuvant vemurafenib in BRAF-V600 as mutant stage III melanomas following complete surgical resection (see **Table 4**).[74] Despite the improvement in disease-free

Table 2
Intralesional and topical therapies

Treatment	Reference	Study Population	Outcomes
Intralesional T-VEC	Anadtbacka et al[60] 2017	Stage IIIB-IV melanoma	Decrease in tumor size by >50% in 64% of injected lesions, 34% of uninjected nonvisceral lesions, and 15% of uninjected visceral lesions
Intralesional IL-2	Byers et al[63] 2014	In-transit melanoma	CRR ranging from 40.7% to 96% (Mean 78%)
Topical Diphencyprone	Damian et al[64] 2014	Locally recurrent, in transit or cutaneously metastatic melanoma	CRR of 46% and partial RR of 38%
Topical Imiquimod	Mora et al[65] 2015	Lentigo maligna	Clinical clearance rate of 76.2% and histologic clearance rate of 78.3%
	Scarfi et al[66] 2020	Local metastatic melanoma	CRR of melanoma mets of 64.3% and partial RR of 17.9%

survival, the NCCN currently does not recommend adjuvant monotherapy with vemurafenib based on rates of AEs and keratinocyte carcinomas.[2,74]

Use of neoadjuvant regimens is also under active investigation with promising results in early trials.[75] One phase II trial enrolled patients with BRAF-V600 K or BRAF-V600 E mutant stage III or IV melanoma to receive neoadjuvant dabrafenib and trametinib before surgery compared with surgery alone.[75] With the use of neoadjuvant targeted therapy the median event-free survival was 19.7 months compared with 2.9 months in the control group.[75]

Neoadjuvant nivolumab showed ORR and pathologic CR rates of 25% in high-risk resectable melanomas.[76] When ipilimumab and nivolumab were used in combination for neoadjuvant therapy the ORR increased to 73% and pathologic CR was 45%.[76] Another trial evaluating different dosing combinations of ipilimumab and nivolumab demonstrated an RFS of 84% at 2 years with neoadjuvant therapy.[77] Importantly, this trial found that patients treated with neoadjuvant immunotherapy who had pathologic response at the time of surgical resection had an RFS of 97% at 2 years compared with 36% of patients without pathologic response.[77]

Further trials assessing the efficacy of both neoadjuvant and adjuvant targeted and immune therapy are ongoing.

Predicting immunotherapy response
Predicting response to immunotherapy is an important future direction for the field. A growing body of research has demonstrated a role for the gut microbiome in response to immunotherapy, including studies on the effect of antibiotic administration prior to immunotherapy and those

Table 3
Phase III trial data for triple targeted therapy and immunotherapy

Trial	Name/Reference	Treatment	PFS (Months)	OS
KEYNOTE-022	Ferrucci et al[67] 2020	Dabrafenib + Trametinib + Pembrolizumab	16.9	Not reached
		Dabrafenib + Trametinib + Placebo	10.7	26.3
NCT02130466	Ascierto et al[68] 2019	Dabrafenib + Trametinib + Pembrolizumab	16.0	
		Dabrafenib + Trametinib + Placebo	10.3	
IMspire150	Gutzmer et al[69] 2020	Vemurafenib + Cobimetinib + Atezolizumab	15.1	
		Vemurafenib + Cobimetinib + Placebo	10.6	

Table 4
Phase III trial data for adjuvant targeted therapy and immunotherapy

Trial	Name/Reference	Treatment	RFS or DFS	OS
EORTC18071	Eggermont et al[70] 2016	Ipilimumab 10 mg/kg	5 y - 41%	5 y - 65%
		Placebo	5 y - 30%	5 y - 54%
CheckMate 238	Weber et al [71]2017	Nivolumab + Placebo	1 y - 71%	–
		Ipilimumab + Placebo	1 y - 61%	–
KEYNOTE-054	Eggermont et al[72] 2018	Pembrolizumab	1 y - 75%	–
		Placebo	1 y - 61%	–
COMBI-AD	Long et al [73]2017	Dabrafenib + Trametinib	3 y - 58%	3 y - 86%
		Placebo	3 y - 39%	3 y - 77%
BRIM8	Maio et al[74]2018	Vemurafenib	2 y - 62%	2 y - 90%
		Placebo	2 y - 53%	2 y - 86%

comparing the biodiversity of microbiome in responders compared with non-responders to immunotherapy.[78] As our understanding of the microbiome grows, it could become another tool to predict and potentially influence response to immunotherapy.[78]

Another emerging biomarker to predict response to immunotherapy is PD-L1 expression. In the CheckMate-067 trial, patients with PD-L1 levels above 5% had improved 4-year survival rates compared with those with levels below 5%.[79] Similar trends were seen in other trials; however, PD-L1 is a dynamic marker and heterogeneity in testing methods limits its routine use.[80] Current recommendations advise not to exclude patients based on PD-L1 expression levels.[2]

Novel agents in development
There are numerous trials exploring new agents to treat melanoma.[58] Some of these treatments include toll-like receptor agonists, CD40 agonists, anti-CD137, and IDO inhibitors amongst others.[81,82] IDO is an enzyme involved in the catalytic pathway of tryptophan which plays a crucial role in immune tolerance and has been shown to be important in tumor immune escape.[83] Studies have begun exploring the utility of IDO-inhibitors in conjunction with immunotherapy.[84]

Future Directions

While targeted and immunotherapy agents have revolutionized treatment options for melanoma, further research is ongoing to improve outcomes. Combinatorial and adjuvant approaches offer promise in fine-tuning systemic therapies for advanced and metastatic disease. Trials are underway analyzing the role of sequential treatment with targeted and immunotherapy. Additionally, developing biomarkers to predict response could help to individualize and personalize treatment

regimens. As our understanding of oncogenesis, molecular profiling, and epigenetics continues to expand it will lead to novel therapeutics and approaches that are more specific, effective, and cause fewer AEs.

CLINICS CARE POINTS

- While more effective than previous options for advanced melanoma, many of the novel medications carry significant side effects.
- Novel agents, combination therapy and adjuvant and neoadjuvant approaches have shown promising results in clinical trials.

DISCLOSURE

D Bolotin Principle Investigator on clinical trial with Replimune Biotech.

REFERENCES

1. Saginala K, Barsouk A, Aluru JS, et al. Epidemiology of Melanoma. Med Sci (Basel) 2021;9(4):63.
2. National Comprehensive Cancer Network. Melanoma: Cutaneous (version 1.2022). 2021. Available at: https://www.nccn.org/professionals/physician_gls/pdf/cutaneous_melanoma.pdf. Accessed December 5, 2021.
3. Cancer Institute National. Melanoma of the Skin-Cancer Stat Facts. Available online: https://seer.cancer.gov/statfacts/html/melan.html. Accessed on December 3, 2021.
4. Chapman PB, Hauschild A, Robert C, et al. Improved survival with vemurafenib in melanoma

with BRAF V600E mutation. N Engl J Med 2011;364: 2507–16.

5. Siegel RL, Miller KD, Jemal A. Cancer Statistics. CA Cancer J Clin 2020;70:7–30.

6. Patel H, Yacoub N, Mishra R, et al. Current Advances in the Treatment of BRAF-Mutant Melanoma. Cancers 2020;12:482.

7. LoRusso PM, Schalper K, Sosman J. Targeted therapy and immunotherapy: Emerging biomarkers in metastatic melanoma. Pigment Cell Melanoma Res 2020;33:390–402.

8. McArthur GA, Chapman PB, Robert C, et al. Safety and efficacy of vemurafenib in BRAF^{V600E} and BRAF^{V600K} mutation-positive melanoma (BRIM- 3): Extended follow-up of a phase 3, randomised, open-label study. Lancet Oncol 2014;15:323–32.

9. Chapman PB, Robert C, Larkin J, et al. Vemurafenib in patients with BRAFV600 mutation- positive metastatic melanoma: Final overall sur- vival results of the random- ized BRIM-3 study. Ann Oncol 2017;28:2581–7.

10. Luke JJ. Comprehensive clinical trial data summation for BRAF-MEK inhibition and checkpoint immunotherapy in metastatic melanoma. Oncologist 2019;24:e1197–211.

11. Hauschild A, Grob JJ, Demidov LV, et al. Dabrafenib in BRAF-mutated metastatic melanoma: A multicentre, open-label, phase 3 randomised controlled trial. Lancet 2012;380:358–65.

12. Dummer R, Ascierto PA, Gogas HJ, et al. Overall survival in patients with BRAF-mutant melanoma receiving encorafenib plus binimetinib versus vemurafenib or encorafenib (COLUMBUS): A multicentre, open-label, randomised, phase 3 trial. Lancet Oncol 2018;19:1315–27.

13. Anforth R, Menzies A, Byth K, et al. Factors influencing the development of cutaneous squamous cell carcinoma in patients on BRAF inhibitor therapy. J Am Acad Dermatol 2015;72:809–15.

14. Sun J, Zager JS, Eroglu Z. Encorafenib/binimetinib for the treatment of BRAF-mutant advanced, unresectable, or metastatic melanoma: design, development, and potential place in therapy. OncoTargets Ther 2018;11:9081.

15. Manzano JL, Layos L, Buges C, et al. Resistant mechanisms to BRAF inhibitors in melanoma. Ann Transl Med 2016;4:237.

16. Hoffner B, Benchich K. Trametinib: a targeted therapy in metastatic melanoma. J Adv Pract Oncol 2018;9:741–5.

17. Flaherty KT, Robert C, Hersey P, et al. Improved survival with MEK inhibition in BRAF-mutated melanoma. N Engl J Med 2012;367:107–14.

18. Schadendorf D, Flaherty KT, Hersey P, et al. Overall survival (OS) update on METRIC (NCT01245062), a randomized phase 3 study to assess efficacy of trametinib (T) compared with chemotherapy (C) in patients (pts) with BRAFV600E/K mutation-positive (+)

advanced or metastatic melanoma (MM). Pigment Cell Melanoma Res 2013;26:997A.

19. Robert C, Flaherty K, Nathan P, et al. Five-year outcomes from a phase 3 METRIC study in patients with BRAF V600 E/K-mutant advanced or metastatic melanoma. Eur J Cancer 2019;109:61–9.

20. Dummer R, Schadendorf D, Ascierto PA, et al. Binimetinib versus dacarbazine in patients with advanced NRAS-mutant melanoma (NEMO): a multicenter, open-label, randomsied, phase 3 trial. Lancet Oncol 2017;18:435–45.

21. Larkin J, Ascierto PA, Dréno B, et al. Combined vemurafenib and cobimetenib in BRAF-mutated melanoma. N Engl J Med 2014;371:1867–76.

22. Ascierto PA, McArthur GA, Dréno B, et al. Cobimetinib combined with vemurafenib in advanced BRAFV600-mutant melanoma (coBRIM):Updated efficacy results from a randomised, double-blind, phase 3 trial. Lancet Oncol 2016;17:1248–60.

23. Dréno B, Ascierto PA, McArthur GA, et al. Efficacy and safety of cobimetinib (C) combined with vemurafenib (V) in patients (pts) with BRAFV600 mutation-positive metastatic melanoma: Analysis from the 4-year extended follow-up of the phase 3 coBRIM study. J Clin Oncol 2018;36(suppl 15): 9522A.

24. Long GV, Stroyakovskiy D, Gogas H, et al. Combined BRAF and MEK inhibition versus BRAF inhibition alone in melanoma. N Engl J Med 2014;71: 1877–88.

25. Long GV, Stroyakovskiy D, Gogas H, et al. Dabrafenib and trametinib versus dabrafenib and placebo for Val600 BRAF-mutant melanoma: A multicentre, double-blind, phase 3 randomsied controlled trial. Lancet 2015;386:444–51.

26. Long GV, Flaherty KT, Stroyakovskiy D, et al. Dabrafenib plus trametinib versus dabrafenib monotherapy in patients with metastatic BRAF V600E/ k-mutant melanoma: Long-term survival and safety analysis of a phase 3 study. Ann Oncol 2017;28: 1631–9.

27. Robert C, Karaszewska B, Schachter J, et al. Improved overall survival in melanoma with combined dabrafenib and trametinib. N Engl J Med 2015;372:30–9.

28. Robert C, Karaszewska B, Schachter J, et al. Three-year estimate of overall survival in COMBI-v, a randomized phase 3 study evaluating first-line dabrafenib (D) + trametinib (T) in patients (pts) with unresectable or metastatic BRAF V600E/k-mutant cutaneous melanoma. Ann Oncol 2016;27(suppl 6):LBA40A.

29. Dummer R, Ascierto PA, Gogas HJ, et al. Results of COLUMBUS part 1: A phase 3 trial of encorafenib (ENCO) plus binimetinib (BINI) versus vemurafenib (VEM) or ENCO in BRAF-mutant melanoma. Oral presentation Annu Soc Melanoma Res Meet 2016.

30. Dummer R, Ascierto PA, Gogas HJ, et al. Encorafenib plus binimetinib versus vemurafenib or encorafenib in patients with BRAF-mutant melanoma (COLUMBUS): A multicentre, open-label, randomised phase 3 trial. Lancet Oncol 2018;19:603–15.

31. Dummer R, Ascierto PA, Gogas H, et al. Results of COLUMBUS part 2: A phase 3 trial of encorafenib (ENCO) plus binimetinib (BINI) versus ENCO in BRAF-mutant melanoma. Ann Oncol 2017;28(suppl 5):1215OA.

32. Sanlorenzo M, Choudhry A, Vujic I, et al. Comparative profile of cutaneous adverse events: BRAF/MEK inhibitor combination therapy versus BRAF monotherapy in melanoma. J Am Acad Dermatol 2014;71(6):1102–9.

33. Peng L, Wang Y, Hong Y, et al. Incidence and relative risk of cutaneous squamous cell carcinoma with single-agent BRAF inhibitor and dual BRAF/MEK inhibitors in cancer patients: A meta-analysis. Oncotarget 2017;8:83280–91.

34. Passarelli A, Mannavola F, Stucci LS, et al. Immune system and melanoma biology: a balance between immunosurveillance and immune escape. Oncotarget 2017;8:106132–42.

35. Onitilo AA, Wittig JA. Principles of immunotherapy in melanoma. Surg Clin North Am 2020;100(1):161–73.

36. Hodi FS, O'Day SJ, McDermott DF, et al. Improved survival with ipilimumab in patients with metastatic melanoma. N Engl J Med 2010;363:711–23.

37. Robert C, Thomas L, Bondarenko I, et al. Ipilimumab plus dacarbazine for previously untreated metastatic melanoma. N Engl J Med 2011;364:2517–26.

38. Robert C, Long GV, Brady B, et al. Nivolumab in previously untreated melanoma without BRAF mutation. N Engl J Med 2015;372:320–30.

39. Weber JS, D'Angelo SP, Minor D, et al. Nivolumab versus chemotherapy in patients with advanced melanoma who progressed after anti-CTLA-4 treatment (CheckMate 037): A randomised, controlled, open-label, phase 3 trial. Lancet Oncol 2015;16:375–84.

40. Weber J, Minor D, D'Angelo S, et al. Overall survival in patients with advanced melanoma who received nivolumab vs investigator's choice chemotherapy in the phase 3 CheckMate 037 trial. Oral presentation Annu Soc Melanoma Res Meet 2016.

41. Robert C, Schachter J, Long GV, et al. Pembrolizumab versus ipilimumab in advanced melanoma. N Engl J Med 2015;372:2521–32.

42. Schachter J, Ribas A, Long GV, et al. Pembrolizumab versus ipilimumab for advanced melanoma: final overall survival results of a multicentre, randomised, open-label phase 3 study (KEYNOTE-006). Lancet 2017;390(10105):1853–62.

43. Long GV, Schachter J, Ribas A, et al. 4-year survival and outcomes after cessation of pembrolizumab (pembro) after 2-years in patients (pts) with ipilimumab (ipi)-naive advanced melanoma in KEYNOTE-006. J Clin Oncol 2018;36(suppl 15):9503A.

44. Keilholz U, Ascierto PA, Dummer R, et al. ESMO Consensus Conference Recommendations on the Management of Metastatic Melanoma: Under the Auspices of the ESMO Guidelines Committee. Ann Oncol 2020;31:1435–48.

45. Robert C, Ribas A, Hamid O, et al. Durable complete response after discontinuation of pembrolizumab in patients with metastatic melanoma. J Clin Oncol 2018;36(17):1668–74.

46. Jansen YJL, Rozeman EA, Mason R, et al. Discontinuation of anti-PD-1 antibody therapy in the absence of disease progression or treatment limiting toxicity: Clinical outcomes in advanced melanoma. Ann Oncol 2019;30:1154–61.

47. Postow MA, Chesney J, Pavlick AC, et al. Nivolumab and ipilimumab versus ipilimumab in untreated melanoma. N Engl J Med 2015;372:2006–17.

48. Larkin J, Chiarion-Sileni V, Gonzalez R, et al. Combined nivolumab and ipilimumab or monotherapy in untreated melanoma. N Engl J Med 2015;373:23–34.

49. Wolchok JD, Chiarion-Sileni V, Gonzalez R, et al. Updated results from a phase III trial of nivolumab (NIVO) combined with ipilimumab (IPI) in treatment-naive patients (pts) with advanced melanoma (MEL) (CheckMate 067). J Clin Oncol 2016;34(suppl 15):9505A.

50. Wolchok JD, Chiarion-Sileni V, Gonzalez R, et al. Overall survival with combined nivolumab and ipilimumab in advanced melanoma. N Engl J Med 2017;377:1345–56.

51. Hodi FS, Chiarion-Sileni V, Gonzalez R, et al. Nivolumab plus ipilimumab or nivolumab alone versus ipilimumab alone in advanced melanoma (CheckMate 067): 4-year outcomes of a multi- centre, randomised, phase 3 trial. Lancet Oncol 2018;19:1480–92.

52. Larkin J, Chiarion-Sileni V, Gonzalez R, et al. Five-year survival with combined nivolumab and ipilimumab in advanced melanoma. N Engl J Med 2019;381:1535–46.

53. National Comprehensive Cancer Network. Management of Immunotherapy-Related Toxicities (version 4.2021). 2021. Available at: https://www.nccn.org/professionals/physician_gls/pdf/immunotherapy.pdf. Accessed December 5, 2021.

54. Simonsen AB, Kaae J, Ellebaek E, et al. Cutaneous adverse reactions to anti-PD-1 treatment-a systematic review. J Am Acad Dermatol 2020;83(5):1415–24.

55. Owen CN, Bai X, Quah T, et al. Delayed immune-related adverse events with anti-PD-1-based immunotherapy in melanoma. Ann Oncol 2021;32:917–25.

56. Puzanov I, Diab A, Abdallah K, et al. Society for Immunotherapy of Cancer Toxicity Management Working Group. Managing toxicities associated with immune checkpoint inhibitors: consensus

recommendations from the Society for Immuno-therapy of Cancer (SITC) Toxicity Management Working Group. J Immunother Cancer 2017;5:95.

57. Hussaini S, Chehade R, Boldt RG, et al. Association between immune-related side effects and efficacy and benefit of immune checkpoint inhibitors—A systematic review and meta-analysis. Cancer Treat Rev 2020;92:102134.

58. Luther C, Swami U, Zhang J, et al. Advanced stage melanoma therapies: detailing the present and exploring the future. Crit Rev Oncol Hematol 2019; 133:99–111.

59. Andtbacka RH, Kaufman HL, Collichio F, et al. Talimogene laherparepvec improves durable response rate in patients with advanced melanoma. J Clin Oncol 2015;33:2780–8.

60. Andtbacka RH, Ross M, Puzanov I, et al. Patterns of clinical response with talimogene laherparepvec (T-VEC) in patients with melanoma treated in the OPTiM phase III clinical trial. Ann Surg Oncol 2016; 23:4169–77.

61. Chesney J, Puzanov I, Collichio F, et al. Randomized, Open-Label Phase II Study Evaluating the Efficacy and Safety of Talimogene Laherparepvec in Combination With Ipilimumab Versus Ipilimumab Alone in Patients With Advanced, Unresectable Melanoma. J Clin Oncol 2017;36(17):9509.

62. Ribas A, Chesney J, Long GV, et al. 1037O MASTERKEY-265: A phase III, randomized, placebo (Pbo)-controlled study of talimogene laherparepvec (T) plus pembrolizumab (P) for unresectable stage IIIB–IVM1c melanoma (MEL). Ann Oncol 2021;32:S868–9.

63. Byers B, Temple-Oberle CF, McKinnon JG, et al. Treatment of in transit melanoma with intra-lesional interleukin-2: A systematic review. Can J Plast Surg 2013;21:142.

64. Damian DL, Saw RP, Thompson JF. Topical immuno-therapy with diphencyprone for in transit and cutaneously metastatic melanoma. J Surg Oncol 2014; 109(4):308–13.

65. Mora AN, Karia PS, Nguyen BM. A quantitative systemic review of the efficacy of imiquimod monotherapy for lentigo maligna and an analysis of factors that affect tumor clearance. J Am Acad Dermatol 2015;73:205–12.

66. Scarfì F, Patrizi A, Veronesi G, et al. The role of topical imiquimod in melanoma cutaneous metastases: a critical review of the literature. Dermatol Ther 2020;1:e14165.

67. Ferrucci PF, Di Giacomo AM, Del Vecchio M, et al. Keynote-022 Part 3: A Randomized, Double-Blind, Phase 2 Study of Pembrolizumab, Dabrafenib, and Trametinib in BRAF-mutant Melanoma. J Immunother Cancer 2020;8:e001806.

68. Ascierto PA, Ferrucci PF, Fisher R, et al. Dabrafenib, trametinib and pembrolizumab or placebo in BRAF-mutant melanoma. Nat Med 2019;25:941–6.

69. Gutzmer R, Stroyakovskiy D, Gogas H, et al. Atezolizumab, vemurafenib, and cobimetinib as first-line treatment for unresectable advanced BRAFV600 mutation-positive melanoma (IMspire150): Primary analysis of the randomised, double-blind, placebo-controlled, phase 3 trial. Lancet 2020;395: 1835–44.

70. Eggermont AMM, Chiarion-Sileni V, Grob J-J, et al. Prolonged survival in stage III melanoma with ipilimumab adjuvant therapy. N Engl J Med 2016;375: 1845–55.

71. Weber J, Mandala M, Del Vecchio M, et al. Adjuvant nivolumab versus ipilimumab in resected stage III or IV melanoma. N Engl J Med 2017;377:1824–35.

72. Eggermont AMM, Blank CU, Mandala M, et al. Adjuvant pembrolizumab versus placebo in resected stage III melanoma. N Engl J Med 2018;378:1789–801.

73. Long GV, Hauschild A, Santinami M, et al. Adjuvant dabrafenib plus trametinib in stage III BRAF-mutated melanoma. N Engl J Med 2017;377: 1813–23.

74. Maio M, Lewis K, Demidov L, et al. Adjuvant vemurafenib in resected, BRAFV600 mutation-positive melanoma (BRIM8): a randomised, double-blind, placebo-controlled, multicentre, phase 3 trial. Lancet Oncol 2018;19:510–20.

75. Amaria RN, Prieto PA, Tetzlaff MT, et al. Neoadjuvant plus adjuvant dabrafenib and trametinib versus standard of care in patients with high-risk, surgically resectable melanoma: a single-centre, open-label, randomised, phase 2 trial. Lancet Oncol 2018; 19(2):181–93.

76. Amaria RN, Reddy SM, Tawbi HA, et al. Neoadjuvant immune checkpoint blockade in high-risk resectable melanoma. Nat Med 2018;24:1649–54.

77. Rozeman EA, Reijers IL, Hoefsmit EP, et al. Twenty-Four months RFS and updated toxicity data from OpACIN-neo: A study to identify the optimal dosing schedule of neoadjuvant ipilimumab (IPI) and nivolumab (NIVO) in stage III melanoma. J Clin Oncol 2020;38:10015.

78. Gopalakrishnan V, Spencer CN, Nezi L, et al. Gut microbiome modulates response to anti -PD-1 immunotherapy in melanoma patients. Science 2018; 359:97–103.

79. Larkin J, Minor D, D'Angelo S, et al. Overall survival in patients with advanced melanoma who received nivolumab versus investigator's choice chemotherapy in CheckMate 037: a randomized, controlled, open-label phase III trial. J Clin Oncol 2018;36(4):383–90.

80. Carlino MS, Long GV, Schadendorf D, et al. Outcomes by line of therapy and programmed death ligand 1 expression in patients with advanced melanoma treated with pembrolizumab or ipilimumab in KEYNOTE-006: a randomised clinical trial. Eur J Cancer 2018;101:236–43.

81. Bajor DL, Mick R, Riese MJ, et al. Abstract CT137: Combination of agonistic CD40 monoclonal antibody CP-870,893 and anti-CTLA-4 antibody tremelimumab in patients with metastatic melanoma. Cancer Res 2015;75:CT137.

82. Segal NH, Logan TF, Hodi FS, et al. Results from an integrated safety analysis of urelumab, an agonist anti-CD137 monoclonal antibody. Clin Cancer Res 2017;23:1929–36.

83. Prendergast GC, Malachowski WP, DuHadaway JB, et al. Discovery of IDO1 Inhibitors: From Bench to Bedside. Cancer Res 2017;77(24):6795–811.

84. Zakharia Y, McWilliams R, Shaheen M, et al. Interim analysis of the phase 2 clinical trial of the IDO pathway inhibitor indoximod in combination with pembrolizumab for patients with advanced melanoma. [AACR abstract CT117]. Cancer Res 2017;77(13):CT117.

Mohs Micrographic Surgery for Melanoma
Evidence, Controversy, and a Critical Review of Excisional Margin Guidelines

David G. Brodland, MD[a,b,c,d,*]

KEYWORDS

- Malignant melanoma • Mohs micrographic surgery • Wide excision
- Excision guidelines for melanoma • Surgical margins of excision • Invasive melanoma
- Melanoma in situ • Lentigo maligna

KEY POINTS

- Mohs surgery has been used for the excision of primary melanoma for over 70 years with mounting clinical research-based evidence showing unequaled low local recurrence rates.
- The unmatched high rate of primary tumor clearance is predicated on histologic evaluation of 100% of peripheral and deep margins using frozen sections with immunostains.
- Mohs surgery for melanoma confirms complete tumor removal on the day of excision and prior to reconstruction.
- Reported recurrence rates for head and neck melanoma are substantially lower for MMS compared with WE, highlighting the lack of evidence supporting the melanoma guidelines universal recommendation for WE to the exclusion of MMS for melanoma.
- The effectiveness of WE is predicated on multiple randomized trials (RT) evaluating predetermined margins of not less than 1 cm. Yet, all guidelines allow excision with narrower margins when there are anatomic or functional concerns, as is very common on head and neck melanomas.

INTRODUCTION

Micrographic surgery (MS) has been used in the treatment of malignant melanoma (MM) for more than 70 years.[1] Dr Fred Mohs' melanoma tumor registry was initiated in 1981.[2] Over the years, refinements to this technique have led to greater acceptance of the procedure, which has been augmented by scientific studies showing excellent efficacy highlighted by unmatched low local recurrence rates.[3–12] The increasing prevalence of melanoma in the population has intensified the focus for safe and efficacious treatments.

Despite virtually uniform findings of excellent efficacy and safety in the literature, Mohs micrographic surgery (MMS) is not recognized in melanoma guidelines as an option in the care of invasive melanoma. The American Academy of Dermatology Melanoma Guidelines recommend wide excision (WE) for noninvasive melanoma but suggest MMS "may be considered" for melanoma in situ, lentigo maligna type "to provide tissue-sparing excision on anatomically constrained sites (e.g. face, ears, scalp)."[13] Furthermore, MMS "may be considered" when WE margins are positive for invasive lentigo maligna

For some things I have to disclose that I am a shareholder in QDP (QualDerm Partners, a private equity company in dermatology). Others do not consider this a confict of interest for such papers.
a Department of Dermatology, University of Pittsburgh; b Department of Otolaryngology, University of Pittsburgh; c Department of Plastic Surgery, University of Pittsburgh; d Z & B Skin Cancer Center, Pittsburgh PA
* 5200 Centre Avenue, Suite 303, Pittsburgh, PA 15232.
E-mail address: davidbrodland@aim.com

Dermatol Clin 41 (2023) 79–88
https://doi.org/10.1016/j.det.2022.07.008
0733-8635/23/© 2022 Elsevier Inc. All rights reserved.

melanoma of the head, neck, hands, and feet. The reason given for not affirming MMS as an alternative treatment to be considered is the lack of high-level evidence. Acknowledged in the guidelines is the lack of any such evidence pertaining to melanoma on the head, neck, hands, and feet for WE. Despite this equal dearth of "high-quality evidence," all guidelines internationally recommend the WE technique for all melanoma, including for locations on the head, neck, hands, and feet. In further contradistinction to the value of high-level evidence, all guidelines recommend that WE margins may be modified (reduced to margins never directly studied) for "functional considerations or anatomic location."[13,14] With this seemingly inconsistent application of scrutiny for the scientific validation of technique, a careful look at the current evidence is important for better insight into key fundamentals in the optimal care of patients with melanoma.

WIDE EXCISION TECHNIQUE AND THE RECOMMENDED SURGICAL MARGIN FOR MELANOMA

Excisional surgery is considered the standard of care for primary melanoma. Excision is performed to ensure complete tumor removal with confirmation of histologically clear margins.[13] The WE technique has been the predominant mode of excision for many years. The technique is based on the identification of the tumor margins by visual inspection, followed by excision of a predetermined, "wide" margin of normal-appearing skin beyond the clinical tumor borders. The essential component of this technique is designating the safe margin of clinically uninvolved skin to be excised. Although this requires potentially unnecessary injury and wounding to the patient, a wide margin of normal skin is needed because visual inspection of margins is inherently inaccurate and often fails to detect subclinical tumor extension. Given this inability of the careful visual inspection to identify true tumor margins accurately, a series of randomized trials (RT) were conducted comparing various predesignated margins of normal skin to be excised. These trials were designed to establish noninferiority for local recurrence and survival.[15–23]

The currently recommended widths of normal skin to be excised are based on these multiple RT comparing the efficacy of wide versus wider margins (Table 1). The consensus, using these results, is that 1-cm margins are as safe as wider margins for invasive melanomas up to 2 mm in thickness with the caveat that melanomas 1 to 2 mm in thickness may be excised with between 1- and 2-cm margins.[13,14] The consensus for melanomas greater than 2 mm in thickness is that 2-cm margins are as safe as wider margins when using the wide local excision technique. This consensus uses data from the RT[15–20,22,23] plus information from a follow-up study of a portion of one of these RT. It is notable that the retrospective data evaluation was only able to assess overall survival (OS) and melanoma-specific survival (MSS). Available data were insufficient to accurately study locoregional recurrence and disease-free survival. Furthermore, the data review could access only a portion of the original randomized cohort.[20,21]

All major guidelines include a statement that a decision to modify these recommended margins "to accommodate anatomic or functional considerations" may be made. This option is not based on any scientific data pertaining to the WE technique and is a departure from evidence-based practice. Given the considerable evidence that a large percentage of MM extends well beyond clinical margins and that margins less than 9 mm would be expected to incompletely excise a significant percentage of tumors, this exception to the margin guidelines is concerning.[24]

Theoretically, in the absence of exhaustive margin evaluation, WE technique with subcentimeter margins may lead to increased incidence of incompletely excised residual melanoma. Indeed, this exception is frequently invoked as suggested by a study showing that the percentage of WE of the head and neck melanoma that conforms to the guideline's recommendations is less than 40%.[25] This may explain the consistently higher local recurrence rates reported for WE of the head and neck melanomas (3%–13%).[11,12,26–31]

Margin guidelines for noninvasive melanoma using WE technique were initially based on expert panel consensus[32] and were set by consensus at 5 mm beyond the clinically visible tumor. There have been no prospective or randomized studies that have established safe margins for WE technique. More recently, a study based on prospectively collected data suggested that 5-mm margins would not provide acceptable levels of histologically tumor-free margins.[24] This study assessed margin adequacy using the incremental, subcentimeter excision method used during MMS. These data found that complete excision of in situ melanoma was accomplished 86% of the time with 6-mm margins and that 9-mm margins provide tumor-free margins in 98.9% of the cases. Based on this information, guidelines were altered to recommend that 5- to 10-mm margins should be excised when using the WE technique.[13,14]

The histologic margin clearance confirmation of WE is quite different from MMS in that traditional

Table 1
Melanoma Margin Guidelines Evidence

Melanoma Margin Guidelines Evidence	
Strengths	• Well-designed trials comparing narrow (1- to 2-cm excision margins) with wide (3- to 5-cm excision margins) • Randomized trials provide data for which confounding factors are minimized • High levels of internal validity • Established safety of narrow margin excision for melanomas • Long-term follow-up • Large cohorts • Multi-institutional studies
Limitations	• Technique specific: Studied wide-excision technique with comparative variable of margins width • Excision margins evaluated with vertical sectioning technique resulting in small percentage of margin evaluation for residual melanoma • Study cohorts limited largely to trunk and extremities • Head, neck, hands, feet, and genitalia excluded (>30% of all melanoma) • Variable exclusion of patients greater that 70–75 years of age (>35% of all melanoma) • No RTs of melanoma in situ • Definition of LR includes "within 2 cm of surgical scar," which may include in-transit metastases • Most studied outcomes of OS but not MSS

Abbreviation: LR, local recurrence.

vertical sectioning technique is used. Vertical sectioning samples the margins with cross-sectional planes of tissue. One advantage of cross-sectioning is that the central portion of the tissue specimen is examined and can provide additional pathologic staging information that may augment what is known from the original biopsy. The disadvantage is that, practically speaking, a very small portion of the entire peripheral margin is actually examined. Estimates are that as little as 0.1% of the entire peripheral margin is examined microscopically.[33] This is at significant variance with the MMS technique, which is designed to examine 100% of the perimetrical margin. The limited extent of pathologic margin examination is thought to be a reason for the higher local recurrence rate of WE compared with MMS.

MOHS MICROGRAPHIC SURGERY TECHNIQUE FOR MELANOMA

MMS is a technique that uniquely determines whether histologically clear margins have been achieved with immediate histologic evaluation that includes the entire deep and lateral perimetrical margins of excision.[5,34] Importantly, the key determinant of tumor clearance is not dependent on the statistical likelihood of tumor extension beyond the clinical margin based on prior studies or margin comparison RT. Rather, the key to MMS is the actual microscopic observance of histologically tumor-free margins. As such, the prescribed margins of normal skin mandated for the WE technique do not have the same critical utility in achieving tumor-free margins for contiguous melanoma. Rather, the size of the excisional margins is determined by the actual subclinical extent of contiguous melanoma. Clear margins can be confidently ascertained using the frozen section technique with immunostains within 2 hours or less of the excision. Reconstruction before achieving clear margins is never recommended with MMS. The challenges of histologic interpretation associated with frozen section histology can be confidently overcome with the use of immunostains (**Table 2**) that highlight melanocytes and simplify the recognition of malignant melanocytic patterns.[35,36]

Comparing the WE and MMS techniques, they are both forms of excision. The incisions are made vertically within clinically normal-appearing skin and extend deeply into the subcutaneous tissue to fascia, beneath the tumor. The major difference is that incisions for MMS may not include the entire 1 to 2 cm of normal skin recommended for WE. However, these margins are extended, as needed, on the day of surgery if they are found histologically to be involved by melanoma. These margin extensions are made specifically where there is occult tumor extension with the precision afforded by the MMS mapping technique. In contrast, at the completion of the WE, the surgeon submits the tissue for pathologic examination to be performed, at minimum, 24 hours later. The decision must be made whether to reconstruct the wound on the same day as the excision or to delay reconstruction until after a pathologist examines the pathologic slides and indicates that the margins appear clear, or not. Typically, the former approach is used. When margins are found to be positive, a reexcision is performed on another day. The location of the residual tumor is typically

Table 2
Most Common Melanoma Immunostains for MMS

	Most Common Melanoma Immunostains of MMS		
	MART 1 (Melanoma Antigen Recognized by T Cells)	MiTF (Microphthalmia Transcription Factor)	SOX 10 (Sry-Related HMB-BOX Gene 10)
Cellular target	Glycoprotein on cytoplasmic melanosomes	Nuclear transcription factor	Nuclear transcription factor
Strengths	• High sensitivityand specificity • Reliable and user-friendly • Easiest to interpret • Rapid protocols available • Useful in metastatic MM • Internal controls inherent due to staining of both normal and malignant melanocytes	• High sensitivity and specificity • Nuclear staining leads to more crisp, clean staining even in chronic sun damage • Stains epithelioid and spindle cell melanoma • Useful for metastatic MM	• High sensitivity and specificity • Nuclear staining leads to more crisp, clean staining even in chronic sun damage • Stains desmoplastic and spindle cell MM • Useful for metastatic MM
Weaknesses	• Does not distinguish benign from malignant melanocytes • Does not reliably stain for desmoplastic or spindle cell melanoma • Keratinocyte pigmentation due to severe sun damage or inflammation can lead to false positives (newer products mitigate this well)	• Poor staining of desmoplastic MM • Staining intensity is less and can be subtitle microscopically	• Does not distinguish benign from malignant melanocytes • Staining intensity is less and can be subtle microscopically

less precisely known, and so, the reexcision will likely have to be more broadly encompassing of marginal tissue. Furthermore, if the reconstruction was performed with a flap and caused anatomic rearrangements of the tissue, precise, selective reexcision is further compromised.

The technique used for MMS of melanomas, although slightly modified from traditional technique used for nonmelanoma skin cancer, allows for 100% of the surgical margin to be evaluated histologically, achieving complete, histologically confirmed tumor clearance on the same day and reconstruction of the tumor-free wound. The technique has been described in detail elsewhere.[5,34]

In brief, an initial circumferential incision is made 6 mm beyond the clinical margin of the melanoma. Inside of this incision, a "debulking" of the tumor is performed with 2 to 3 mm of normal-appearing skin extending to the junction of the dermis, and subcutaneous tissue is then removed and submitted for permanent section pathology. This debulking specimen can also be processed using frozen section technique with vertical sectioning concurrently

with the MMS sections, if desired.[5] Next, the initial incision made 6 mm from the clinical margin is deepened at a 90° angle to the level of the deep subcutaneous tissue above fascia to include the full thickness of the fat. Orientation hash marks are made on the skin surface perpendicular to the incision line. These hash marks will be visible microscopically on the frozen section slides as well as at the edge of the incisional wound on the patient. After maintaining orientation of the specimen, it is grossly sectioned to separate the epidermis, dermis, and a thin layer of subcutaneous fat from the horizontal deep fat margin. All edges of the sections are inked, and a map is drawn, representing the gross tissue sections and corresponding tissue stains. Once grossly sectioned and inked, the tissue is presented to the MMS histotechnologist who is then carefully apprised of the correct orientation of the tissue. Tissue sectioning is carried out using the standard MMS histotechnique with an emphasis on creating complete, yet very thin sections to optimize staining with immunohistochemical stains.[35,36]

MOHS SURGERY AND THE CONTROVERSY OF SUBCENTIMETER EXCISION MARGINS

The advantages of MMS in achieving histologically confirmed tumor-free margins conveniently, with same-day reconstruction carried out on verified tumor-free margins, are evident. However, critics of MMS express concern that the 10- to 20-mm margins of excision that are recommended for the WE technique are rarely achieved by MMS unless contiguous or noncontiguous metastatic tumor is present and extends to, or beyond, these margins. Their concern is that this could place the patient with invasive melanoma at risk because of a failure to excise the full 1 to 2 cm of skin. It is the contention that in-transit micrometastases may exist in this unexcised tissue. If not excised, the theory is that "failure to excise *both* the primary and subclinically locally metastatic disease could result in a local recurrence, which in reality is better termed 'local metastasis'."[37] This theory contends that not excising the additional few millimeters for a total of 1 cm in invasive melanomas 2 mm or less, or the additional 1 cm for tumors greater than 2 mm thick, will result in a potential "lost opportunity" and failure to *cure* patients with in-transit metastases that exist within this perimeter.[38] The theory further presumes that micrometastatic tumor within 1 or 2 cm of the tumor margin, if excised, would be curative in a significant proportion of patients and improve survival. In contrast, this theory also contends that excisions wider than 2 cm are not clinically helpful in removing metastases beyond the 2-cm margin. Although this could theoretically be true, it has never been directly proven to be the case. In fact, there are arguments against this hypothesis of surgical salvage for in-transit metastatic melanoma through the use of wider excisions.

The first argument is that in order for surgical salvage of in-transit metastatic disease to occur, the hypothesis would contend that often a metastatic event is limited and solitary, located within the 1- or 2-cm excision margin and that other metastases beyond the margin do not exist. The result is surgical salvage of the patient through extirpation of solitary local metastases. Animal models of metastasis generally do not support this concept. Rather, when metastasis occurs, it occurs in large numbers and widely beyond the primary tumor.[39–43] The concept that metastases could exist 1 or 2 cm from the primary tumor, but not beyond, is best supported by the Halstedian theory of metastasis in which metastatic disease arises in a single location followed by local tumor progression. Eventually, the tumor migrates to regional lymph nodes and then to more distant organs in a stepwise fashion.[44] Because many cancers do not conform to this rather organized, stepwise metastasis theory, another theory, the Fisher theory, postulates that metastatic disease is systemic by the time it is detectable. Finally, the Hellman theory suggests that for each cancer there are multiple paths of metastasis.[45] Suffice to say that many favor the Fisher paradigm for melanoma, although the Hellman theory is also very plausible.

The second argument against the plausibility of significant surgical salvage of in-transit metastatic melanoma accomplished by 1- or 2-cm excision margins is based on the fact that the RT performed for WE showed no definitive difference in either marginal recurrence rates or 5-year OS rates between the narrow and the wider margin cohorts. It is not illogical to think that if surgical salvage of in-transit metastases leading to survival benefit is possible, all of the wider margin cohorts would likely show some additional survival benefit. However, it is only a solitary study[21] that was an extension of one of the RT,[20] which performed, retrospectively, a long-term follow-up analysis on a portion of the original cohort that suggested a worse outcome in the narrow margin group.[21] In this delayed analysis, the narrower 1-cm margin showed a lower MSS than the 3-cm margin but no difference in the OS. Thus, the investigators concluded that 1-cm margins for melanoma greater than 2 mm in thickness is inadequate. The decision to recommend 2-cm margins for tumors greater than 2 mm in thickness was deductive using a prior RT that had shown 2-cm margins to be equal in efficacy to 4-cm margins for thick melanomas.[22] All of this historical explanation is to say that the consensus to use 2-cm margins for tumors deeper than 2 mm and up to 2-cm margins for tumors between 1 and 2 mm in thickness is not made based directly on an RT, but rather on a synthesis of several study results.

The controversy surrounding the use of subcentimeter margins in cases whereby the guidelines would recommend 1- or 2-cm margins arises if one concludes that the evidence unequivocally suggests that successful surgical salvage of in-transit metastases occurs by virtue of the wider excision. That presumption entails the hypothesis that in-transit metastases occur within 1 cm of the primary tumor less than 2 mm in thickness. For deep tumors 2 mm or greater, in-transit metastases are thought to occur within 2 cm of the primary tumor in contrast to less-invasive melanoma. The extension of this logic is that meaningful metastases beyond 1 or 2 cm do not occur to any significant degree, or if they do, their removal by wider excision margins is, for some reason, not beneficial to the patient. Furthermore, if MMS excises a 6-mm margin, then the patient will be harmed because of the 4 or 14 mm of skin peripheral to the primary tumor that was not removed, and therefore, the opportunity for successful salvage is lost. Of course, this anticipated harm to the patient would be expected for WE as well when guidelines are not followed.

A third argument is that if this tenet is true, then studies with large cohorts of patients with melanoma treated with MMS should readily show a decrease in MSS and OS, not to mention a higher rate of in-transit metastases. Numerous large retrospective cohort studies as well as studies utilizing prospectively collected databases have been done and are reviewed in later discussion.

When subcentimeter margins are used to treat invasive melanomas, such as is often the case with MMS, the theory favoring wider excision would predict diminished survival rates along with increased development of in-transit metastasis, which would lead to increased nodal metastases and, ultimately, systemic metastases. Given the aggressive nature of melanoma and if the theory of unresected in-transit metastases resulting from narrow margins of excision is true, these consequences should be easily demonstrated in the cohorts treated with MMS. There are large, prospectively collected databases, systematic reviews, and large retrospective studies that have been recorded for MMS-treated melanoma cohorts.[1,8,9,46–52] In each of these studies, both risk of metastasis and long-term survival rates were at least equivalent to historical controls treated with WE. None of these results confirm a measurable risk to subcentimeter excision when micrographic margins are obtained.

These are real-world studies of the treatment of melanoma. They are heavily weighted toward head, neck, hands, and feet melanoma, filling a knowledge gap regarding specialty site melanoma. The low local recurrence rate and excellent survival metrics of these studies are especially notable because the studies for WE on head and neck melanoma would suggest that these sites may be particularly prone to poorer outcomes compared with trunk and extremity melanoma.[26–31] The validity of these studies is bolstered by the uniformity of findings, that true local recurrence is extraordinarily low and that survival is excellent, and by all measures, equal to WE.

One explanation for the fact that survival is not documented as worse in the MMS studies and that survival is not unequivocally better with wide versus narrow excision in WE studies is that meaningful surgical salvage of in-transit metastasis does not occur. The only way this is possible is if nearby in-transit metastases rarely occur as a solitary event enabling a cure that is achieved by the removal of these solitary metastases. As outlined earlier, this possibility is consistent with both the Fischer and the Hellman theories of metastasis.

In support of the findings for MMS of noninferior local recurrence and survival, when studies carefully looking for microscopic evidence of micrometastases are reviewed, it is not surprising that the studies of MMS do not show evidence of unresected micrometastases. Pathologic evidence of in-transit metastases detected in WE specimens are very rare, ranging between 3% and 4.3%.[37,53] Of those metastases identified, only 7.4% are found 7 to 20 mm from the primary melanoma, and the mean distance from the primary tumor was 3.25 mm. Microsatellites a mean of 3.25 mm from the clinical margin would be included within standard MMS margins. In addition, in-transit metastases were likely associated with very deeply invasive melanomas with the mean Breslow depth of 5.02 mm. Therefore, the number of in-transit metastases not removed with subcentimeter excisions would be expected to be exceedingly small.

DISCUSSION

The optimal care of primary melanoma should be accomplished using the most efficacious surgical modalities available and should be focused on accomplishing this with great regard to minimizing the injury and morbidity for the patient. The importance of complete removal of contiguous melanoma is unquestioned. MMS is well supported to be the ideal technique to achieve this most basic of tenets a very high percentage of the time. An entirely different issue is the excision of nearby, isolated, metastatic tumor. Of course, inclusion of all tumor within excision margins would be the ideal. However, the prevalence of such isolated metastases is unknown. If it occurs, it is likely very rare.

Although evidence supporting this type of metastasis is tenuous, critics of the 6-mm margin initially taken by MMS for melanoma maintain that the excision of a 1- or 2-cm margin of clinically normal skin is essential for surgical salvage of solitary in-transit metastases. There are currently no credible or compelling data that using the MS technique with exhaustive margin examination and subcentimeter excision margins worsens prognosis or causes measurable harm to patients. The hypothetical possibility of surgical salvage with 4- to 14-mm wider margins that underscore these concerns have not been verified in real-world studies of MMS. In fact, what has been found is improved LLR and no indication of diminished survival with its subcentimeter margins.

Without compelling data that MMS places the patient at risk, it seems rational to offer it as a reasonable treatment option to patients with primary melanoma. All studies show that MMS provides dramatically lower true marginal recurrence rates with similar MSS, OS, and in-transit metastasis rates. Along with LLR, surgery is completed on the same day with reconstruction of histologically confirmed tumor-free margins and often with less complex reconstructions of the smaller wounds. These advantages are very obvious for specialty site tumors[54] but also for outlier tumors on the trunk and extremities.[6,49] In trunk and extremity melanoma, the advantages are in part attenuated because there is less downside to larger excision margins. However, the other advantages of smaller wounds and histologically confirmed tumor-free margins before reconstruction remain significant.

Given the significant difference of reported LLR between MMS and WE, and that untreated residual melanoma remains capable of progression, important concerns for the patient's well-being arise. Indeed, residual, incompletely excised melanoma does progress and is often of greater depth at the time of the clinical discovery.[55] These factors should be considered by the clinician when choosing excision type for MM removal and included in the patient's informed consent process.

Current guidelines endorse unproven reductions in WE margins when they are inconvenient given "anatomic or functional considerations." The desire to minimize tissue loss in critical sites is, appropriately, a concern to all. Not only does local recurrence lead to reoperations and the possibility of clinical progression, but it is the biggest concern of patients who have a melanoma removed.[56] Given the potential for MMS to safely decrease tissue loss in areas where anatomic or functional considerations are an issue, the melanoma guidelines would be well served by eliminating the recommendation to reduce WE margins to less than 1 cm. MMS, with its exhaustive margin evaluation, would be a more logical choice in those melanomas in tissue constrained areas, rather than using unproven subcentimeter margins with WE technique.

SUMMARY

Change in medicine is difficult. Margins for melanoma were set at no less than 5 cm for almost a century and were based on a single case report by Handley.[57] The available evidence does not support the currently held sovereignty of WE for melanoma to the exclusion of other techniques. The evidence supports the safety of Mohs for melanoma. Because of its potential benefits to the patient in terms of low-recurrence rates and same-day histologic confirmation of tumor removal with reconstruction of tumor-free margins of potentially smaller wounds, it should be one of the excision techniques considered. The informed consent process for the patient should not be complete without discussion of the attributes of Mohs surgery for melanoma.

RECOMMENDATIONS
Summary/discussion/future directions

Key to future treatment refinements is the clarification of exactly what the realistic goals of excision of the primary melanoma is. The belief that "wider" excisions benefit the patient not only in removal of the primary lesion, but also by removing nearby in transit or satellite lesions is archaic and unproven. Inferences of it's justification by randomized trials are not supported by the data. The solitary valid goal of excisional treatment is the complete removal of the entire contiguous tumor. Exhaustive margin evaluation greatly improves the rates of primary tumor extirpation. When such procedures are not available or practical, wide excision should be employed using RT confirmed margins of normal skin and not less until subcentimeter WE has been proven safe. Complete informed consent should include MMS for most patients. The advantages for the patient of excision with same day histologically confirmed tumor free margins using exhaustive microscopic evaluation with immunohistochemical staining and mapping are worth considering in all cases. In the future, melanoma guidelines would be enhanced by including MMS as an option for all melanomas given the extensive evidence of lower local recurrence and overall patient safety.

CLINICS CARE POINTS

- Current melanoma guidelines are based on randomized trials and retrospective studies limited to the WE technique and largely overlook extensive evidence affirming safety and effectiveness of other surgical techniques such as MMS.

- Same day histologically confirmed tumor free margins using exhaustive microscopic evaluation with immunohistochemical staining and mapping is valuable in the care of patients with melanoma.

- The universal recommendations of melanoma guidelines to allow subcentimeter wide excision for "anatomic or funcitonal considerations" is not evidence based.
- While all melanoma excisions would benefit from exhaustive margin evaluation, those in areas with anatomic or functional considerations, or with other features portending subclinical extension should be considered candidates for MMS.

ACKNOWLEDGMENT

Our research is mostly self funded and recently has been funded through a 501c3, Skin Cancer Trust for Independent Research and Education.

REFERENCES

1. Mohs FE. Chemosurgical treatment of melanoma; a microscopically controlled method of excision. Arch Dermatol Symphilol 1950;62(2):269–79.
2. Snow SN, Mohs FE, Oriba HA, et al. Cutaneous malignant melanoma treated by Mohs surgery review of the treatment results of 179 cases from the Mohs melanoma registry. Dermatol Surg 1997;23(11):1055–60.
3. Bienert TN, Trotter MJ, Arlette JP. Treatment of cutaneous melanoma of the face by Mohs micrographic surgery. J Cutan Med Surg 2003;7:25–30.
4. Bhardwaj SS, Tope WD, Lee PK. Mohs micrographic surgery for lentigo maligna and Lentigo maligna melanoma using Mel-5 immunostaining: University of Minnesota experience. Dermatol Surg 2006;32:690–6 [discussion: 96-7].
5. Etzkorn JR, Sobanko JF, Elenitsas R, et al. Low recurrence rates for in situ and invasive melanomas using Mohs micrographic surgery with melanoma antigen recognized by T cells 1 (MART-1) immunostaining: tissue processing methodology to optimize pathologic staging and margin assessment. J Am Acad Dermatol 2015;72:840–50.
6. Stigall LE, Brodland DG, Zitelli JA. The use of Mohs micrographic surgery (MMS) for melanoma in situ (MIS) of the trunk and proximal extremities. J Am Acad Dermatol 2016;75:1015–21.
7. Zalla MJ, Lim KK, Dicaudo DJ, et al. Mohs micrographic excision of melanoma using immunostains. Dermatol Surg 2000;26:771–84.
8. Valentin-Nogueras SM, Brodland DG, Zitelli JA, et al. Mohs micrographic surgery using MART-1 immunostain in the treatment of invasive melanoma and melanoma in situ. Dermatol Surg 2016;42:733–44.
9. Zitelli JA, Brown CD, Hanusa BH. Surgical margins for excision of primary cutaneous melanoma. J Am Acad Dermatol 1997;37:422–9.
10. Demer AM, Vance KK, Cheraghi N, et al. Benefit of Mohs micrographic surgery over wide local excision for melanoma of the head and neck: a rational approach to treatment. Dermatol Surg 2019;45:381–9.
11. Theunissen CCW, Lee MH, Murad FG, et al. Systematic review of the role of Mohs micrographic surgery in the management of early-stage melanoma of the head and neck. Dermatol Surg 2021;47(9):1185–9.
12. Pride RLD, Miller CJ, Murad MH, et al. Local recurrence of melanoma is higher after wide local excision versus Mohs micrographic surgery or staged excision: A systemic review of meta-analysis. Dermatol Surg 2022;48:164–70.
13. Swetter SM, Tsao H, Wyatt S, et al. Guidelines of care for the management of primary cutaneous melanoma. J Am Acad Dermatol 2018;80:208–50.
14. National comprehensive Cancer Network. NCCN clinical practice guidelines in oncology: melanoma (version 2.2022. January 26, 2022.
15. Veronesi U, Cascinelli N, Adamus J, et al. Thin stage I primary cutaneous malignant melanoma. Comparison of excision with margins of 1 or 3 cm. N Engl J Med 1988;318:1159–62.
16. Veronesi U, Cascinelli N. Narrow Excision (1-cm margin). A safe procedure for thin cutaneous melanoma. Arch Surg 1991;126(4):438–41.
17. Cohn-Cedermark G, Rutqvist LE, Andersson R, et al. Long term results of a randomized study by the Swedish Melanoma Study Group on 2-cm versus 5-cm resection margins for patients with cutaneous melanoma with a tumor thickness of 0.8-2.0 mm. Cancer 2000;89(7):1495–501.
18. Balch CM, Soong SJ, Smith T, et al. Long-term results of a prospective surgical trial comparing 2 cm vs 4 cm excision margins for 740 patients with 1-4 mm melanomas. Ann Surg Oncol 2001;8(2):101–8.
19. Khayat D, Rixie O, Martin G, et al. French Group of Research on Malignant Melanoma. Surgical margins in cutaneous melanoma (2 cm versus 5 cm for lesions measuring less than 2.1 mm thick). Cancer 2003;97(8):1941–6.
20. Thomas JM, Newton-Bishop J, A'Hern R, et al. Excisions Margins in high risk malignant melanoma. N Engl J Med 2004;350:757–66.
21. Hayes AJ, Maynard L, Coombes G, et al. Wide versus narrow excision margins for high-risk, primary cutaneous melanomas: long-term follow-up of survival in a randomized trial. Lancet Oncol 2016;17(2):184–92.
22. Gillgren P, Drzewiecki KT, Niin M, et al. 2-cm versus 4-cm surgical excision margins for primary cutaneous melanoma thicker than 2 mm: a randomized, multicentre trial. Lancet 2011;378:1635–42.
23. Utjes D, Malmstedt J, Teras J, et al. 2-cm versus 4-cm surgical excision margins for primary cutaneous melanoma thicker than 2 mm: long-term follow-up of

a multicentre, randomized trial. Lancet 2019;394:471–7.

24. Kunishige JH, Brodland DG, Zitelli JA. Surgical margins for melanoma in situ. J Am Acad Dermatol 2012;66:438–44.

25. Trofymenko O, Bordeaux JS, Zeitouni NC, et al. Melanoma of the face and Mohs micrographic surgery: nationwide mortality data analysis. Dermatol Surg 2018;(4):481–92.

26. Bittar PG, Bittar JM, Etzkorn JR, et al. Systemic review and meta-analysis of local recurrence rates of head and neck cutaneous melanomas after wide local excision, Mohs micrographic surgery, or staged excision. Dermatol Surg 2021;85(3):681–92.

27. Urist MM, Balch CM, Soong SJ, et al. The influence of surgical margins and prognostic factors predicting the risk of local recurrence in 3445 patients with primary cutaneous melanoma. Cancer 1985;55:1398–402.

28. O'Brien CJ, Coates AS, Peterson-Schaefer K, et al. Experience with 998 cutaneous melanomas of the head and neck over 30 years. Am J Surg 1991;162:310–4.

29. Anderson AP, Gottlieb J, Drzewlecki KT, et al. Skin melanoma of the head and neck. Prognostic factors and recurrence-free survival in 512 patients. Cancer 1992;69:1153–6.

30. Rawlani R, Rawlani V, Qureshi HA, et al. Reducing Margins of Wide Local excision in hand and neck melanoma for function and cosmesis: 5-Year local recurrence free survival. J Surg Oncol 2015;111:795–9.

31. Sullivan S, Liu DZ, Mathes DW, et al. Head and neck malignant melanoma: local recurrence rate following wide local excision and immediate reconstruction. Ann Plast Surg 2012;68(1):33–6.

32. Goldsmith LA, Askin FB, Chang AE, et al. Nation Institutes of Health Consensus Development Conference statement on diagnosis and treatment of early melanoma. Am J Dermatopathol 1993;15(1):34–43.

33. Abide JM, Nahai F, Bennett RG. The meaning of surgical margins. Plast Reconstr Surg 1984;73:492–7. Evidence-Based Procedural Dermatology. Second Edition.

34. Panther D, Brodland DG. Invasive melanoma. Switzerland AG: Springer Nature; 2012. p. 1095.

35. Bricca GM, Brodland DG, Zitelli JA. Immunostaining melanoma frozen sections: the one hour protocol. Dermatol Surg 2004;30:403–8.

36. Hendi A, Brodland DG, Zitelli JA. Melanocytes in longstanding sun-exposed skin. Arch Dermatol 2006;142:871–6.

37. Balch CM. Microscopic satellites around a primary melanoma: another piece of the puzzle in melanoma staging. Ann Surg Oncol 2009;16:1092–4.

38. Ross MI, Balsh CM. Excision margins of melanoma make a difference: new data support an old paradigm. Ann Surg Oncol 2016;23:1053–6.

39. Brodland DG, Zitelli JA. Mechanisms of metastasis. J Am Acad Dermatol 1992;27(1):1–8.

40. Poste G, Fider IJ. The pathogenesis of cancer metastasis. Nature 1980;283:1139–46.

41. Weiss L, Harlos JP, Elkin G, et al. Mechanisms for the biomechanical destruction of L1210 leukemia cells: a rate regulator for metastasis. Cell Biophys 1990;16:149–59.

42. Fidler IJ, Gersten DM, Hart IR. The biology of cancer invasion and metastasis. Adv Cancer Res 1978;28:149–250.

43. Poste G. Experimental systems for analysis of malignant phenotype. Cancer Metastasis Rev 1982;1:141–99.

44. Welch HG, Gorski DH, Albertsen PC. Trends in metastatic breast and prostate cancer – lessons in cancer dynamics. N Engl J Med 2015;373:18 1685–1687.

45. Hellman S. Natural history of small breast cancers. J Clin Oncol 1994;12:2229–34.

46. Bricca GM, Brodland DG, Ren D, et al. Cutaneous head and neck melanoma treated with Mohs micrographic surgery. J Am Acad Dermatol 2005;52(1):92–100.

47. Demer AM, Hanson JL, Maher IA, et al. Association of Mohs micrographic surgery vs wide local excision with overall survival outcomes for patients with melanoma of the trunk and extremities. JAMA Dermatol 2021;157(1):84–9.

48. Hanson J, Demer A, Liszewski W, et al. Improved overall survival of melanoma of the head and neck treated with Mohs micrographic surgery versus wide location excision. J Am Acad Dermatol 2019;82(1):149–55.

49. Burnett ME, Brodland DG, Zitelli JA. Long-term outcomes of Mohs micrographic surgery for invasive melanoma of the trunk and proximal extremities. J Am Acad Dermatol 2020;84(3):1–8.

50. Degesys CA, Powell HB, Hsia LB, et al. Outcomes for invasive melanomas treated with Mohs micrographic surgery: a retrospective cohort study. Dermatol Surg 2019;45:223–8.

51. Namin AW, Oudin EM, Tassone PT, et al. Treatment of cutaneous melanoma of the head and neck with wide local excision versus Mohs. Laryngoscope 2021;131(11):2490–6.

52. Bednar ED, Zon M, Abu-Hilal M. Morbidity and mortality of melanoma on the trunk and extremities treated with Mohs surgery versus wide excision: A systematic review. Dermatol Surg 2022;48:1–6.

53. Niebling MG, Haydu LE, Lo SN, et al. The prognostic significance of microsatellites in cutaneous melanoma. Mod Pathol 2020;13:1369–79.

54. Rzepecki AK, Hwang CD, Etzkorn JR, et al. The rule of 10s versus the rule of 2s: high complication rates after conventional excision with postoperative margin assessment of specialty site versus trunk and proximal extremity melanomas. J Am Acad Dermatol 2021;85(2):442–52.

55. DeBloom JR, Zitelli JA, Brodland DG. The invasive growth potential of residual melanoma and melanoma in situ. Dermatol Surg 2010;36(8):1251–7.

56. Etzkorn JR, Tuttle SD, Lim I, et al. Patients prioritize local recurrence risk over other attributes for surgical treatment of facial melanomas – Results of a stated preference survey and choice-based conjoint analysis. J Am Acad Dermatol 2018; 79(2):210–9.

57. Handley WS. The pathology of melanotic growths in relation to their operative treatment. Lancet 1907;1: 996–1003.

Gene Expression Profiles in Cutaneous Oncology

Bo M. Kitrell, BS[a], Elliot D. Blue, MD[b], Alfredo Siller Jr, MD[b], Marissa B. Lobl, PhD[a],
Tyler D. Evans, MD[b], Melodi Javid Whitley, MD, PhD[b], Ashley Wysong, MD, MS[b],*

KEYWORDS

- Gene expression profile(s) • Gene expression profiling • Squamous cell carcinoma
- Cutaneous melanoma • Prognostic • Diagnostic

KEY POINTS

- The sizable and growing burden of skin cancer underscores the importance of personalizing current diagnostic, prognostic, and treatment modalities to improve patient outcomes.
- Skin cancer treatment has advanced through the discovery of pertinent genes influencing pathogenesis and further revolutionized by the advent of specific gene expression profiles.
- Gene expression profiling is a laboratory method used to elucidate patterns of genes expressed in specific cells or tissues that are actively transcribing messenger RNA under certain circumstances.
- Gene expression profiling is rapidly being developed and adopted in dermatology and oncology as a clinical and research tool.
- Significant work is needed to validate and expand these next-generation diagnostic and prognostic tools and to identify where they can make the greatest impact on patient care.

INTRODUCTION

Cutaneous malignancies, specifically cutaneous melanoma (CM) and non-melanoma skin cancers (NMSCs), are the most common forms of cancer in the United States.[1] In 2012, the incidence of NMSC was documented to be 3 times greater than all other forms of cancer combined.[2] Furthermore, the prevalence and treatment costs for cutaneous malignancy are steadily rising.[3] Although most patients with early-stage cutaneous malignancies have high rates of cure, those who develop locally advanced or metastatic disease historically have poor outcomes and limited treatment options. The sizable and growing burden of skin cancer further underscores the importance of refining current diagnostic, prognostic, and treatment modalities to improve patient outcomes and lower costs. In recent years, skin cancer treatment has been advanced by the discovery of pertinent genes influencing pathogenesis and the development of specific gene expression profiles (GEPs).

Gene expression profiling is a laboratory method used to elucidate patterns of gene expression in specific cells or tissues by measuring messenger RNA (mRNA). Traditionally, microarrays have been used; however, RNA sequencing has become a popular technique to identify which specific genes are expressed (Fig. 1). In cancer, the expression of specific genetic signatures ("profiles"), or groups of genes, have been shown to correlate diagnostically or prognostically in several malignancies. When developed and validated to predict specific diagnoses or outcomes, GEPs have the potential to provide physicians with biological characteristics of an individual patient's tumor that can assist in diagnosis, risk profiling, and patient management (Fig. 2). To date, GEPs have been developed and are used

[a] College of Medicine, University of Nebraska Medical Center, 985645 Nebraska Medical Center, Omaha, NE, USA; [b] Department of Dermatology, University of Nebraska Medical Center, 985645 Nebraska Medical Center, Omaha, NE, USA
* Corresponding author.
E-mail address: ashley.wysong@unmc.edu

Dermatol Clin 41 (2023) 89–99
https://doi.org/10.1016/j.det.2022.07.018
0733-8635/23/© 2022 Elsevier Inc. All rights reserved.

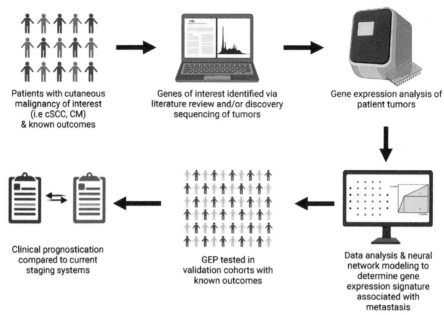

Fig. 1. Developing a gene expression profile (GEP). A discovery cohort of patients with the cutaneous malignancy of interest and known outcomes is assembled. Genes of interest are identified through literature review and/or discovery sequencing. Gene expression analysis of patient tumors is performed with subsequent data analysis and neural network modeling to delineate a gene expression signature associated with a known diagnostic or prognostic outcome. The GEP is tested in a new cohort with known outcomes and the diagnostic or prognostic ability of the GEP is validated. (*Created with BioRender.com.*)

in the characterization of various solid tumors such as breast and prostate,[4,5] and most recently, cutaneous malignancies such as CM and cutaneous squamous cell carcinoma (cSCC).[6,7] The purpose of this article was to give a high-level overview of GEPs in cSCC and CM and to illustrate the potential benefits, risks, and future applications.

Cutaneous Squamous Cell Carcinoma

The incidence of cSCC is approximately 1 million cases annually in the United States.[2] The metastatic risk of cSCC is estimated at 3% to 5% overall with the number of deaths per year similar to or exceeding melanoma.[8] Because metastatic risk

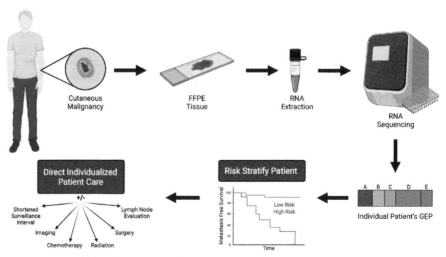

Fig. 2. Gene expression profiling clinical workflow. Individual patient tumor is sampled. RNA is extracted from the formalin-fixed paraffin-embedded (FFPE) tissue and undergoes RNA sequencing. An individual's tumor GEP is ascertained, and the patient is placed into a high- or low-risk classification.[14,51,75] (*Created with BioRender. com.*)

correlates so strongly with survival outcomes, identification of high-risk patients with cSCC is crucial.[9] The National Comprehensive Cancer Network (NCCN) guidelines designate patients in very high-, high-, or low-risk groups based on clinicopathologic features and provide broad recommendations for surgical interventions and treatment regimens.[10] In addition to the NCCN guidelines, other well-used stratification and staging systems exist for cSCC, such as the Brigham and Women's Hospital (BWH) and American Joint Committee on Cancer (AJCC) Staging Manual.[10–12] The challenge that clinicians experience when characterizing an individual cSCC lesion is that many of these high-risk features are not seen on initial biopsy, making treatment planning without the knowledge of these high-risk features difficult.[13] This has led to the development of prognostic GEPs in cSCC to provide additional information on tumor biology and metastatic risk of an individual cSCC tumor.

A major advance in cSCC GEPs was published by Wysong and colleagues[6] in 2020, in which a 40-gene genetic signature (40-GEP) was developed and validated with the ability to risk stratify individual tumors by their risk for regional or distant metastasis (Table 1). The 40-GEP test identifies 3 classes (classes 1, 2A, and 2B) of patients with cSCC and predicts the likelihood of developing metastasis within 3 years of diagnosis. The algorithm was developed using a cohort of 122 patients, 13 of whom had regional/distant metastasis and validated in a separate cohort of 321 patients, 52 of whom had documented metastasis.[6] Patients with class 2A and 2B GEP results were associated with a significant increase in both risk for metastasis (hazard ratio [HR] 2.44, $P < 0.01$; HR 10.15, $P < 0.0001$, respectively) and disease-specific death (HR 5.4, $P < .05$; HR 8.8, $P < 0.01$, respectively).[6] The 40-GEP was shown to be an individual predictor of metastatic risk apart from the BWH and AJCC guidelines with a larger positive predictive value (PPV) (60% vs 35.1% and 32.8%, respectively), while upholding similar values for negative predictive value (NPV), sensitivity, and specificity (Table 2).[6]

Although the 40-GEP is an independent predictor of metastatic risk in cSCC, combining GEP results with T-stage has clinical utility to improve risk-management decisions. In a study conducted by Farberg and colleagues,[14] the 40-GEP was combined with T-stage guidelines from either BWH or AJCC and were compared with known patient outcomes in a clinical validation cohort. A cohort of 300 NCCN-defined high-risk patients were placed into 3 metastatic risk bins corresponding to low- (<10%), moderate- (10%–49%),

or high- (≥50%) intensity risk-directed management.[14] The management intensity categories showed statistically significant differences in 3-year metastasis-free survival (MFS) rates when combined with both BWH (low: 92.5%, moderate: 80.6%, high: 41.7%) and AJCC (low: 92.5%, moderate: 82.1%, high: 41.7%) staging systems.[14] The 40-GEP has also been shown to impact management decisions when coupled with AJCC T-stage and other tumor characteristics.[14,15] In 2 separate survey studies of clinicians, the 40-GEP was presented alongside patient vignettes that included information about other high-risk features such as age, sex, tumor location, size and depth of lesion, margin status, histologic differentiation, and AJCC T-stage.[14,15] When a vignette was combined with a class 2B result, clinicians increased recommendations for SLNB, adjuvant chemotherapy, adjuvant radiation, and nodal imaging.[14] A class 1 GEP result was associated with a significant reduction in recommendations for SLNB, chemotherapy, and adjuvant radiation, as well as a tendency to increase the follow-up period.[15]

Regional lymph node spread is an important prognostic factor in cSCC, as it has shown to significantly increase the risk of recurrence and mortality.[16] Haisma and colleagues[17] found that patients with lymph node metastasis had a 5-year disease-specific survival (DSS) rate of 37.3% and overall survival (OS) rate of 22.5%, compared with a 5-year DSS of 98.8% and OS of 71.4% in patients without lymph node metastasis ($P < 0.001$). There are currently no consensus recommendations regarding when to perform SLNB or nodal staging in patients with high-risk tumor features. SLNB is not recommended in patients with clinically apparent lymph nodes due to low sensitivities compared with lymph node dissections, but in non-clinically apparent lymph nodes, the value of SLNB is unknown.[18–20] In a quantitative review of 260 cases of patients with cSCC defined as high-risk, not oropharyngeal in location, and without clinically apparent lymph nodes, 14.6% of patients were found to have positive SLNB.[20] Predicting tumor behavior through GEPs may aid clinicians in deciding which patients may benefit from SLNB or nodal staging, although additional studies are needed.

GEPs may have the opportunity to help guide decisions regarding radiation therapy for patients with cSCC; however, there are some unique considerations. A preclinical study of head and neck oropharyngeal SCC cells found that cells that were sensitive versus resistant to radiotherapy had upregulated expression of genes involved with DNA repair, cell cycle, and cellular stress.[21] Radiation has been demonstrated to modulate

Table 1
Currently available gene expression profiles (GEPs) for cutaneous malignancies

Tumor Type	Prognostic/Diagnostic	Currently Available GEP	Classification System	Validation Cohorts
BCC	N/A	None	N/A	N/A
SCC	Prognostic	40-GEP	Class 1 (Low Risk) Class 2A & 3B (Increased Risk for Metastasis & DSD)	321 Patients, 52 with Documented metastasis[6] 300 patients[14] 420 cases[75]
Melanoma	Prognostic	31-GEP	Class 1A & 1B (Low Risk) Class 2A & 2B (High Risk)	26 patients[51] 323 patients[52] 1479 patients[53] 157 Primary tumors[54] 159 patients[55] 523 patients[56] 322 patients[57] 205 tumors[44] 690 patients[60] 86 patients[76] 256 patients[77]
		CP-GEP	Low Risk High Risk	210 patients[67] 837 patients[78]
		MelaGenix	Low Risk High Risk	203 tumors[68] 245 patients[69] 88 tumors[79]
	Diagnostic	2-GEP pigmented lesion assay (PLA)	Melanoma Not Melanoma	555 lesions[36] 3416 lesions[37] 2104 PLA-negative lesions[39]
		3-GEP pigmented lesion assay (PLAplus)	Melanoma Not melanoma	103 lesions[40]
		23-GEP	Melanoma Not melanoma	437 lesions[41] 1400 lesions[42]

Abbreviations: BCC, basal cell carcinoma; CP-GEP, clinicopathological and gene expression profile; DSD, disease-specific death; N/A, not applicable; PLA, pigmented lesion assay; SCC, squamous cell carcinoma.

gene expression in both normal and tumor cells.[22] Therefore, cSCCs arising in areas of previous radiation exposure or those that have had previous radiation therapy may have altered GEPs. Future GEP studies analyzing cSCCs that respond compared with those that do not respond to radiation may help clinicians determine which patients are good candidates for radiation therapy.

Table 2
Comparison of metastatic risk prediction in cSCC by the 40-GEP and established staging systems

	40-GEP (Class 2B vs 1/2A)[6]	AJCC8 (T3/T4 vs T1/T2)[6]	BWH (T2b/T3 vs T1/T2a)[6]
Sensitivity (%)	28.8	38.5	25.0
Specificity (%)	96.3	84.8	91.1
PPV (%)	60.0	32.	35.1
NPV (%)	87.5	87.7	86.3

Abbreviations: AJCC8, American Joint Committee on Cancer, Cancer Staging Manual eighth edition; BWH, Brigham and Women's Hospital; GEP, gene expression profile; NPV, negative predictive value; PPV, positive predictive value.

Adapted from Wysong A, Newman JG, Covington KR, Kurley SJ, Ibrahim SF, Farberg AS, Bar A, Cleaver NJ, Somani AK, Panther D, Brodland DG, Zitelli J, Toyohara J, Maher IA, Xia Y, Bibee K, Griego R, Rigel DS, Meldi Plasseraud K, Estrada S, Sholl LM, Johnson C, Cook RW, Schmults CD, Arron ST. Validation of a 40-gene expression profile test to predict metastatic risk in localized high-risk cutaneous squamous cell carcinoma. J Am Acad Dermatol. 2021 Feb;84(2):361 to 369.

In other cancers, GEPs have been correlated with tumor response to chemotherapy and immunotherapy. In colorectal cancer, GEPs identify patients who may not benefit from cetuximab, an epidermal growth factor receptor–targeted therapy that is also used off-label for cSCC.[23] A study of pancreatic ductal adenocarcinomas identified tumors with an "immunogenic" GEP that may indicate a superior response to immunotherapy.[24] As immunotherapies, cemiplimab and pembrolizumab are now approved by the Food and Drug Administration for cSCC and have objective response rates of 44% and 34.3%, respectively; GEPs may prove useful in identifying which patients might benefit from immunotherapy.[25,26]

In addition to improving selection of patients for existing therapeutics, differentially expressed genes discovered in GEP studies may lead to the development of novel therapeutics. One example is podoplanin, which is a differentially expressed gene in the 40-GEP. Although no therapeutics targeting podoplanin are currently available, a monoclonal antibody targeting the extracellular domain of podoplanin (SZ168) has been shown to inhibit pulmonary metastasis of melanoma.[27] Although GEPs provide insight into genes correlated with clinical behavior, additional studies evaluating DNA mutations, RNA expression, and protein function in high-risk cSCC are likely to lead to novel therapeutic targets. Immunosuppressed patients (ISPs), in particular organ transplant recipients (OTRs), are at 65 to 100 times increased risk of developing cSCC compared with the general population.[28] In addition, cSCCs from OTRs have a metastatic rate of 7.3% to 11.0%.[29] A GEP of cSCC demonstrated distinct differences between immunocompetent patients (ICPs) and ISPs, with 48 genes differentially expressed.[30] ISPs have also been found to have fewer UV-induced mutations compared with ICPs, suggesting a lower threshold for mutagenesis.[31] In addition, alterations of tumor microenvironments have been demonstrated in ISPs, particularly in hBD1 and psoriasin expression.[32] The initial cohort used to create the 40-GEP included 76 ISPs (67 OTRs), allowing this test to be used in this population.[6] Because of the more aggressive nature of cSCC in OTRs, further studies are necessary to understand prognostic differences and management implications for GEPs between ISPs and ICPs.

Melanoma

CM carries more morbidity and a higher mortality rate than all other forms of skin cancer. Although rarer than NMSC, the incidence rate of CM has been rising faster than any other malignancy.[33,34]

To improve patient outcomes, accurate diagnosis and staging of CM is vital to predict patient prognosis and drive treatment decisions.

Diagnostic

Discordance in the histologic diagnosis of melanocytic lesions is common, thus there has been a focus on the development of diagnostic tools, including GEPs, to aid in the diagnosis of pigmented lesions (see **Table 1**).[35] A 2-GEP for CM, known as the pigmented lesion assay (PLA), was created using the genes PRAME (PReferentially expressed Antigen in MElanoma) and LINC (LINC00518, Long Intergenic Non-Coding RNA 518) and can be obtained using a noninvasive adhesive patch.[36] This PLA was validated in 389 samples, 87 of which were melanoma, with a sensitivity of 91% and a specificity of 69%.[36] This noninvasive test may benefit clinicians regarding difficult biopsy decisions. In fact, Brouha and colleagues[37] studied a registry of 3418 lesions clinically suspicious for melanoma that underwent 2-GEP testing and compared genomic and histopathologic results in 316 biopsied lesions; 18.7% of these biopsied 2-GEP–positive lesions were confirmed to be melanoma in situ or invasive melanoma.[37] This is more than 4 times greater than the 4.7% of lesions biopsied based on visible atypia, underscoring the clinical utility of the 2-GEP in the decision to biopsy suspicious pigmented lesions.[37,38] The use of the PLA to rule out melanoma has also been studied. In a cohort of 1233 PLA-negative patients, fewer than 1% of patients had early-stage melanoma on initial biopsy (NPV = 99.2%).[39] A total of 302 of these initially negative lesions were PLA tested an average of 15.3 months later and 34 resulted PLA-positive. Three of these 34 lesions were identified as melanoma in situ by biopsy, confirming an NPV > 99% of the original test.[39] To increase the clinical utility, Jackson and colleagues[40] combined additional genes with the PLA to enhance the test's sensitivity and discovered that the addition of the TERT protein improved the ability to rule out CM, with sensitivity increased from 93% to 97% in their study of 103 lesions. This 3-GEP, or PLAplus, also showed a 62% specificity leading to an NPV of 99.7%.[40] Further studies in an independent cohort are needed to validate the PLAplus, but the initial findings are promising.

Another notable diagnostic GEP in CM is the 23-GEP (see **Table 1**). At the time of development, this GEP was found to classify melanocytic lesions as benign or malignant with a sensitivity of 89% and specificity of 93% in a cohort of 464 samples and was subsequently validated on 437 samples with a sensitivity of 90% and specificity of 91%.[41] In 2017, the 23-GEP was independently and prospectively validated in 1400 melanocytic lesions, showing the ability to differentiate benign nevi from malignant melanoma with a sensitivity of 91.5% and a specificity of 92.5%.[42] Diagnostic GEPs may be an increasingly useful tool for clinicians in the accurate diagnosis of CM and future research should be completed to define their role in routine patient care.

Prognostic

The most used staging system for melanoma is the AJCC, which is based on clinicopathologic features of CM to determine different melanoma-specific survival (MSS) estimates.[43] This staging system guides decisions about sentinel lymph node (SLN) mapping, biopsy, frequency and intensity of screening, and use of adjuvant therapy. However, because of the prevalence of low-risk AJCC patients, 2 of 3 patients who die of CM are stage I or IIA at initial diagnosis.[44] This emphasizes the need for further exploration into alternative methods for identifying high-risk disease not predicted by AJCC staging. Multiple large-scale gene expression studies have been conducted to investigate whether genes in CM could predict its metastatic capabilities.[45–50] Based on the culmination of these study results, an advancement was made using known genes involved in melanoma metastasis through the development of a 31-GEP in order to better predict local recurrence and metastatic risk for patients with CM.[7]

The 31-GEP has 4 prognostic categories of increasing risk of local recurrence and 5-year metastatic risk: Class 1A and 1B (low risk) and class 2A and 2B (high risk) (see **Table 1**).[7] High-risk 31-GEP classification is associated with thicker Breslow depth, AJCC stage greater than IIB, and ulceration.[51] The 31-GEP has been validated as an independent predictor of patient outcomes (see **Table 1**).[51–56] Patients with a class 2 result had significantly lower recurrence-free survival (RFS), distant metastasis-free survival (DMFS), and OS at 3 years and had higher sensitivity and NPV than AJCC high-risk stages alone (**Table 3**).[52] This was further validated retrospectively in a meta-analysis of 1479 patients with a mean follow-up time of 3.3 years.[53] This study suggested that the 31-GEP can independently and robustly predict the risk of MFS in patients with melanoma despite differences in study design and cohorts ($P < 0.0001$).[53] The 31-GEP for CM has also been validated prospectively with the high- and low-risk GEP classes significantly correlating with RFS, DMFS, and OS.[52,55,57]

SLN status remains an important factor when assessing prognosis and treatment strategies for patients with CM. In patients with clinical stage I/II melanoma, SLN status has been shown to be the strongest predictor of survival.[58] Although SLNB is considered a minimally invasive procedure, it still poses risk.[59] In a meta-analysis of 1479 patients with CM, the 31-GEP was found to be more sensitive and demonstrated a higher NPV for predicting distant metastasis and recurrence than SLNB, while exhibiting comparable specificity and PPVs.[53,54] When the 31-GEP and SLNB were considered together, both the sensitivity and NPV for DMFS improved.[53] The addition of the 31-GEP test to customary staging may provide complementation of node status and help identify patients at high risk for metastasis among SLNB-negative patients who could benefit from more aggressive surveillance and therapeutic interventions. Despite these emerging data, GEPs for melanoma require further investigation across large prospective studies. The NCCN recommends that currently available GEPs should not replace pathologic staging procedures, be used to determine SLNB eligibility, or guide clinical decision making.[59]

Although the 31-GEP has been validated to be an independent predictor of CM patient outcomes, the 31-GEP may be used in conjunction with AJCC staging for additional prognostic information.[44,52,54,57] The GEP may complement AJCC staging to identify patients at high risk of metastasis in low-risk AJCC groups.[56,57,60] One study assessed the 31-GEP's performance on low-stage AJCC tumors and found that patients with AJCC stage I-IIA CM and a class 2 31-GEP (high risk) have similar 3-year survival outcomes to patients with AJCC stage IIB-III CM.[52] Therefore, patients in this cohort may benefit from increased surveillance. In a study analyzing primary melanoma tumors from 523 patients, the 31-GEP identified 70% of patients who eventually developed metastasis in patients classified as AJCC stage I and II.[56] Through multivariate analysis, the 31-GEP was shown to be the strongest and only predictor of RFS, DMFS, and MSS in patients with AJCC stage I to IIA.[60] To study the clinical utility of the 31-GEP used in concordance with low-risk AJCC staging, a meta-analysis of 7 studies was conducted in patients with AJCC stage I and stage II disease showing that, of the patients with a melanoma recurrence, most who were incorrectly classified as low-risk by GEP were stage I (rather than stage II).[61] Additional studies are needed to define the clinical utility of the 31-GEP in patients with stage I-III melanoma.

As the understanding and utilization of the 31-GEP increases, the management of CM is bound

Table 3
***Comparison of metastatic risk prediction in CM by available prognostic GEPs and established staging systems**

	31-GEP (DMFS, Stage I-III CM)[52]	CP-GEP (T1-T3 Nodal Metastasis)[67]	MelaGenix (Relapse Prediction, Stage I-II)[80]	AJCC8 (DMFS, Stage I-III CM)[52]
Sensitivity (%)	64	91.5	32–76	62
Specificity (%)	82	29.7	43–77	83
PPV (%)	25	32.3	-	24
NPV (%)	97	90.5	-	96

Abbreviations: AJCC8, American Joint Committee on Cancer, Cancer Staging Manual eighth edition; CM, cutaneous melanoma; GEP, gene expression profile; NPV, negative predictive value; PPV, positive predictive value.
*Data from Hsueh et al. 2021,[52] Mulder et al. 2021,[67] Reschke et al. 2021.[80]

to evolve. The 31-GEP used in conjunction with other staging criteria has been shown to alter management decisions.[62–65] In a study involving 6 institutions, changes in management were seen after receipt of the 31-GEP results.[63] Documented changes were observed in 53% of class 2 patients (increased management) compared with 37% of class 1 patients (decreased management).[63] In patients with AJCC stage I and II melanoma, GEP results significantly altered management of patients in conjunction with node status.[64] Patients with a negative SLNB who were labeled class 2 by the GEP prompted more physicians to have more aggressive follow-up and management as compared with class 1.[64] Ulceration and Breslow thickness of >0.5 mm were both shown to cause a statistically significant increase in physicians who recommended the 31-GEP test.[62] A negative SLNB was not a significant provocation for physicians to order a 31-GEP, even though two-thirds of patients with CM who develop metastasis have a negative SLNB.[62]

Because of vast improvements in melanoma care over the past several years, identification of high-risk patients is extremely relevant when weighing the risks and benefits of adjuvant or neo-adjuvant therapies.[58,66] Although current studies have investigated the ability of the 31-GEP to predict metastasis and recurrence compared with SLNB, no studies have addressed the 31-GEP's ability to predict response to systemic therapies. However, the 31-GEP could help identify high-risk patients in whom the benefits of adjuvant therapy would outweigh the risks. Further studies are needed to evaluate the 31-GEP in the context of adjuvant therapy.

Additional GEPs for melanoma have been developed, such as the clinicopathological and gene expression profile (CP-GEP) model (see **Table 1**).[67] This model includes age and Breslow thickness alongside 8 pathologic target genes in primary

melanoma. The CP-GEP was created to identify patients with T1-T3 CM that had low risk of nodal metastasis. It was validated with tumor tissue obtained by full excision rather than microdissection, a significant benefit to clinicians due to the time-consuming process of microdissection. The CP-GEP model was validated as an independent predictor of nodal metastasis and identified patients with low risk of nodal metastasis with an NPV of 90.5% while maintaining a high sensitivity of 91.5% (see **Table 3**). This test indicated that the CP-GEP could decrease the number of SLN-negative biopsies performed in patients with T2 or T3 melanomas with low risk of metastasis.[67] Although this GEP prognosticates nodal metastasis with high sensitivity and NPV without the requirement of microdissection, future prospective studies are needed to further analyze its predictive ability.

A third GEP for melanoma known as MelaGenix has also been created (see **Table 1**). This 8-GEP test focuses on 7 protective genes and 1 high-risk gene found in a cohort of 125 patients with CM.[68] Validation studies revealed that the test's gene expression risk score (GRS) complements AJCC7 in predicting MSS and that combining the GRS with SLN status improved prognostic performance. A study by Amaral and colleagues[69] showed that in patients with stage II disease, a high GRS was associated with decreased RFS, DMFS, and MSS. Additional studies are needed to further evaluate the clinical utility of MelaGenix; however, studies thus far suggest the GRS may add value to AJCC classification in defining both low-risk and high-risk patients.[70]

Despite increasing data for the diagnostic and prognostic value of GEPs in CM, national consensus guidelines recommend against routine use of GEPs.[58,71] Concerns surrounding the use of GEPs in melanoma include the questions of which tumors should be tested, to what degree should results affect patient care, and does the benefit justify the cost.[72] Of note, the 31-GEP was developed to predict local recurrence and metastasis in melanoma, in contrast to the 40-GEP, which was developed to predict metastasis alone in cSCC. This is an important distinction, as local recurrence likely reflects surgical failure rather than tumor biology and may alter the prognostic algorithm. In addition, barriers to implementing GEPs have been noted, including general resistance to change and abandoning familiar practices.[72] In 2020, the Melanoma Prevention Working Group (MPWG) published a review on the use of GEPs in melanoma and, while noting optimism for its future use, cited current limitations to patients with stage I disease and lack of studies comparing results in context of all relevant clinicopathologic factors. The MPWG recommended that retrospective studies be completed before turning attention to costly prospective studies, with the ultimate recommendation of avoiding routine GEP testing until prospective studies prove their utility.[70]

SUMMARY

Gene expression profiling is quickly being developed and adopted in the fields of dermatology and oncology as a research tool and in the care of patients with cutaneous malignancy. Data from GEPs are versatile with potential applications including the development of diagnostic and prognostic tools as well as the identification of genes in cutaneous malignancy that may serve as targets for novel pharmacotherapy. Further, the characterization of tumor profiles with an ability to portend individual tumor-level behavior can be used in combination with staging systems, such as the AJCC and BWH staging systems, to help predict MFS and ultimately guide clinical practice.[14,15,44,52,54,57]

Future directions of GEPs in cutaneous malignancy involve continued development and validation of currently available profiles. In addition, the identification of new mutational profiles and genetic signatures (both diagnostic and/or prognostic) in other high-risk cutaneous tumors (i.e., Merkel cell carcinoma, cutaneous lymphomas, cutaneous sarcomas, etc.) may be beneficial. There are also populations at increased risk for developing skin cancer such as the immunosuppressed (i.e., OTRs, human immunodeficiency virus, leukemia/lymphoma, etc.) where the innate biological characteristics of the tumors and the tumor microenvironment may differ from the general population.[73] Additional analysis of currently available GEP tests or development of new genetic signatures in these specialized populations may provide useful data with clinical management implications. Our group has shown somatic mutational differences among Asian, Hispanic, and Caucasian patients with basal cell carcinoma, highlighting that gene expression may vary by race and ethnicity.[74] Continued research into potential differences in genetic mutations and expression profiles across different racial and ethnic populations is an important future direction of research.

Overall, the growth of GEPs in cutaneous malignancies signals an exciting and potentially game-changing tool to be used in the care of patients. Significant work is needed to validate and expand these next-generation tools; however, the future of cutaneous oncology diagnostics and treatment continues to advance in an exciting direction.

DISCLOSURE

Ashley Wysong is the recipient of an Institutional Research Grant for Castle Biosciences. There were no incentives or transactions, financial or otherwise, relevant to this article.

REFERENCES

1. Apalla Z, et al. Skin cancer: epidemiology, disease burden, pathophysiology, diagnosis, and therapeutic approaches. Dermatol Ther (Heidelb) 2017; 7(Suppl 1):5–19.
2. Rogers HW, et al. Incidence estimate of nonmelanoma skin cancer (keratinocyte carcinomas) in the us population, 2012. JAMA Dermatol 2015;151(10): 1081–6.
3. Guy GP, et al. Prevalence and costs of skin cancer treatment in the U.S., 2002-2006 and 2007-2011. Am J Prev Med 2015;48(2):183–7.
4. Rashmi Kumar N, et al. NCCN Guidelines Version 2.2022 Breast Cancer. 2021. Available at: https:// www.nccn.
5. Freedman-Cass D, et al. NCCN Guidelines Version 3.2022 Prostate Cancer. 2022. Available at: https:// www.nccn.org/home/.
6. Wysong A, et al. Validation of a 40-gene expression profile test to predict metastatic risk in localized high-risk cutaneous squamous cell carcinoma. J Am Acad Dermatol 2020. https://doi.org/10.1016/ j.jaad.2020.04.088.
7. Gerami P, et al. Development of a prognostic genetic signature to predict the metastatic risk associated with cutaneous melanoma. Clin Cancer Res 2015;21(1):175–83.
8. Joseph MG, et al. Squamous cell carcinoma of the skin of the trunk and limbs: the incidence of metastases and their outcome. Aust N Z J Surg 1992; 62(9):697–701.

9. Brougham NDLS, et al. The incidence of metastasis from cutaneous squamous cell carcinoma and the impact of its risk factors. J Surg Oncol 2012; 106(7):811–5.

10. Mai Nguyen N, et al. NCCN Squamous Cell Skin Cancer Guidelines Version 1.2022. 2021. Available at: https://www.nccn.org/home/member-.

11. Amin MB, et al. In: Amin MB, Edge SB, Greene FL, et al, editors. AJCC cancer staging manual. 8th edition. Springer International Publishing; 2017.

12. Jambusaria-Pahlajani A, et al. Evaluation of AJCC tumor staging for cutaneous squamous cell carcinoma and a proposed alternative tumor staging system. JAMA Dermatol 2013;149(4):402–10.

13. Farberg AS, Fitzgerald AL, Ibrahim SF, et al. Current methods and caveats to risk factor assessment in cutaneous squamous cell carcinoma (cSCC): a narrative review. Dermatol Ther (Heidelb) 2022; 12(2):267–84.

14. Farberg AS, et al. Integrating gene expression profiling into NCCN high-risk cutaneous squamous cell carcinoma management recommendations: impact on patient management. Curr Med Res Opin 2020;36(8):1301–7.

15. Litchman GH, et al. Impact of a prognostic 40-gene expression profiling test on clinical management decisions for high-risk cutaneous squamous cell carcinoma. Curr Med Res Opin 2020;36(8):1295–300.

16. Mullen JT, et al. Invasive squamous cell carcinoma of the skin: defining a high-risk group. Ann Surg Oncol 2006;13(7):902–9.

17. Haisma MS, et al. Multivariate analysis of potential risk factors for lymph node metastasis in patients with cutaneous squamous cell carcinoma of the head and neck. J Am Acad Dermatol 2016;75(4): 722–30.

18. Waldman A, et al. Cutaneous squamous cell carcinoma. Hematol Oncol Clin North Am 2019;33(1): 1–12.

19. Edkins O, et al. Does sentinel lymph node biopsy have a role in node-positive head and neck squamous carcinoma? S Afr J Surg 2013;51(1):22–5.

20. Ahadiat O, et al. SLNB in cutaneous SCC: a review of the current state of literature and the direction for the future. J Surg Oncol 2017;116(3):344–50.

21. Michna A, et al. Transcriptomic analyses of the radiation response in head and neck squamous cell carcinoma subclones with different radiation sensitivity: time-course gene expression profiles and gene association networks. Radiat Oncol 2016;11(1). https://doi.org/10.1186/s13014-016-0672-0.

22. Chaudhry MA. Analysis of gene expression in normal and cancer cells exposed to γ-radiation. J Biomed Biotechnol 2008;2008(1). https://doi.org/10.1155/2008/541678.

23. Baker JB, et al. Tumour gene expression predicts response to cetuximab in patients with KRAS wild-type metastatic colorectal cancer. Br J Cancer 2011;104(3):488–95.

24. Bailey P, et al. Genomic analyses identify molecular subtypes of pancreatic cancer. Nature 2016; 531(7592):47–52.

25. Migden MR, et al. Cemiplimab in locally advanced cutaneous squamous cell carcinoma: results from an open-label, phase 2, single-arm trial. Lancet Oncol 2020;21(2):294–305.

26. Grob JJ, et al. Pembrolizumab monotherapy for recurrent or metastatic cutaneous squamous cell carcinoma: a single-arm phase II trial (KEYNOTE-629). J Clin Oncol 2020;38:2916–25.

27. Xu M, et al. Blocking podoplanin suppresses growth and pulmonary metastasis of human malignant melanoma. BMC Cancer 2019;19(1). https://doi.org/10.1186/s12885-019-5808-9.

28. Lindelöf B, et al. Incidence of skin cancer in 5356 patients following organ transplantation. Br J Dermatol 2000;143(3):513–9.

29. Genders RE, et al. Metastasis of cutaneous squamous cell carcinoma in organ transplant recipients and the immunocompetent population: is there a difference? A systematic review and meta-analysis. J Eur Acad Dermatol Venereol 2019;33(5):828–41.

30. Feldmeyer L, et al. Differential T-cell subset representation in cutaneous squamous cell carcinoma arising in immunosuppressed versus immunocompetent individuals. Exp Dermatol 2016;25(3). https://doi.org/10.1111/exd.12878.

31. Lobl MB, et al. The correlation of immune status with ultraviolet radiation–associated mutations in cutaneous squamous cell carcinoma: a case-control study. J Am Acad Dermatol 2020;82(5):1230–2.

32. Muehleisen B, et al. Distinct innate immune gene expression profiles in non-melanoma skin cancer of immunocompetent and immunosuppressed patients. PLoS One 2012;7(7). https://doi.org/10.1371/journal.pone.0040754.

33. Ali Z, et al. Melanoma epidemiology, biology and prognosis. EJC Suppl 2013;11(2):81–91.

34. Dooley TP, et al. Biomarkers of human cutaneous squamous cell carcinoma from tissues and cell lines identified by DNA microarrays and qRT-PCR. Biochem Biophysical Res Commun 2003;306(4):1026–36.

35. Elmore JG, et al. Pathologists' diagnosis of invasive melanoma and melanocytic proliferations: observer accuracy and reproducibility study. BMJ (Online) 2017;357. https://doi.org/10.1136/bmj.j2813.

36. Gerami P, et al. Development and validation of a noninvasive 2-gene molecular assay for cutaneous melanoma. J Am Acad Dermatol 2017;76(1): 114–20.e2.

37. Brouha B., Ferris L., Skelsey M., et al., Genomic atypia to enrich melanoma positivity in biopsied lesions: gene expression and pathology findings from a

large US registry study, *SKIN J Cutan Med Surg*, 5 (1), 2021, 13-18.

38. Nault A, et al. Biopsy use in skin cancer diagnosis: comparing dermatology physicians and advanced practice professionals. JAMA Dermatol 2015; 151(8):899–902.

39. Skelsey M, Brouha B, Rock J, et al. Non-Invasive Detection of Genomic Atypia Increases Real-World NPV and PPV of the Melanoma Diagnostic Pathway and Reduces Biopsy Burden. SKIN J Cutan Med Surg 2021;5(5):512–23.

40. Cullison S.R., Jansen B., Yao Z., et al., Risk Stratification of Severely Dysplastic Nevi by Non-Invasively Obtained Gene Expression and Mutation Analyses, SKIN J Cutan Med Surg, 4 (2), 2020, 124-129.

41. Clarke LE, et al. Clinical validation of a gene expression signature that differentiates benign nevi from malignant melanoma. J Cutan Pathol 2015;42(4): 244–52.

42. Clarke LE, et al. An independent validation of a gene expression signature to differentiate malignant melanoma from benign melanocytic nevi. Cancer 2017; 123(4):617–28.

43. Gershenwald JE, et al. Melanoma staging: evidence-based changes in the American Joint Committee on Cancer eighth edition cancer staging manual. CA: A Cancer J Clinicians 2017;67(6): 472–92.

44. Ferris LK, et al. Identification of high-risk cutaneous melanoma tumors is improved when combining the online American Joint Committee on Cancer Individualized Melanoma Patient Outcome Prediction Tool with a 31-gene expression profile–based classification. J Am Acad Dermatol 2017;76(5):818–25.e3.

45. Jaeger J, et al. Gene expression signatures for tumor progression, tumor subtype, and tumor thickness in laser-microdissected melanoma tissues. Clin Cancer Res 2007;13(3):806–15.

46. Bittner M, et al. Molecular classification of cutaneous malignant melanoma by gene expression profiling. Nature 2000;406(6795):536–40.

47. Smith AP, et al. Whole-genome expression profiling of the melanoma progression pathway reveals marked molecular differences between nevi/melanoma in situ and advanced-stage melanomas. Cancer Biol Ther 2005;4(9):1018–29. https://doi.org/10.4161/cbt.4.9.2165.

48. Haqq C, et al. The gene expression signatures of melanoma progression. Proc Natl Acad Sci U S A 2005;102(17):6092–7.

49. Mauerer A, et al. Identification of new genes associated with melanoma. Exp Dermatol 2011;20(6): 502–7.

50. Scatolini M, et al. Altered molecular pathways in melanocytic lesions. Int J Cancer 2010;126(8):1869–81.

51. Scott AM, et al. Integration of a 31-gene expression profile into clinical decision-making in the treatment of cutaneous melanoma. Am Surg 2020;86(11): 1561–4.

52. Hsueh EC, et al. Long-term outcomes in a multi-center, prospective cohort evaluating the prognostic 31-gene expression profile for cutaneous melanoma. JCO Precis Oncol 2021;5(PO.20):00119.

53. Greenhaw BN, et al. Molecular risk prediction in cutaneous melanoma: a meta-analysis of the 31-gene expression profile prognostic test in 1,479 patients. J Am Acad Dermatol 2020;83(3):745–53.

54. Gastman BR, et al. Performance of a 31-gene expression profile test in cutaneous melanomas of the head and neck. Head and Neck 2019;41(4): 871–9.

55. Keller J, et al. Prospective validation of the prognostic 31-gene expression profiling test in primary cutaneous melanoma. Cancer Med 2019;8(5): 2205–12.

56. Zager JS, et al. Performance of a prognostic 31-gene expression profile in an independent cohort of 523 cutaneous melanoma patients. BMC Cancer 2018;18(1). https://doi.org/10.1186/s12885-018-4016-3.

57. Hsueh EC, et al. Interim analysis of survival in a prospective, multi-center registry cohort of cutaneous melanoma tested with a prognostic 31-gene expression profile test. J Hematol Oncol 2017;10(1). https://doi.org/10.1186/s13045-017-0520-1.

58. National Comprehensive Cancer Network. NCCN Clinical Practice Guidelines in Oncology Melanoma: Cutaneous. 2022. Available at: www.nccn.org/patients.

59. Swetter SM, et al. Melanoma: cutaneous, version 2.2021 featured updates to the NCCN guidelines. JNCCN J Natl Compr Cancer Netw 2021;19(4): 364–76.

60. Gastman BR, et al. Identification of patients at risk of metastasis using a prognostic 31-gene expression profile in subpopulations of melanoma patients with favorable outcomes by standard criteria. J Am Acad Dermatol 2019;80(1):149–57.e4.

61. Marchetti MA, et al. Performance of gene expression profile tests for prognosis in patients with localized cutaneous melanoma: a systematic review and meta-analysis. JAMA Dermatol 2020;156(9):953–62.

62. Svoboda RM, et al. Factors affecting dermatologists' use of a 31-gene expression profiling test as an adjunct for predicting metastatic risk in cutaneous melanoma. J Drugs Dermatol 2018;17(5):544–7.

63. Berger AC, et al. Clinical impact of a 31-gene expression profile test for cutaneous melanoma in 156 prospectively and consecutively tested patients. Curr Med Res Opin 2016;32(9):1599–604.

64. Mbbs DS, et al. Impact of gene expression profiling on decision-making in clinically node negative melanoma patients after surgical staging. J Drugs Dermatol 2018;17(2):196–9.

65. Farberg AS, et al. Impact of a 31-gene expression profiling test for cutaneous melanoma on dermatologists' clinical management decisions. J Drugs Dermatol 2017;16(5):428–31.

66. Eggermont AMM, et al. Prolonged survival in Stage III melanoma with ipilimumab adjuvant therapy. New Engl J Med 2016;375(19):1845–55.

67. Mulder EEAP, et al. Validation of a clinicopathological and gene expression profile model for sentinel lymph node metastasis in primary cutaneous melanoma. Br J Dermatol 2021;184(5):944–51.

68. Gambichler T, et al. Gene-signature based prediction of relapse-free survival in melanoma patients with known sentinel lymph node status. J Clin Oncol 2017;35(15_suppl):e21037.

69. Amaral TMS, et al. Clinical validation of a prognostic 11-gene expression profiling score in prospectively collected FFPE tissue of patients with AJCC v8 stage II cutaneous melanoma. Eur J Cancer 2020;125:38–45.

70. Grossman D, et al. Prognostic gene expression profiling in cutaneous melanoma: identifying the knowledge gaps and assessing the clinical benefit. JAMA Dermatol 2020;156(9):1004–11.

71. Swetter SM, et al. Guidelines of care for the management of primary cutaneous melanoma. J Am Acad Dermatol 2019;80(1):208–50.

72. Grossman D, et al. Prognostic gene expression profiling in melanoma: necessary steps to incorporate into clinical practice. Melanoma Management 2019;6(4):MMT32.

73. Inman GJ, et al. The genomic landscape of cutaneous SCC reveals drivers and a novel azathioprine associated mutational signature. Nat Commun 2018; 9(1):3667.

74. Lobl M, et al. Basal cell carcinoma gene mutations differ between Asian, Hispanic, and Caucasian patients: a pilot study. J Drugs Dermatol 2021;20(5):504–10.

75. Ibrahim SF, et al. Enhanced metastatic risk assessment in cutaneous squamous cell carcinoma with the 40-gene expression profile test. Future Oncol 2021. https://doi.org/10.2217/fon-2021-1277. Published online November 25.

76. Podlipnik S, et al. Early outcome of a 31-gene expression profile test in 86 AJCC stage IB-II melanoma patients. A prospective multicentre cohort study. J Eur Acad Dermatol Venereol 2019;33(5):857–62.

77. Greenhaw BN, et al. Estimation of prognosis in invasive cutaneous melanoma: an independent study of the accuracy of a gene expression profile test. Dermatol Surg 2018;44(12):1494–500.

78. Eggermont AMM, et al. Identification of stage I/IIA melanoma patients at high risk for disease relapse using a clinicopathologic and gene expression model. Eur J Cancer 2020;140:11–8.

79. Koelblinger P, et al. A prognostic gene-signature based identification of high-risk thin melanomas. J Clin Oncol 2018;36(15_suppl):e21575.

80. Reschke R, et al. Identifying high-risk tumors within AJCC stage IB-III melanomas using a seven-marker immunohistochemical signature. Cancers (Basel) 2021;13(12):2902.

Merkel Cell Carcinoma

Daniel J. Lewis, MD[a],*, Joseph F. Sobanko, MD[b], Jeremy R. Etzkorn, MD, MS[b],
Thuzar M. Shin, MD, PhD[b], Cerrene N. Giordano, MD[b], Stacy L. McMurray, MD[b],
Joanna L. Walker, MD[b], Junqian Zhang, MD[b], Christopher J. Miller, MD[b],
H. William Higgins II, MD, MBE[b]

KEYWORDS

- Merkel cell carcinoma • Merkel cell polyomavirus • Wide local excision
- Mohs micrographic surgery • Sentinel lymph node biopsy • Radiation therapy
- Immune checkpoint inhibitors

KEY POINTS

- Merkel cell carcinoma (MCC) is a rare malignancy, but its incidence is rapidly increasing, with 0.79 cases occurring per 100,000 person-years. Most cases of MCC are linked to the Merkel cell polyomavirus (MCPyV). Ultraviolet radiation exposure, immunosuppression, and increased age are other important risk factors.
- Treatment of the primary tumor includes wide or narrow margin excision or Mohs micrographic surgery; adjuvant radiation therapy is administered after narrow excision and can be considered after wide excision or Mohs surgery.
- MCC has a high risk of nodal metastasis, so sentinel lymph node biopsy is recommended in all patients with clinically negative nodes to determine prognosis and to plan comprehensive therapy.
- Immunotherapy has replaced chemotherapy as first-line therapy for metastatic MCC. Avelumab and pembrolizumab inhibit the programmed cell death-1 pathway and are approved by the Food and Drug Administration for MCC.
- Long-term surveillance with MCPyV oncoprotein antibody levels and imaging are recommended due to the high risk of local, regional, and distant recurrence.

INTRODUCTION

Merkel cell carcinoma (MCC) is a rare neuroendocrine carcinoma with high rates of local recurrence and metastasis. Five-year survival rates are 51% for local disease, 35% for nodal disease, and 14% for distant disease.[1] National Comprehensive Cancer Network (NCCN) guidelines for MCC are evolving rapidly. We discuss the epidemiology and pathogenesis of MCC and provide an evidence-based approach to diagnosis, staging, therapy, and surveillance.[2]

EPIDEMIOLOGY AND RISK FACTORS

The incidence of MCC has steadily risen over the past 30 years.[3] Analysis of the Surveillance, Epidemiology, and End Results (SEER) registry in the United States revealed an incidence of 0.79 cases per 100,000 person-years in 2011, or approximately 1600 new cases each year, a 95% annual increase since 2000.[3] European countries, Australia, and China have also seen increasing incidence of MCC over the past several decades.[4–6]

This increase has been primarily attributed to the rising proportion of the worldwide population older than 65 years, as MCC incidence is highest during the eighth decade of life, likely due to immunosenescence as well as higher cumulative exposure to ultraviolet (UV) radiation.[3,7] The rise is also likely partly due to increased reporting as well as improved diagnostics, namely cytokeratin-20

[a] Department of Dermatology, University of Pennsylvania, Hospital of the University of Pennsylvania, 3600 Spruce Street, 2 Maloney, Philadelphia, PA 19104-4283, USA; [b] Department of Dermatology, University of Pennsylvania, 3400 Civic Center Boulevard, Suite 1-330S, Philadelphia, PA 19104, USA
* Corresponding author.
E-mail address: daniel.lewis@pennmedicine.upenn.edu

Dermatol Clin 41 (2023) 101–115
https://doi.org/10.1016/j.det.2022.07.015

(CK-20) immunohistochemical staining, which was introduced in 1992.[8]

The prevalence of MCC varies significantly with geography, race, and sex. UV radiation is a risk factor for MCC; therefore, MCC preferentially affects individuals living in geographic areas with high UVB radiation indices.[9] MCC is also approximately 25-fold more common in white than in other ethnic groups and affects men more than women.[10] Immunosuppressed patients, such as those with hematologic malignancy, human immunodeficiency virus infection, or history of solid organ transplantation, are also at higher risk for MCC.[11]

PATHOGENESIS
Merkel Cell Polyomavirus (Virus-Positive Pathway)

Discovered in 2008, the Merkel cell polyomavirus (MCPyV) is ubiquitous, with 60% to 80% of the population infected based on serology and initial exposure likely occurring during childhood.[12–14] Despite the high incidence of MCPyV infection, MCC is rare likely because of adequate immunosurveillance in the large majority of individuals.[15] Nearly 80% of MCC in the United States is attributed to MCPyV, compared with only 25% in Australia.[16]

In the evolution of MCC, MCPyV DNA is clonally integrated into the host cell genome, resulting in the expression of 2 oncoproteins: small T-antigen (T-Ag) and large T-Ag.[12,17] The small T-Ag promotes transcription and gene expression to transform fibroblasts and is postulated to initiate tumorigenesis.[17] Meanwhile, the large T-Ag inhibits the tumor suppressor genes retinoblastoma (Rb) and p53, producing uncontrolled MCC cell proliferation.[17,18] Notably, the mutational burden of virus-positive MCC is the lowest among all cancers.[19]

Ultraviolet Radiation (Virus-Negative Pathway)

The remaining cases of MCC are attributed to UV exposure, accounting for roughly 20% of cases in the United States and most cases in Australia.[16] MCPyV-negative MCC cells show the highest burden of UV-associated mutations and neoantigen expression of any malignancy, including melanoma and cutaneous squamous cell carcinoma (cSCC).[20,21] An array of loss-of-function mutations in tumor suppressor, DNA repair, and activating genes have been implicated in MCPyV-negative MCC, including inactivation of Rb and p53.[20,21]

Cell of Origin

The cell of origin in MCC remains unidentified and controversial. It is likely derived from a cell population such as dermal fibroblasts that enter the Merkel cell differentiation pathway before or during neoplastic transformation.[22–24] MCPyV can infect dermal fibroblasts, whereas UV radiation likely stimulates the expression of genes in fibroblasts that encode matrix metalloproteinases, driving MCC development.[25,26] Investigators have recently suggested that MCC may encompass 2 tumors: a neuroendocrine carcinoma related to MCPyV integration derived from fibroblasts and a UV-related squamous cell carcinoma (SCC) with neuroendocrine differentiation derived from keratinocytes or epidermal stem cells.[27] Others have argued that the term MCC is a misnomer and that the cell of origin is a pre-B lymphocyte rather than a Merkel cell.[24]

DIAGNOSIS
Clinical Presentation

The primary lesion in MCC classically manifests as a solitary erythematous or violaceous papulonodule or plaque on sun-exposed skin (**Fig. 1**), most commonly on the head and neck followed by the extremities.[28] It is usually firm and nontender, and it may ulcerate and grow rapidly after it first appears, often doubling in size within 1 to 3 months. Metastatic MCC with no known primary tumor can also occur and accounts for 4% of all cases.[1]

Common features of MCC are captured in the acronym "AEIOU": asymptomatic, expanding rapidly, immunosuppression, older than age 50, and ultraviolet radiation.[28] This acronym is sensitive in that 89% of patients with MCC have at least 3 of these 5 characteristics, but it is not specific.[28] The nonspecific clinical appearance of MCC can have a broad clinical differential diagnosis, including a cyst, lipoma, dermatofibroma, cSCC, basal cell carcinoma (BCC), or amelanotic melanoma.[29] Biopsy is necessary for diagnosis.

Histopathology and Immunohistochemistry

Histopathology often exhibits nodular growth in the dermis and subcutis (**Fig. 2**A) of undifferentiated small, round blue cells with large nuclei containing granular chromatin, scant cytoplasm, high mitotic figures, apoptotic bodies, and necrosis (**Fig. 2**B).[30] The histopathologic differential diagnosis includes BCC, melanoma, Ewing sarcoma, neuroblastoma, leukemia cutis, and metastatic small-cell lung carcinoma.[30] MCC in situ, in which neoplastic cells are confined to the epidermis or

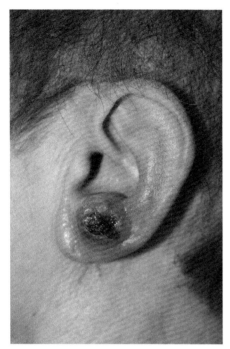

Fig. 1. Classic clinical appearance and anatomic location of MCC: a pink, erythematous nodule with central ulceration on the left ear.

follicular epithelium, may mimic pagetoid intraepidermal neoplasms such as SCC in situ, melanoma in situ, or extramammary Paget disease.[31] Last, a small-cell variant of MCC may share histopathologic features with cutaneous lymphoma.[32]

Immunohistochemistry with neurofilament, CK-20, CK-7, and thyroid transcription factor-1 (TTF-1) exhibits high sensitivity and specificity in distinguishing MCC from common histopathologic mimics (**Table 1**).[30] CK-20 stains MCC in both a diffuse cytoplasmic and a perinuclear dot pattern with 75% sensitivity, with the latter more specific for MCC (**Fig. 2**C).[8,33] Neurofilament promotes detection of CK-20-negative tumors and also

frequently exhibits a perinuclear dot pattern.[34] Most MCC lesions are CK7-negative, but a minority of cases demonstrate partial CK-7 positivity.[35] TTF-1 is typically negative and assists in differentiating MCC from metastatic small-cell lung carcinoma.[36] Expression of neuroendocrine markers such as synaptophysin, chromogranin, CD56, and neuron-specific enolase is also characteristic of MCC, but their specificity is low.[34] Lymphovascular invasion can be assessed with D2-40 or CD31 staining.

STAGING AND PROGNOSIS
American Joint Committee on Cancer Staging

In addition to biopsy of the primary MCC, physical examination, imaging, and lymph node (LN) sampling are necessary to stage patients (**Fig. 3**) to determine prognosis, treatment, and eligibility for clinical trials. Updated in 2018, the American Joint Committee on Cancer (AJCC) 8th Edition staging system implemented changes to stratify patients by prognosis more accurately (**Table 2**).[37] The revision distinguishes between clinical and pathologic staging for LNs and distant metastases, an important distinction, as pathology provides more accurate prognostication than clinical assessment.[38] It also now stratifies patients with nodal disease based on whether the primary tumor is known or unknown, because metastases with unknown primary tumors have better prognoses.[38]

Other Prognostic Factors

Additional factors affect prognosis but are not currently reflected in the AJCC 8th Edition staging. Multiple studies have shown that patient-specific factors, such as male sex, immunosuppression, and increasing age at diagnosis, are associated with decreased survival and increased recurrence rates.[39,40] Infiltrative growth on microscopy has

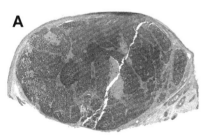
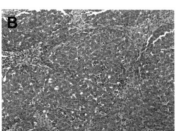
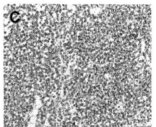

Fig. 2. Typical histopathologic appearance of MCC. (*A*) Nodular collection of monotonous, round blue cells in the dermis; hematoxylin and eosin, original magnification ×25. (*B*) High-power magnification shows atypical cells with round nuclei with finely granular chromatin, scant eosinophilic cytoplasmic rims, and numerous mitotic figures and apoptotic cells; hematoxylin and eosin, original magnification ×150. (*C*) Immunohistochemistry with cytokeratin-20 shows positivity with a characteristic perinuclear dot pattern; magnification ×150.

Table 1
Immunohistochemical staining of Merkel cell carcinoma and histopathologic mimics

Stain	MCC	SCLC	Neuroblastoma	Ewing Sarcoma
Cytokeratin-7	−[a]	+/−	−	−
Cytokeratin-20	+	−	−	−
Thyroid transcription factor-1	−	+	−	−
Neuron-specific enolase	+	+	+	+/−
Chromogranin A	+	+	+	−
Synaptophysin	+	+	+	+/−
Neurofilament	+	−	+	+
CD56	+	+	+	+/−

Abbreviations: CD, cluster of differentiation; MCC, Merkel cell carcinoma; SCLC, small-cell lung cancer.
[a] Cytokeratin-7 (CK-7) is typically negative in MCC; however, a small subset of CK7-positive cases has been described.[36]

also been associated with decreased survival compared with a nodular pattern; evidence remains contradictory on whether Breslow depth affects prognosis.[1] Last, detectable antibodies to T-Ag at diagnosis correlate with lower recurrence rates and increased survival.[41,42]

Baseline Imaging

Up to 13% of patients may exhibit clinically occult metastatic disease on baseline imaging.[43] Therefore, NCCN guidelines now recommend considering baseline imaging at diagnosis for all patients before surgery.[2] PET–computed tomography (PET-CT) is recommended over CT,

because PET-CT is twofold more sensitive (17% vs 7%) in upstaging patients.[2,43]

Regional Lymph Nodes

In addition to imaging, clinical assessment of the regional LNs should be performed. Patients with palpable nodes or nodal disease on imaging should undergo fine-needle aspiration, core-needle biopsy, or excisional biopsy.[2] Excisional biopsy should be considered if needle aspiration or core biopsy is negative to exclude a false-negative biopsy result.[2,44] For those with no clinical or radiologic nodal involvement, sentinel lymph node biopsy (SLNB) should be performed,

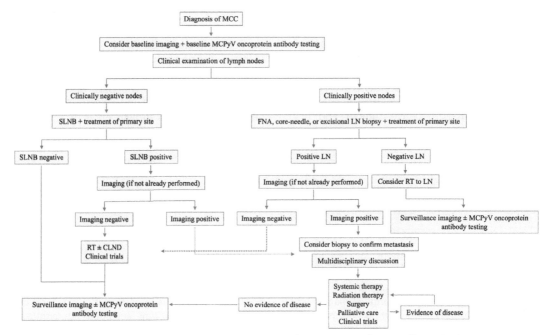

Fig. 3. Overview of evaluation, treatment, and monitoring for MCC. FNA, fine-needle aspiration.

Table 2
American Joint Committee on Cancer 8th Edition staging system for Merkel cell carcinoma

Stage	Method	Primary Tumor	Lymph Node	Metastasis
0	Pathologic	In situ (within epidermis only)	No regional lymph node metastasis	No distant metastasis
I	Clinical[a]	Tumor ≤2 cm in maximum dimension	Negative nodes on clinical exam only (no pathology performed)	No distant metastasis
	Pathologic[b]	Tumor ≤2 cm in maximum dimension	Negative nodes by pathology	No distant metastasis
IIA	Clinical	Tumor ≥2 cm in maximum dimension	Negative nodes on clinical examination only (no pathology performed)	No distant metastasis
	Pathologic	Tumor ≥2 cm in maximum dimension	Negative nodes by pathology	No distant metastasis
IIB	Clinical	Tumor invasion into muscle, fascia, bone, or cartilage	Negative nodes on clinical examination only (no pathology performed)	No distant metastasis
	Pathologic	Tumor invasion into muscle, fascia, bone, or cartilage	Negative nodes by pathology	No distant metastasis
III	Clinical	Any tumor size or invasion	Negative nodes on clinical examination only (no pathology performed)	No distant metastasis
IIIA	Pathologic	Any tumor size or invasion	Positive nodes on pathology only (negative nodes on clinical examination)	No distant metastasis
	Pathologic	Not detected (unknown primary)	Positive nodes on clinical examination and confirmed via pathology	No distant metastasis
IIIB	Pathologic	Any tumor size or invasion	Positive nodes on clinical examination and confirmed via pathology OR in-transit metastasis[c]	No distant metastasis
IV	Clinical	Any tumor size or invasion or unknown primary	Presence or absence of regional nodal disease	Distant metastasis detected via clinical examination
	Pathologic	Any tumor size or invasion or unknown primary	Presence or absence of regional nodal disease	Distant metastasis confirmed via pathology

[a] Clinical detection of nodal or metastatic disease includes inspection, palpation, and imaging.
[b] Pathologic detection of nodal disease includes sentinel lymph node biopsy, fine-needle aspiration, core-needle biopsy, or excisional biopsy. Pathologic confirmation of metastatic disease is via biopsy of the suspected metastasis.
[c] In-transit metastasis represents a tumor distinct from the primary lesion and is located either (1) between the primary lesion and the regional lymph node basin or (2) distal to the primary lesion.

except when contraindicated due to comorbidities.[2,45] All pathologic analysis of nodal tissue should include immunohistochemistry for improved sensitivity.[2]

SLNB is recommended based on evidence that 25% to 30% of patients without lymphadenopathy have occult regional nodal metastasis.[2,46,47] Even patients with small primary tumors have a significant risk of nodal disease: a 0.5-cm tumor confers a 14% risk of regional nodal disease.[1,47,48] In addition, for patients with no nodal disease on imaging, SLNB is still recommended, as PET-CT is less sensitive in detecting micrometastasis and does not replace SLNB as a staging tool.[43] Factors associated with SLNB positivity include large tumor size and pathologic features such as increased thickness, high mitotic rate, and infiltrative growth.[47,49,50]

The effect of SLNB status on survival, particularly disease-specific survival (DSS), remains unclear. Several studies have shown SLNB status to be a strong predictor of DSS and overall survival (OS).[40,51–53] In some studies, a positive SLNB was associated with a 5-year OS of 50% to 62%, compared with 60% to 80% with a negative SLNB.[1,46] A negative SLNB, compared with negative clinical nodal assessment alone, has been associated with lower rates of recurrence (11% vs 44%) and improved 5-year OS (97% vs 75%).[1,46] However, other single-center studies showed no association between DSS and SLNB status.[49,52] Analysis of 4543 patients with MCC from the SEER registry found a correlation between improved DSS and use of SLNB on univariate but not multivariate analysis.[40] Although the precise effects on DSS remain unclear, SLNB aids in identifying patients who can benefit from therapies for regional control that may improve survival.[54]

Distant Metastasis

Although clinical examination may sometimes detect skin and LN metastases, imaging is often necessary to detect visceral metastases. Although PET-CT should be considered at baseline in all patients, those with pathologic nodal disease should be evaluated for distant metastasis, preferentially with whole-body PET-CT or alternatively with CT with contrast of the neck, chest, abdomen, and pelvis.[2] Imaging is also warranted in patients with unresectable disease or whenever metastasis is suspected based on signs or symptoms.[2] MRI of the brain may be considered for suspected intracranial metastasis.[2] Biopsy may be necessary to confirm metastasis when imaging detects suspicious lesions.

TREATMENT
Primary Tumor Bed

Surgical excision
Surgical excision of the primary tumor is the initial step in treating local MCC (**Fig. 4**). The main objective is to obtain negative microscopic margins when surgically feasible.[2] Regardless of surgical approach, excision should be coordinated with and occur synchronously with or following SLNB, if indicated, to avoid altering lymphatic drainage patterns.[44,54] Reconstruction involving extensive undermining or adjacent tissue rearrangement should be performed only after negative margins are confirmed.[54] Complex reconstruction, especially staged flaps and grafts, also should be avoided in cases in which adjuvant radiation therapy (RT) is planned, as these repair approaches require prolonged postoperative care that may delay RT.[44]

Wide versus narrow margin excision Although the requisite depth of excision is usually to fascia or periosteum, the optimal surgical margin remains poorly defined and typically ranges from 1 to 3 cm.[32] Current NCCN guidelines recommend excision with individualized margins.[2] Margin size should be based on multiple factors: (1) whether adjuvant RT is being considered, (2) associated surgical morbidity, and (3) ability to close the surgical defect based on the margin size.[46,55,56] Some studies have suggested that wide margins of 1 to 2 cm confer lower rates of local recurrence, whereas others have shown no difference in local recurrence with wide (>1 cm) versus narrow (<1 cm) margins.[46,57,58] Importantly, these studies did not account for whether or not adjuvant RT was administered.

Wide local excision (WLE) is the standard and most common surgical method of treating the primary tumor.[2,57] Rates of local recurrence after WLE range are 25% to 40% without adjuvant RT.[57,59,60] However, recent evidence has supported narrow margins if adjuvant RT is planned.[61] In patients with stage I to III disease undergoing surgery without radiation of the primary tumor, local recurrence rate was lower after wide (>1 cm) versus narrow (<1 cm) excision.[62] However, in patients receiving adjuvant RT after excision, local control was excellent with a 1% local recurrence rate regardless of margin size, including patients with positive microscopic margins.[62] Thus, adjuvant RT is powerful in controlling narrow or even positive surgical margins. Based on these findings, NCCN guidelines now recommend either narrow or wide margin excision, allowing the surgical margin to be based on whether adjuvant RT will be administered.[2] Histologically negative margins are recommended when clinically feasible, but surgical margins should be balanced with morbidity of surgery.[2]

Mohs micrographic surgery Mohs micrographic surgery (MMS) represents another surgical approach outlined in NCCN guidelines (**Fig. 5**).[2] Compared with conventional excision, MMS permits complete peripheral and deep margin evaluation before reconstruction, whereas standard excision confers the risk of positive margins from incomplete excision, which occur as often as 10.4% following WLE, or false-negative margins from examination of less than 1% of the surgical margin.[63] The ability to confirm microscopic clearance of the tumor along all margins with MMS may reduce the need for adjuvant RT.[64] MMS also maximizes sparing of normal tissue, a notable benefit in MCC, given it commonly affects cosmetically sensitive areas on the head and neck.

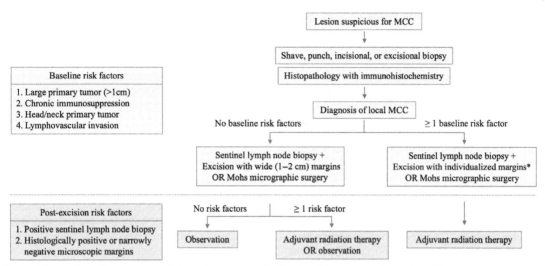

Fig. 4. Diagnosis and treatment of the primary tumor in local MCC. *Narrow (<1 cm) excision margins minimize morbidity, and microscopically positive margins are acceptable when followed by adjuvant RT to the primary site.

MMS for MCC typically involves the intraoperative use of CK-20 immunohistochemistry on frozen section pathology to aid in visualizing tumor cells at the margins and oftentimes within a central debulk specimen. Nevertheless, the central tumor debulk should also be sent for permanent sections for microstaging.[65] Retrospective studies have shown that MMS is effective; however, prospective trials comparing MMS and WLE have not been performed.[63,65,66] Local recurrence rates after MMS are lower than with WLE, ranging from 0% to

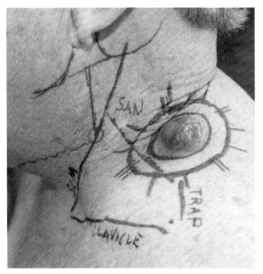

Fig. 5. Preoperative marking during MMS for an MCC on the left neck showing planned incisions for the debulk and initial stage as well as the approximate course of the spinal accessory nerve using surface topographic landmarks.

22%, whereas survival outcomes are comparable based on limited studies.[59,63,65–67] To ensure accurate LN staging, SLNB is performed first, followed by MMS and reconstruction of the primary tumor in a subsequent operative session.[65]

Radiation therapy

Radiation monotherapy Radiation monotherapy is an alternative to surgery in patients who are poor surgical candidates or who have primary tumor in an anatomic site where excision would produce significant functional compromise.[68] NCCN guidelines recommend higher doses if RT is administered as monotherapy; specifically, 60 to 66 Gy with a field that includes a wide (5-cm) margin around the tumor.[2] However, outcome data on radiation monotherapy remain limited. Although in-field control rates range from 75% to 100%, rates of distant recurrence are increased, and DSS and OS are lower compared with excision.[69] However, these rates are likely influenced by factors unrelated to therapy, because patients selected for radiation monotherapy often have inoperable tumors or comorbidities precluding surgery that may lower OS.

Adjuvant radiation therapy Approximately 50% of patients with MCC in the United States receive local adjuvant RT.[70] Adjuvant RT to the tumor bed provides superb local control, even after narrow excision or positive microscopic margins, and is associated with a trend toward improved disease-free survival (DFS) in multiple retrospective studies.[71,72] Adjuvant RT is indicated in a number of scenarios: (1) narrowly negative microscopic surgical margins, (2) positive microscopic surgical margins, (3) grossly positive surgical margins when additional surgery is not possible, and (4) in the setting of adverse microscopic features such as lymphovascular invasion.[2,44] NCCN guidelines also recommend adjuvant RT in patients with one or more of the following risk factors: large (>1 cm) primary tumors, head or neck tumors, chronic immunosuppression, and positive SLNB.[2]

Adjuvant RT should be administered within 2 months of surgery to minimize local recurrence.[44] Conventionally fractionated RT consists of 50 to 66 Gy delivered in 25 to 33 fractions.[44] However, this regimen is associated with substantial toxicity, including radiation dermatitis, mucositis, and chronic fibrosis, and requires several treatments over 4 to 6 weeks.[44,73] Preliminary evidence suggests that 8-Gy single-fraction RT (SFRT) provides a high rate of durable local control (94%) while minimizing toxicity.[73,74] SFRT may be considered for tumors with a lower risk of local recurrence, especially those in areas such as the head and neck where higher morbidity associated with RT is anticipated.[44]

The use of adjuvant RT in patients with clear surgical margins remains controversial. Adjuvant RT was not associated with improved local control after margin-negative WLE in one study, and another study failed to show a significant difference in OS, relapse-free survival, or DFS after clear pathologic margins after MMS.[46,64]

Lymph nodes The optimal treatment after assessing LN status has not been defined. Evidence suggests that patients with pathologically negative nodes can be safely observed without adjuvant RT given the low incidence of same nodal basin recurrence after negative SLNB.[75] However, adjuvant RT can be considered in patients at risk for false-negative SLNB, cases in which the primary tumor is located on the head and neck, where SLNB is less accurate due to the complex lymphatic drainage in this region, or in which excision is performed before SLNB, altering lymphatic drainage patterns.[2] Adjuvant RT to regional nodes can also be considered in clinically node-negative patients who decline SLNB.[71,72]

For patients with confirmed nodal disease without distant metastasis, treatment options include complete lymph node dissection (CLND), definitive nodal RT, or both.[44] Patients with SLN-positive disease who undergo either CLND or RT have OS and DSS similar to patients with SLN-negative disease, highlighting the importance of treating the nodal basin.[52] However, data comparing treatment options remain limited. In patients with clinically evident nodal disease, RT provides excellent regional control and has been reported to lower regional recurrence rates; however, it is unclear if these findings apply to occult nodal disease detected by SLNB.[76] Overall, rates of regional recurrence after RT or CLND appear comparable, with no additional benefit derived from RT following CLND.[52] CLND offers the advantage of pathologic evaluation of the entire nodal basin, which may guide the planning of additional RT fields.

NCCN guidelines recommend RT to the nodal basin after CLND in patients with multiple involved nodes or pathologic evidence of extracapsular tumor extension.[2] However, until further evidence and more specific guidelines become available, treatment options for managing nodal disease should be discussed with the patient and may vary based on site-specific morbidity, tumor characteristics, and patient comorbidities.[2,54] At present, systemic agents are not considered first-line for nodal disease.[2] However, guidelines may change as data emerge on immunotherapy in the neoadjuvant setting.[2,77]

Metastatic disease For patients with metastatic disease, consensus guidelines recommend multidisciplinary tumor board discussion of options such as systemic therapy, RT, and palliative care based on the clinical scenario.[2,78] Immunotherapy is now considered first-line therapy for metastatic MCC.[2]

Immunotherapy There is significant rationale for the use of immunotherapy in MCC given the host immune system plays an essential role in controlling the malignancy. Immunosuppressed patients have a 10-fold higher incidence of MCC, and a robust CD8+ T-cell infiltrate within MCC tumors is an excellent prognostic factor associated with no reported MCC-related deaths.[41,42] Oncogenic mutations in MCC tumor cells upregulate the programmed death receptor-1 (PD-1)/programmed death ligand-1 (PD-L1) pathway, promoting local immune evasion via impaired T-cell activation. Furthermore, tumor-infiltrating lymphocytes and circulating MCPyV-specific T cells appear exhausted in MCC.[79–81] PD-1 or PD-L1 blockade with immune checkpoint inhibitors (ICIs) reinvigorates exhausted T cells and stimulates the antitumor response. Response rates with ICIs are approximately 50% to 70% for treatment-naïve disease and 30% for refractory disease, with 70% to 80% response durability at 2 years in both groups.[82–87]

Avelumab, a monoclonal antibody inhibiting PD-L1, was approved by the US Food and Drug Administration (FDA) in 2017 as first-line therapy for metastatic MCC based on the JAVELIN Merkel 200 trial.[85] This trial was a phase II, open-label, multicenter study in which avelumab was given intravenously every 2 weeks in 88 patients with stage IV disease refractory to chemotherapy.[85] Twenty-eight (33%) patients responded to therapy, with an 11% complete response (CR) rate and with 82% of responses persisting over 10.4 months of follow-up.[85] Median OS was 12.6 months, with a 5-year OS rate of 26%.[87]

Pembrolizumab, an anti-PD-1 monoclonal antibody, was FDA-approved in 2018 for recurrent locally advanced or metastatic MCC. A multicenter phase II trial investigated intravenous pembrolizumab as first-line systemic therapy every 3 weeks for up to 2 years.[83,86] The overall response rate was 58% in 50 patients with metastatic or recurrent locoregional MCC.[83,86] Median progression-free survival (PFS) was 16.8 months and PFS at 3 years was 39%.[83,86]

Nivolumab, another PD-1 inhibitor, is currently under investigation, particularly in combination with ipilimumab, an antibody that inhibits cytotoxic T-lymphocyte associated antigen-4 (CTLA-4).[88,89] Like PD-1/PD-L1, CTLA-4 inhibits T-cell activation, and its blockade can potentiate an antitumor response. Ipilimumab may be particularly useful, either as monotherapy or in combination with a PD-1/PD-L1 inhibitor, in patients in whom PD-1 blockade remains or becomes ineffective.

Use of ICIs as neoadjuvant and adjuvant therapy is a novel approach in MCC actively being studied. In the neoadjuvant setting, a recent trial studied 39 patients with higher-risk local or regional disease treated with 2 doses of nivolumab followed by definitive excision.[77] Approximately 50% patients demonstrated CR, and recurrence-free survival significantly correlated with disease response at the time of surgery.[77] With additional study, neoadjuvant therapy may reduce the extent of therapy to the tumor bed in select patients.

Although the success of ICIs remains encouraging overall, more than 50% of patients demonstrate no response or develop progressive disease after an initial response.[44] In addition, patients receiving immunosuppression for a solid organ transplant or with severe autoimmune disease are poor candidates for ICIs because of the risk of transplant failure or worsened autoimmune disease.

Chemotherapy With the adoption of immunotherapy, chemotherapy is now reserved for palliative therapy or for patients who cannot receive immunotherapy. Common regimens include etoposide with carboplatin or cyclophosphamide, doxorubicin, and vincristine.[90,91] These regimens lead to tumor regression in 53% to 76% of patients but fail to produce a lasting response and lack an OS benefit.[90,91] The duration of response is often as short as 3 months, and median PFS is a mere 3 to 8 months, with fewer than 5% of responders continuing to benefit at 2 years after starting therapy.[90,91] Chemotherapy is also associated with a high risk of toxicity, particularly in patients older than 65, including myelosuppression, renal injury, and sepsis.[90,91]

Radiation therapy A brief course of RT as palliative therapy may be considered in patients with oligometastatic disease. Reported regimens consist of 8 Gy administered as a single fraction or via 3 fractions.[74,92] Regardless of the specific regimen, short-course RT is well-tolerated and may yield response rates as high as 94% with an in-field control rate of 77% at 8 months.[74,92] Combinations of hypofractionated RT and immunotherapy are under active investigation in clinical trials based on the immunologic rationale that radiation induces the release of tumor antigens, essentially priming the cytotoxic T cells reinvigorated by immunotherapy.[93]

Future therapies Other treatment modalities under investigation as either single or adjuvant therapy include immunostimulatory agents such as Toll-like receptor agonists, interleukin-12, MCPyV vaccination, and talimogene laherparepvec.[94–97] Targeted molecular therapies such as Ataxia telangiectasia mutated and Rad3-related kinase inhibitors, double minute 2 protein inhibitors, and histone deacetylase inhibitors are also being studied.[98–100] These molecular therapies may become especially relevant for patients who are poor candidates for immunotherapy.

SURVEILLANCE
Risk of Recurrence

MCC is associated with a high risk of local, regional, and distant recurrence, estimated to be approximately 40% across multiple studies.[25] However, this risk varies by stage: 20% for stage I disease to 75% for stage III disease and by patient-specific factors such as age, sex, tumor location, MCPyV seropositivity, and immunosuppression.[25,44] The median time to recurrence is 7 to 9 months, with 80% to 90% of cases manifesting within the first 2 years.[101] In local disease, recurrence tends to occur locally or in the nodal basin (40%–60%), whereas distant recurrence occurs frequently (80%) in advanced-stage disease.[44]

Follow-Up and Imaging

Prompt recognition of recurrence allows for earlier initiation of therapy. Follow-up visits with complete skin and nodal examination and review of systems can be considered every 3 to 6 months for 2 to 3 years, and every 6 to 12 months thereafter in disease-free patients.[2,44] Immunosuppressed patients are at a higher risk for recurrence and, as such, more frequent follow-up may be indicated.[44] Immunosuppressive agents should be minimized as clinically feasible.

Surveillance studies should be based on patient-specific risk factors or symptoms, as no guidelines exist.[2,54] A personalized, web-based risk calculator (https://merkelcell.org/recur/) integrating the aforementioned patient risk factors, may assist in quantifying the risk of recurrence and guiding the frequency of surveillance studies. Routine surveillance imaging with PET-CT or CT, with the former exhibiting higher sensitivity, warrants consideration in patients with high-risk tumor features, nodal disease, or immunosuppression.[54] Surveillance imaging may not be necessary in immunocompetent patients with low-risk tumors and negative SLNB.[54]

Merkel Cell Polyomavirus Oncoprotein Antibody Testing

Antibodies targeting MCPyV oncoproteins are detected in approximately 50% of patients with MCC.[102,103] Baseline MCPyV oncoprotein antibody titers can assist with risk stratification and subsequent detection of disease recurrence. An immunologic response to the MCPyV T-Ag oncoprotein appears protective, as seropositive patients have a better prognosis and a 30% lower rate of recurrence than seronegative patients.[102,103] In addition, in patients who are seropositive at baseline, changes in titers over time reflect changes in MCC disease burden, making MCPyV oncoprotein antibodies a useful serum tumor marker for surveillance.[102,103] These titers can be measured via an anti-Merkel cell panel available through the University of Washington.

NCCN guidelines recommend MCPyV oncoprotein antibody titers as part of initial workup and for surveillance in seropositive patients.[2] A baseline level should be obtained ideally within 3 months of initiating therapy.[44] For seropositive patients, levels can then be repeated every 3 months.[2,44] Two consecutive increasing titers of greater than 20% have a 99% positive predictive value for disease recurrence and should prompt imaging studies to evaluate for recurrence.[44] An increase in titers enables detection of 90% of recurrences within 45 days of the first elevated titer.[44] Conversely, a decreasing titer by more than 20% is associated with a 99% negative predictive value for clinically residual disease.[44] For seronegative

patients, surveillance should be centered around imaging studies, although the recent emergence of a circulating tumor DNA assay may offer a more sensitive method of surveillance in these patients.[104]

SUMMARY

The past 2 decades have produced advances in cancer biology, molecular genetics, and immunology that have further characterized the pathophysiology of MCC and expanded our therapeutic armamentarium. New immunotherapies such as those targeting the PD-1/PD-L1 pathway have shown promise in yielding durable responses in nearly half of patients with advanced disease and are now first-line agents for advanced-stage MCC. In addition to offering greater efficacy, therapy for MCC has shifted to a less toxic approach, including narrower excision margins, lower doses of RT, and limited use of chemotherapy. Furthermore, discovery of the MCPyV and its role in pathogenesis has led to the introduction of MCPyV oncoprotein antibody testing, the first serologic tool for surveillance in most patients with MCC. However, there is an ongoing need for continued investigation because survival rates, although improved, remain modest. As further studies enhance our understanding and treatment of MCC, guidelines for managing this aggressive malignancy will continue to evolve.

CLINICS CARE POINTS

- Surgical treatment of the primary MCC tumor consists of individualized margin (wide versus narrow) excision or Mohs micrographic surgery. Adjuvant radiation therapy is recommended after narrow excision and can be considered after wide excision or Mohs surgery.

- Sentinel lymph node biopsy is recommended in all patients without clinically apparent nodal disease or distant metastasis and should be performed prior to surgical treatment of the primary tumor.

- MCC is highly immunogenic and thus PD-1/PD-L1 inhibitors such as avelumab and pembrolizumab are now first-line agents for metastatic MCC.

- MCPyV oncoprotein antibody testing can indicate prognosis at time of diagnosis and can be used to monitor for recurrence following treatment.

AUTHOR CONTRIBUTIONS

D. Lewis: Conceptualization, visualization, and original draft preparation.

J. Sobanko: Review and editing.

J. Etzkorn: Review and editing.

T. Shin: Review and editing.

C. Giordano: Review and editing.

S. McMurray: Review and editing.

J. Walker: Review and editing.

J. Zhang: Review and editing.

C. Miller: Project administration, supervision, review and editing.

H. William Higgins: Conceptualization, methodology, project administration, supervision, review and editing.

Data curation, formal analysis, funding acquisition, investigation, resources, software, validation: not applicable.

DISCLOSURES

The authors have nothing to disclose. This research did not receive any specific grant from funding agencies in the public, commercial, or not-for-profit sectors.

REFERENCES

1. Harms KL, Healy MA, Nghiem P, et al. Analysis of prognostic factors from 9387 Merkel cell carcinoma cases forms the basis for the new 8th edition AJCC staging system. Ann Surg Oncol 2016; 23(11):3564–71.

2. National Comprehensive Care Network Clinical Practice Guidelines in Oncology (NCCN Guidelines): Merkel Cell Carcinoma, Version 1.2021. 2021.

3. Paulson KG, Park SY, Vandeven NA, et al. Merkel cell carcinoma: current US incidence and projected increases based on changing demographics. J Am Acad Dermatol 2018;78(3): 457–463 e452.

4. Kieny A, Cribier B, Meyer N, et al. Epidemiology of Merkel cell carcinoma. A population-based study from 1985 to 2013, in northeastern of France. Int J Cancer 2019;144(4):741–5.

5. Youlden DR, Soyer HP, Youl PH, et al. Incidence and survival for Merkel cell carcinoma in Queensland, Australia, 1993-2010. JAMA Dermatol 2014; 150(8):864–72.

6. Song PI, Liang H, Wei WQ, et al. The clinical profile of Merkel cell carcinoma in mainland China. Int J Dermatol 2012;51(9):1054–9.

7. Aw D, Silva AB, Palmer DB. Immunosenescence: emerging challenges for an ageing population. Immunology 2007;120(4):435–46.

8. Moll R, Lowe A, Laufer J, et al. Cytokeratin 20 in human carcinomas. A new histodiagnostic marker detected by monoclonal antibodies. Am J Pathol 1992;140(2):427–47.

9. Agelli M, Clegg LX, Becker JC, et al. The etiology and epidemiology of Merkel cell carcinoma. Curr Probl Cancer 2010;34(1):14–37.

10. Albores-Saavedra J, Batich K, Chable-Montero F, et al. Merkel cell carcinoma demographics, morphology, and survival based on 3870 cases: a population based study. J Cutan Pathol 2010; 37(1):20–7.

11. Paulson KG, Iyer JG, Blom A, et al. Systemic immune suppression predicts diminished Merkel cell carcinoma-specific survival independent of stage. J Invest Dermatol 2013;133(3):642–6.

12. Feng H, Shuda M, Chang Y, et al. Clonal integration of a polyomavirus in human Merkel cell carcinoma. Science 2008;319(5866):1096–100.

13. Chen T, Hedman L, Mattila PS, et al. Serological evidence of Merkel cell polyomavirus primary infections in childhood. J Clin Virol 2011;50(2): 125–9.

14. Tolstov YL, Pastrana DV, Feng H, et al. Human Merkel cell polyomavirus infection II. MCV is a common human infection that can be detected by conformational capsid epitope immunoassays. Int J Cancer 2009;125(6):1250–6.

15. Church CD PN. How does the Merkel polyomavirus lead to a lethal cancer? Many answers, many questions, and a new mouse model. J Invest Dermatol 2015;135(5):1221–4.

16. Garneski KM, Warcola AH, Feng Q, et al. Merkel cell polyomavirus is more frequently present in North American than Australian Merkel cell carcinoma tumors. J Invest Dermatol 2009;129(1):246–8.

17. Starrett GJ, Marcelus C, Cantalupo PG, et al. Merkel cell polyomavirus exhibits dominant control of the tumor genome and transcriptome in virus-associated Merkel cell carcinoma. mBio 2017;8(1). e02079–16.

18. Hesbacher S, Pfitzer L, Wiedorfer K, et al. RB1 is the crucial target of the Merkel cell polyomavirus large T antigen in Merkel cell carcinoma cells. Oncotarget 2016;7(22):32956–68.

19. Harms PW, Vats P, Verhaegen ME, et al. The distinctive mutational spectra of polyomavirus-negative Merkel cell carcinoma. Cancer Res 2015;75(18):3720–7.

20. Goh G, Walradt T, Markarov V, et al. Mutational landscape of MCPyV-positive and MCPyV-negative Merkel cell carcinomas with implications for immunotherapy. Oncotarget 2016;7(3):3403–15.

21. Wong SQ, Waldeck K, Vergara IA, et al. UV-associated mutations underlie the etiology of mcv-negative Merkel cell carcinomas. Cancer Res 2015;75(24):5228–34.

22. Tilling T, Wladykowski E, Failla AV, et al. Immunohistochemical analyses point to epidermal origin of

human Merkel cells. Histochem Cell Biol 2014; 141(4):407–21.

23. Szeder V, Grim M, Halata Z, et al. Neural crest origin of mammalian Merkel cells. Dev Biol 2003; 253(2):258–63.

24. Zur Hausen A, Rennspiess D, Winnepenninckx V, et al. Early B-cell differentiation in Merkel cell carcinomas: clues to cellular ancestry. Cancer Res 2013;73(16):4982–7.

25. Becker JC. Merkel cell carcinoma. Ann Oncol 2010;21(Suppl 7):vii81–5.

26. Liu W, MacDonald M, You J. Merkel cell polyomavirus infection and Merkel cell carcinoma. Curr Opin Virol 2016;2016(20):20–7.

27. Nirenberg A, Steinman H, Dixon J, et al. Merkel cell carcinoma update: the case for two tumours. J Eur Acad Dermatol Venereol 2020;34(7):1425–31.

28. Heath M, Jaimes N, Lemos B, et al. Clinical characteristics of Merkel cell carcinoma at diagnosis in 195 patients: the "AEIOU" features. J Am Acad Dermatol 2008;58(3):375–81.

29. Svensson H, Paoli J. Merkel cell carcinoma is still an unexpected diagnosis. J Eur Acad Dermatol Venereol 2021;35(12):e883–4.

30. Tetzlaff MT, Nagarajan P. Update on Merkel cell carcinoma. Head Neck Pathol 2018;12(1):31–43.

31. Jour G, Aung PP, Rozas-Munoz E, et al. Intraepidermal Merkel cell carcinoma: a case series of a rare entity with clinical follow up. J Cutan Pathol 2017;44(8):684–91.

32. Coggshall K, Tello TL, North JP, et al. Merkel cell carcinoma: an update and review: pathogenesis, diagnosis, and staging. J Am Acad Dermatol 2018;78(3):433–42.

33. Chan JK, Suster S, Wenig BM, et al. Cytokeratin 20 immunoreactivity distinguishes Merkel cell (primary cutaneous neuroendocrine) carcinomas and salivary gland small cell carcinomas from small cell carcinomas of various sites. Am J Surg Pathol 1997;21(2):226–34.

34. Fantini F, Johansson O. Neurochemical markers in human cutaneous Merkel cells. An immunohistochemical investigation. Exp Dermatol 1995;4(6): 365–71.

35. Calder KB, Coplowitz S, Schlauder S, et al. A case series and immunophenotypic analysis of CK20-/ CK7+ primary neuroendocrine carcinoma of the skin. J Cutan Pathol 2007;34(12):918–23.

36. Bobos M, Hytiroglou P, Kostopoulos I, et al. Immunohistochemical distinction between Merkel cell carcinoma and small cell carcinoma of the lung. Am J Dermatopathol 2006;28(2):99–104.

37. Amin MB, Gress DM, Meyer Vega LR, et al. AJCC Cancer Staging Manual. Eighth Edition. 2018.

38. Amin MB, Greene FL, Edge SB, et al. The Eighth Edition AJCC Cancer Staging Manual: continuing to build a bridge from a population-based to a more "personalized" approach to cancer staging. CA Cancer J Clin 2017;67(2):93–9.

39. Tarantola TI, Vallow LA, Halyard MY, et al. Prognostic factors in Merkel cell carcinoma: analysis of 240 cases. J Am Acad Dermatol 2013;68(3): 425–32.

40. Sridharan V, Muralidhar V, Margalit DN, et al. Merkel cell carcinoma: a population analysis on survival. J Natl Compr Canc Netw 2016;14(10):1247–57.

41. Paulson KG, Iyer JG, Simonson WT, et al. CD8+ lymphocyte intratumoral infiltration as a stage-independent predictor of Merkel cell carcinoma survival: a population-based study. Am J Clin Pathol 2014;142(4):452–8.

42. Paulson KG, Iyer JG, Tegeder AR, et al. Transcriptome-wide studies of Merkel cell carcinoma and validation of intratumoral CD8+ lymphocyte invasion as an independent predictor of survival. J Clin Oncol 2011;29(12):1539–46.

43. Singh N, Alexander NA, Lachance K, et al. Clinical benefit of baseline imaging in Merkel cell carcinoma: analysis of 584 patients. J Am Acad Dermatol 2021;84(2):330–9.

44. Park SY, Doolittle-Amieva C, Moshiri Y, et al. How we treat Merkel cell carcinoma: within and beyond current guidelines. Future Oncol 2021;17(11): 1363–77.

45. Lewis DJ, Fathy RA, Nugent S, et al. Sentinel lymph node biopsy in Merkel cell carcinoma: Rates and predictors of compliance with the National Comprehensive Cancer Network guidelines. J Am Acad Dermatol 2022. https://doi.org/10.1016/j. jaad.2022.05.054.

46. Allen PJ, Bowne WB, Jaques DP, et al. Merkel cell carcinoma: prognosis and treatment of patients from a single institution. J Clin Oncol 2005;23(10): 2300–9.

47. Schwartz JL, Griffith KA, Lowe L, et al. Features predicting sentinel lymph node positivity in Merkel cell carcinoma. J Clin Oncol 2011;29(8):1036–41.

48. Iyer JG, Storer BE, Paulson KG, et al. Relationships among primary tumor size, number of involved nodes, and survival for 8044 cases of Merkel cell carcinoma. J Am Acad Dermatol 2014;70(4):637–43.

49. Fields RC, Busam KJ, Chou JF, et al. Recurrence and survival in patients undergoing sentinel lymph node biopsy for Merkel cell carcinoma: analysis of 153 patients from a single institution. Ann Surg Oncol 2011;18(9):2529–37.

50. Conic RRZ, Ko J, Saridakis S, et al. Sentinel lymph node biopsy in Merkel cell carcinoma: predictors of sentinel lymph node positivity and association with overall survival. J Am Acad Dermatol 2019;81(2): 364–72.

51. Lemos BD, Storer BE, Iyer JG, et al. Pathologic nodal evaluation improves prognostic accuracy in Merkel cell carcinoma: analysis of 5823 cases as

the basis of the first consensus staging system. J Am Acad Dermatol 2010;63(5):751–61.

52. Sims JR, Grotz TE, Pockaj BA, et al. Sentinel lymph node biopsy in Merkel cell carcinoma: the Mayo Clinic experience of 150 patients. Surg Oncol 2018;27(1):11–7.

53. Gupta SG, Wang LC, Penas PF, et al. Sentinel lymph node biopsy for evaluation and treatment of patients with Merkel cell carcinoma: the Dana-Farber experience and meta-analysis of the literature. Arch Dermatol 2006;142(6):685–90.

54. Cornejo C, Miller CJ. Merkel cell carcinoma: updates on staging and management. Dermatol Clin 2019;37(3):269–77.

55. Perez MC, de Pinho FR, Holstein A, et al. Resection margins in Merkel cell carcinoma: is a 1-cm margin wide enough? Ann Surg Oncol 2018;25(11): 3334–40.

56. Gillenwater AM, Hessel AC, Morrison WH, et al. Merkel cell carcinoma of the head and neck: effect of surgical excision and radiation on recurrence and survival. Arch Otolaryngol Head Neck Surg 2001;127(2):149–54.

57. Gollard R, Weber R, Kosty MP, et al. Merkel cell carcinoma: review of 22 cases with surgical, pathologic, and therapeutic considerations. Cancer 2000;88(8):1842–51.

58. Yiengpruksawan A, Coit DG, Thaler HT, et al. Merkel cell carcinoma. Prognosis and management. Arch Surg 1991;126(12):1514–9.

59. Singh B, Qureshi MM, Truong MT, et al. Demographics and outcomes of stage I and II Merkel cell carcinoma treated with Mohs micrographic surgery compared with wide local excision in the National Cancer Database. J Am Acad Dermatol 2018;79(1):126–134 e123.

60. O'Connor WJ, Roenigk RK, Brodland DG. Merkel cell carcinoma. Comparison of Mohs micrographic surgery and wide excision in eighty-six patients. Dermatol Surg 1997;23(10):929–33.

61. Harrington C, Kwan W. Radiotherapy and conservative surgery in the locoregional management of Merkel cell carcinoma: the British Columbia Cancer Agency experience. Ann Surg Oncol 2016;23(2): 573–8.

62. Tarabadkar ES, Fu T, Lachance K, et al. Narrow excision margins are appropriate for Merkel cell carcinoma when combined with adjuvant radiation: Analysis of 188 cases of localized disease and proposed management algorithm. J Am Acad Dermatol 2021;84(2):340–7.

63. Terushkin V, Brodland DG, Sharon DJ, et al. Mohs surgery for early-stage Merkel cell carcinoma (MCC) achieves local control better than wide local excision +/- radiation therapy with no increase in MCC-specific death. Int J Dermatol 2021;60(8): 1010–2.

64. Boyer JD, Zitelli JA, Brodland DG, et al. Local control of primary Merkel cell carcinoma: review of 45 cases treated with Mohs micrographic surgery with and without adjuvant radiation. J Am Acad Dermatol 2002;47(6):885–92.

65. Shaikh WR, Sobanko JF, Etzkorn JR, et al. Utilization patterns and survival outcomes after wide local excision or Mohs micrographic surgery for Merkel cell carcinoma in the United States, 2004-2009. J Am Acad Dermatol 2018;78(1):175–177 e173.

66. Carrasquillo OY, Cancel-Artau KJ, Ramos-Rodriguez AJ, et al. Mohs micrographic surgery versus wide local excision in the treatment of merkel cell carcinoma: a systematic review. Dermatol Surg 2021;48(2):176–80.

67. Su C, Bai HX, Christensen S. Relative survival analysis in patients with stage I-II Merkel cell carcinoma treated with Mohs micrographic surgery or wide local excision. J Am Acad Dermatol 2018. S0190-9622(18)30816-8. Epub ahead of print.

68. Harrington C, Kwan W. Outcomes of Merkel cell carcinoma treated with radiotherapy without radical surgical excision. Ann Surg Oncol 2014; 21(11):3401–5.

69. Veness M, Howle J. Radiotherapy alone in patients with Merkel cell carcinoma: the Westmead Hospital experience of 41 patients. Australas J Dermatol 2015;56(1):19–24.

70. Bhatia S, Storer BE, Iyer JG, et al. Adjuvant radiation therapy and chemotherapy in Merkel cell carcinoma: survival analyses of 6908 cases from the national cancer data base. J Natl Cancer Inst 2016;108(9):djw042.

71. Takagishi SR, Marx TE, Lewis C, et al. Postoperative radiation therapy is associated with a reduced risk of local recurrence among low risk Merkel cell carcinomas of the head and neck. Adv Radiat Oncol 2016;1(4):244–51.

72. Mojica P, Smith D, Ellenhorn J. Adjuvant radiation therapy is associated with improved survival in Merkel cell carcinoma of the skin. J Clin Oncol 2007;25(9):1043–7.

73. Cook MM, Schaub SK, Goff PH, et al. Postoperative, single-fraction radiation therapy in Merkel cell carcinoma of the head and neck. Adv Radiat Oncol 2020;5(6):1248–54.

74. Iyer JG, Parvathaneni U, Gooley T, et al. Single-fraction radiation therapy in patients with metastatic Merkel cell carcinoma. Cancer Med 2015;4(8): 1161–70.

75. Grotz TE, Joseph RW, Pockaj BA, et al. Negative sentinel lymph node biopsy in Merkel cell carcinoma is associated with a low risk of same-nodal-basin recurrences. Ann Surg Oncol 2015;22(12): 4060–6.

76. Fang LC, Lemos B, Douglas J, et al. Radiation monotherapy as regional treatment for lymph node-positive Merkel cell carcinoma. Cancer 2010;116(7):1783–90.

77. Topalian SL, Bhatia S, Amin A, et al. Neoadjuvant nivolumab for patients with resectable Merkel cell carcinoma in the checkmate 358 trial. J Clin Oncol 2020;38(22):2476–87.

78. Prieto I, Perez de la Fuente T, Medina S, et al. Merkel cell carcinoma: an algorithm for multidisciplinary management and decision-making. Crit Rev Oncol Hematol 2016;98:170–9.

79. Iyer JG, Afanasiev OK, McClurkan C, et al. Merkel cell polyomavirus-specific CD8(+) and CD4(+) T-cell responses identified in Merkel cell carcinomas and blood. Clin Cancer Res 2011;17(21):6671–80.

80. Lyngaa R, Pedersen NW, Schrama D, et al. T-cell responses to oncogenic Merkel cell polyomavirus proteins distinguish patients with Merkel cell carcinoma from healthy donors. Clin Cancer Res 2014;20(7):1768–78.

81. Afanasiev OK, Yelistratova L, Miller N, et al. Merkel polyomavirus-specific T cells fluctuate with Merkel cell carcinoma burden and express therapeutically targetable PD-1 and Tim-3 exhaustion markers. Clin Cancer Res 2013;19(19):5351–60.

82. D'Angelo SP, Russell J, Lebbe C, et al. Efficacy and safety of first-line avelumab treatment in patients with stage IV metastatic Merkel cell carcinoma: a preplanned interim analysis of a clinical trial. JAMA Oncol 2018;4(9):e180077.

83. Nghiem PT, Bhatia S, Lipson EJ, et al. PD-1 blockade with pembrolizumab in advanced Merkel-cell carcinoma. N Engl J Med 2016;374(26):2542–52.

84. Ngheim P, Bhatia S, Lipson EJ, et al. Durable tumor regression and overall survival in patients with advanced Merkel cell carcinoma receiving pembrolizumab as first-line therapy. J Clin Oncol 2019;37(9):693–702.

85. Kaufman HL, Russell J, Hamid O, et al. Avelumab in patients with chemotherapy-refractory metastatic Merkel cell carcinoma: a multicentre, single-group, open-label, phase 2 trial. Lancet Oncol 2016;17(10):1374–85.

86. Nghiem P, Bhatia S, Lipson EJ, et al. Three-year survival, correlates and salvage therapies in patients receiving first-line pembrolizumab for advanced Merkel cell carcinoma. J Immunother Cancer 2021;9(4):e002478.

87. D'Angelo SP, Bhatia S, Brohl AS, et al. Avelumab in patients with previously treated metastatic Merkel cell carcinoma (JAVELIN Merkel 200): updated overall survival data after >5 years of follow-up. ESMO Open 2021;6(6):100290.

88. Glutsch V, Kneitz H, Gesierich A, et al. Activity of ipilimumab plus nivolumab in avelumab-refractory Merkel cell carcinoma. Cancer Immunol Immunother 2021;70(7):2087–93.

89. Khaddour K, Rosman IS, Dehdashti F, et al. Durable remission after rechallenge with ipilimumab and nivolumab in metastatic Merkel cell carcinoma refractory to avelumab: any role for sequential immunotherapy? J Dermatol 2021;48(2):e80–1.

90. Iyer JG, Blom A, Doumani R, et al. Response rates and durability of chemotherapy among 62 patients with metastatic Merkel cell carcinoma. Cancer Med 2016;5(9):2294–301.

91. Voog E, Biron P, Martin JP, et al. Chemotherapy for patients with locally advanced or metastatic Merkel cell carcinoma. Cancer 1999;85(12):2589–95.

92. Cimbak N, Barker CA Jr. Short-course radiation therapy for Merkel cell carcinoma: relative effectiveness in a "radiosensitive" tumor. Int J Radiat Oncol 2016;96(2):S160.

93. Lee Y, Auh SL, Wang Y, et al. Therapeutic effects of ablative radiation on local tumor require CD8+ T cells: changing strategies for cancer treatment. Blood 2009;114(3):589–95.

94. Bhatia S, Miller NJ, Lu H, et al. Intratumoral G100, a TLR4 agonist, induces antitumor immune responses and tumor regression in patients with Merkel cell carcinoma. Clin Cancer Res 2019;25(4):1185–95.

95. Bhatia S, Longino NV, Miller NJ, et al. Intratumoral delivery of plasmid IL12 via electroporation leads to regression of injected and noninjected tumors in Merkel cell carcinoma. Clin Cancer Res 2020;26(3):598–607.

96. Westbrook BC, Norwood TG, Terry NLJ, et al. Talimogene laherparepvec induces durable response of regionally advanced Merkel cell carcinoma in 4 consecutive patients. JAAD Case Rep 2019;5(9):782–6.

97. Joshi TP, Farr MA, Hsiou DA, et al. Therapeutic targets for vaccination in polyomavirus-driven Merkel cell carcinoma. Dermatol Ther 2022;35(7):e15580.

98. Goff PH, Bhakuni R, Pulliam T, et al. Intersection of two checkpoints: could inhibiting the DNA damage response checkpoint rescue immune checkpoint-refractory cancer? Cancers (Basel) 2021;13(14):3415.

99. Park DE, Cheng J, Berrios C, et al. Dual inhibition of MDM2 and MDM4 in virus-positive Merkel cell carcinoma enhances the p53 response. Proc Natl Acad Sci U S A 2019;116(3):1027–32.

100. Song L, Bretz AC, Gravemeyer J, et al. The HDAC inhibitor domatinostat promotes cell-cycle arrest, induces apoptosis, and increases immunogenicity of Merkel cell carcinoma cells. J Invest Dermatol 2021;141(4):903–912 e904.

101. Bichakjian CK, Lowe L, Lao CD, et al. Merkel cell carcinoma: critical review with guidelines for multi-disciplinary management. Cancer 2007;110(1): 1–12.
102. Samimi M, Molet L, Fleury M, et al. Prognostic value of antibodies to Merkel cell polyomavirus T antigens and VP1 protein in patients with Merkel cell carcinoma. Br J Dermatol 2016;174(4):813–22.
103. Paulson KG, Lewis CW, Redman MW, et al. Viral oncoprotein antibodies as a marker for recurrence of Merkel cell carcinoma: a prospective validation study. Cancer 2017;123(8):1464–74.
104. Riethdorf S, Hildebrandt L, Heinzerling L, et al. Detection and characterization of circulating tumor cells in patients with Merkel cell carcinoma. Clin Chem 2019;65(3):462–72.

Adnexal and Sebaceous Carcinomas

Edward W. Seger, MD, MS[a], Brett C. Neill, MD[b], Stanislav N. Tolkachjov, MD[b,c,d,e,*]

KEYWORDS

- Adnexal • Carcinoma • Eccrine • Apocrine • Sebaceous • Mohs micrographic surgery
- Skin cancer

KEY POINTS

- Adnexal and sebaceous neoplasms are rare and collectively represent a small percentage of non-melanoma skin cancers.
- Distinction of these neoplasms is essential, as many individual subtypes carry aggressive clinical courses with metastatic potential or may be similar to metastases.
- Surgical treatment is the first line of treatment for nearly all of these neoplasms, with Mohs micrographic surgery an emerging option that may offer superior outcomes given intraoperative margin control.

INTRODUCTION

Adnexal carcinomas (AC) and sebaceous neoplasms are rare malignant neoplasms that are derived from eccrine and apocrine sweat glands or the pilosebaceous unit.[1] Despite the extensive subtypes, they collectively represent a small percentage of non-melanoma skin cancers (NMSC).[2] Distinction of these neoplasms is essential, as many individual subtypes carry aggressive clinical courses with metastatic potential or may be similar to metastases.[2,3] Treatment of these neoplasms varies, with surgical excision being most common.[4] Mohs micrographic surgery (MMS) is increasingly recognized as an effective option and may minimize the risk of recurrence.[4] For this review, apocrine, eccrine, follicular, and sebaceous neoplasms are discussed. For each neoplasm, a review of clinical presentation, classic histologic findings, and management recommendations is provided. The histopathologic characteristics of each neoplasm are outlined in **Table 1** (apocrine and eccrine neoplasms) and **Table 3** (Follicular and Sebaceous Neoplasms). In addition, a summary of management and further workup is provided in **Table 2** (apocrine and eccrine neoplasms) and in **Table 4** (follicular and sebaceous neoplasms).

Malignant Apocrine and Eccrine Tumors

Extramammary Paget disease

Extramammary Paget disease (EMPD) is an adnexal neoplasm of unclear origin; however, Toker cells may represent a benign precursor.[5] EMPD is defined as either primary or secondary, with secondary most often arising from gastrointestinal or urogenital malignancy.[6] Average age of diagnosis is 65 years, and the genital and perianal locations represent most EMPD cases.[7-9] EMPD often presents as a white to red "strawberries and cream" thin plaque that enlarges over time and may be associated with pruritis or burning.[7] MMS is the treatment of choice (TOC), and appropriate screening for underlying malignancy should be performed in confirmed cases.[6,10-12] Overall survival can vary dramatically if associated with underlying malignancy, but appropriately treated primary EMPD has an excellent prognosis.[13]

Funding: None.
[a] Division of Dermatology, University of Kansas Medical Center, Kansas City, KS, USA; [b] Epiphany Dermatology, Dallas, TX, USA; [c] Baylor University Medical Center, Dallas, TX, USA; [d] Texas A&M School of Medicine, Dallas, TX, USA; [e] Derpartment of Dermatology, University of Texas at Southwestern, Dallas, TX, USA
* Corresponding author. Epiphany Dermatology, 1640 FM 544 Suite 100, Lewisville, TX 75056.
E-mail address: stan.tolkachjov@gmail.com

Dermatol Clin 41 (2023) 117–132
https://doi.org/10.1016/j.det.2022.07.010
0733-8635/23/© 2022 Elsevier Inc. All rights reserved.

Table 1
Key histopathologic characteristics of malignant apocrine and eccrine tumors

Tumor	Figure	Histopathologic Characteristics
EMPD	**Fig. 1**	Paget cells are concentrated in lower epidermis, within hair follicles, sweat ducts, and secretory coils. Hyperplastic epidermis with occasional fibroepithelioma-like changes; Intraepidermal acantholytic clefts may be seen.[7]
MAC	**Fig. 2**	Superficial keratinous cysts, small islands, or cords of basaloid and squamous epithelium. Dense hyalinized stroma with smaller nests and strands and frequent perineural invasion.[17]
HAC	**Fig. 3**	Dermal-based basaloid neoplasm comprised of nodules with keloidal and hyalinized stroma and infiltrative borders. Stromal hyalinization and clear cells typical of hidradenoma class of tumors.[22]
EPC	**Fig. 4**	Dermal-based neoplasm comprised of basaloid tumor nodules with ductal differentiation and deep invasion. Poroid cells with partial squamatization, focal tumor necrosis, and ductal formation.[27]
PCMC	**Fig. 5**	Basaloid tumor islands "floating in a lake of mucin." Dermal or subcutaneous mucinous nodule with small epithelial islands.[4]
CC	**Fig. 6**	Asymmetric dermal tumor lacking epidermal connection. Tube-like, duct-forming rows and clear vacuolated tumor cells. May have a prominent vascular component. Periphery may present as a typical cylindroma "jigsaw pattern" of tumor cells with surrounding hyalinized membrane.[54]
MES	**Fig. 7**	Basophilic polygonal neoplastic cells with variable atypia. May have infiltration into subcutaneous fat, central necrosis, and lymphovascular invasion. Periphery may present as typical spiradenoma with nested and trabecular growth and ductal differentiation.[4,55]
ADPA	-	Non-encapsulated basaloid micronodular tumor with solid and cystic components. Papillary projections, tubular, and ductal structures seen. May have focal squamous metaplasia and clear cell change, variable atypia.[56,57]
PCACC	**Fig. 8**	Basophilic neoplastic cells with distinct adenoid or cribriform pattern in mid to reticular dermis. True lumina is surrounded by modified myoepithelial cells with a prominent basement membrane. Cystic spaces occupied by mucin. Frequent perineural invasion.[58]
CMT	-	Well circumscribed tumor in the dermis or subcutis with possible peripheral lymphocytes satellite lesions. Epithelial composed mainly of simple monolayered tubular elements embedded in a myxohyaline and cartilaginous stroma.[59]
PCSC	-	Neoplastic cells densely aggregating in dermis and subcutaneous tissue. Intraductal and invasive components comprised of epithelial cells with bland nuclei and lumina with bubbly eosinophilic secretion. Various growth patterns including solid, tubular, microcystic, and papillary.[47,48]

(continued on next page)

Table 1 (continued)		
Tumor	Figure	Histopathologic Characteristics
AA	Fig. 9	Dermal-based poorly differentiated tumor without epidermal connection. Sheets of severely atypical epithelioid cells that show prominent nucleoli and ductal differentiation.[60] May mimic breast metastasis.
CCC	-	Well circumscribed non-encapsulated dermal nodule with sieve-like spaces at low power. Cribriform and tubular structures are major architectural patterns. Cribriform patterns variable. Variable necrosis which can be focal or en masse, and scarce desmoplastic stroma. No lymphovascular or perineural involvement.[53,61]

Abbreviations: AA, apocrine adenocarcinoma; ADPA, aggressive digital papillary adenocarcinoma; CC, cylindrocarcinoma; CCC, cutaneous cribriform carcinoma; CMT, malignant cutaneous mixed tumor; EMPD, Extramammary Paget disease; EPC, eccrine porocarcinoma; HAC, hidradenocarcinoma; MAC, microcystic adnexal carcinoma; MES, malignant eccrine spiradenoma; PCACC, primary cutaneous adenoid cystic carcinoma; PCMC, primary cutaneous mucinous carcinoma; PCSC, primary cutaneous secretory carcinoma

Microcystic adnexal carcinoma

Microcystic adnexal carcinoma (MAC) is derived from a pluripotent adnexal keratinocyte and has an indolent locally aggressive course with frequent perineural invasion.[14] The average patient is diagnosed in the 7th decade of life, and the head and neck region (HNR), particularly centrofacial area, is the most common site.[15] MAC presents as a skin-colored to yellow slow-growing nodule or plaque which may have associated paresthesia or anesthesia due to frequent perineural invasion.[16–18] MMS is the TOC, as the tumor often extends beyond clinical margins, and recurrence with wide local excision (WLE) is high.[4] Recurrence with MAC is most often local, and metastasis is rare, with disease-specific mortality likely very low.[4,19]

Hidradenocarcinoma

Hidradenocarcinoma (HAC) is of eccrine and apocrine derivation and has a propensity for local recurrence and metastasis.[20,21] Most patients diagnosed with HAC are older, and the scalp has historically been reported as a common site.[4] HAC often presents as a nonspecific skin-colored solitary papule or nodule which may arise from a preexisting hidradenoma.[22–24] Excision is TOC (WLE or MMS), and the utility of sentinel lymph node biopsy (SLNB) or additional imaging is unclear given its rarity.[22,23,25] Adjuvant radiation therapy (RT) is sometimes considered for perineural invasion, as well as for extensive and recurrent tumors.[23] 5-year survival for HAC is 93%; however, disease-specific mortality is unknown.[2]

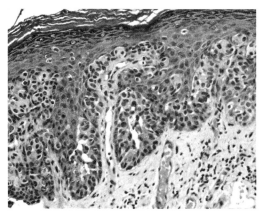

Fig. 1. Extramammary Paget disease. (*Courtesy of* Cary Chisholm, MD, Waco, TX.)

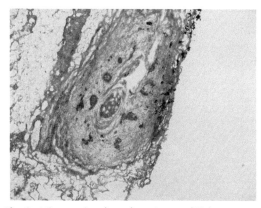

Fig. 2. Microcystic adnexal carcinoma (10x).

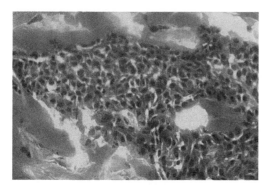

Fig. 3. Hidradenocarcinoma (40x).

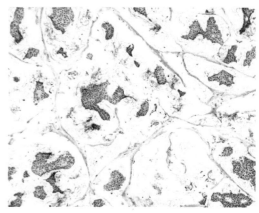

Fig. 5. Primary cutaneous mucinous carcinoma (10x).

Eccrine porocarcinoma

Eccrine porocarcinoma (EPC) is derived from the acrosyringium and may arise de novo or via malignant degeneration of a preexisting eccrine poroma.[26] EPC is often seen in older patients as a pearly pink papule (similar to a basal cell carcinoma) on the lower extremities.[27,28] Excision (WLE or MMS) is TOC, and imaging (ultrasound [US], computed tomography [CT], or Magnetic resonance imaging (MRI) of the regional lymph node [LN] basins) can be considered for higher risk sites such as the trunk, extremities, and genitalia.[27,29] The efficacy of SLNB is unclear; however, it can be considered in larger lesions and those with high mitotic activity.[27,30] Disease-specific survival is unknown, but 5-year overall survival has been reported at 68.8%.[31]

Primary cutaneous mucinous carcinoma

Primary cutaneous mucinous carcinoma (PCMC) is believed to be of eccrine origin and most often follows an indolent course with rare metastasis.[32–34] It is important to distinguish PCMC from cutaneous metastasis (reported from the breast, GI tract, ovary, prostate, or lung) at the time of diagnosis.[4,35] Most patients with PCMC are older, and the periorbital region is the most common site of involvement.[33,34] PCMC is typically a painless erythematous nodule, cyst, or ulcer.[4,34] Surgical excision (WLE or MMS) is the TOC, and MMS may be superior given its tissue-sparing nature and PCMC's propensity for periocular involvement.[4,34] Prognosis is excellent, with 98% of cases localized to the skin at diagnosis; however, close follow-up and age-appropriate cancer screenings should be performed given difficulty differentiating from cutaneous metastasis.[36]

Other adnexal neoplasms

Adnexal neoplasms encompass a diverse group of malignancies that are often differentiated primarily based on histologic variables. A comprehensive

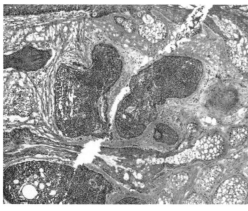

Fig. 4. Eccrine porocarcinoma (10x).

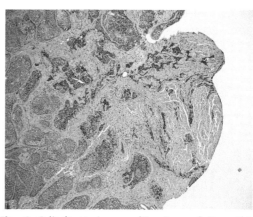

Fig. 6. Cylindrocarcinoma. (*Courtesy of* Cary Chisholm, MD, Waco, TX.)

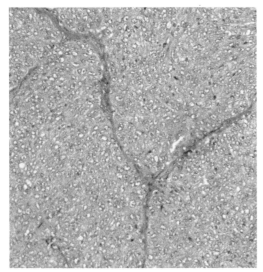

Fig. 7. Malignant eccrine spiradenoma (20x).

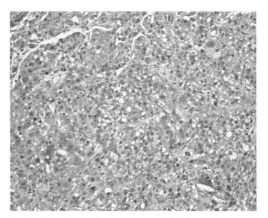

Fig. 9. Apocrine adenocarcinoma (20x).

review of additional adnexal neoplasms, including histology, treatment, and additional management recommendations is included in **Tables 1** and **2** Among these include Endocrine mucin-producing sweat gland carcinoma (EMPSGC) which is distinct from the non-neuroendocrine PCMC and historically more similar to solid papillary

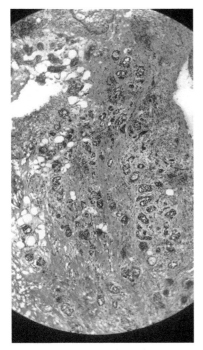

Fig. 8. Primary cutaneous adenoid cystic carcinoma (10x).

carcinoma of the breast.[37] Cylindrocarcinoma (CC) and Malignant eccrine Spiradenoma (MES) exist on a spectrum and may be seen more often in patients with Brook Spiegler Syndrome who are more predisposed to the development of their benign counterparts.[38,39] Aggressive digital papillary adenocarcinoma (ADPA) is most often seen in men and frequently treated with WLE including amputation given high rates of local recurrence and distant metastasis.[40,41] Primary cutaneous adenoid cystic carcinoma (PCACC) presents as a solid to a cystic nodule on the HNR (particularly the scalp) and must be distinguished from cutaneous metastasis from distant gland-bearing organs which are much more common.[42–44] Malignant cutaneous mixed tumor (CMT) is more often seen on the extremities of middle-aged females as an indurated plaque or nodule.[45,46] CMT follows an unpredictable course with recurrence rates over 50% and mortality rates reported at 26%.[45,46] Primary cutaneous secretory carcinoma (PCSC) is most often seen in the axilla as a dermal or subcutaneous nodule. Prognosis is excellent following surgical excision, without reported cases of metastasis or LN involvement.[47,48] Apocrine adenocarcinoma (AA) is hypothesized to arise from apocrine hyperplasia and is seen in apocrine-rich areas such as the axilla as a slow-growing nontender nodule or plaque.[49,50] Surgery is TOC; however, over half of the patients have regional LN involvement at the time of diagnosis.[50,51] AA must be distinguished from other cutaneous metastasis (such as breast or GI) and additional workup should be considered. Cutaneous cribriform carcinoma (CCC) is seen most often in middle-aged females as a subcutaneous nodule on the extremities.[52] Surgery (WLE or MMS) is TOC, and recurrence is rare without reported cases of metastasis.[52,53]

Table 2
Management of malignant apocrine and eccrine tumors

Tumor	Treatment	Associations	SLNB	Further Workup	Follow-up
EMPD	Excision with MMS is TOC.[12,62] Consider scouting biopsies before surgery.	May be associated with internal malignancy (GI, urogenital, breast, among others).[12]	No published guidelines. Some reports suggest considering for all except cases restricted to epidermis on complete histologic examination.[63]	Complete PE including LN, DRE (males), Breast examination (females), urine cytology, colonoscopy, and age-appropriate cancer screenings.[12] Consider imaging (CT, PET) based on clinical suspicion.[12]	No published guidelines.[a]
MAC	Excision with MMS is TOC.[4]	None.	Not routinely recommended for staging.[64]	Complete PE including LN and neurologic examination. Consider CT or MRI based on location and index of suspicion (clinically evident LN, extensive periocular involvement, neurologic symptoms suggestive of bony involvement).[64]	Complete history, PE, and LN examination every 6–12 mo for 5 y[64]
HAC	Excision is TOC (WLE or MMS).[22] Adjunct RT can be considered for perineural involvement.[23]	May arise from benign hidradenoma.	No published guidelines. Some reports advocate for SLNB given high rates of metastasis.[23,25]	No published guidelines. Authors recommend complete PE including LN. Consider imaging if high index of suspicion.	No published guidelines.[a]
EPC	Excision is TOC (MMS or WLE).[4] Margins of 3–5 mm advocated for MMS based on subtype.[65]	May arise from preexisting eccrine poroma.[66]	No published guidelines. Consider in tumors > 7 mm depth and high mitotic rates.[27,30]	No published guidelines. Consider US, CT, MRI of regional lymph node basin for primary tumors on the trunk, extremities, and genitalia/buttock. May consider PET-CT scan for genital/buttock primary tumors given highest rates of distance metastasis.[67]	No published guidelines.[a]

PCMC	Excision is TOC (WLE or MMS).[4,34]	Must distinguish from cutaneous metastasis (including breast, GI, ovary, prostate, and lung).[4]	No published guidelines. Unclear impact on survival. FNA may be useful adjunct in diagnosis.[35]	No published guidelines. Must rule out cutaneous metastasis before diagnosis of PCMC.[68] Consider additional imaging to rule out cutaneous metastasis (mammography, PET-CT, colonoscopy)	No published guidelines.[a] Age-appropriate cancer screenings given risk of underlying malignancy.
EMPSGC	Excision is TOC (WLE or MMS).[37]	Distinct entity from PCMC. Histologically similar to solid papillary carcinoma of breast.[37]	No published guidelines. Likely not needed as no cases of metastasis reported.[37]	Screening mammogram (+/– additional imaging) to rule out metastatic solid papillary carcinoma of breast.[37]	No published guidelines.[a]
CC	Excision is TOC (WLE or MMS).[69,70]	May arise from preexisting cylindroma, particularly in patients with multiple cylindromas (Brooke-Spiegler Syndrome).[38]	No published guidelines. Unclear impact on survival given rare nature of tumor.	No published guidelines. Authors recommend complete PE including LN.	No published guidelines.[a]
MES	Excision is TOC (WLE or MMS).[4,71]	May arise from preexisting spiradenoma, particularly in patients with multiple spiradenomas (Brooke-Spiegler Syndrome).[39]	No published guidelines. Unclear impact on survival given rare nature of tumor.	No published guidelines. Authors recommend complete PE including LN.	No published guidelines.[a]
ADPA	Excision is TOC (WLE or MMS).[41,57] Amputation is common but controversial.[41]	None.	No published guidelines. Unclear impact on survival; however, cases of positive SLNB have been reported.[72,73]	No published guidelines. Reports recommend imaging staging of regional LN's, lung, and abdomen.[57]	No published guidelines.[a]
PCACC	WLE with proposed 2 cm margins given propensity for perineural invasion.[42] Unclear benefit of MMS.	Must distinguish from cutaneous metastasis from gland bearing organs (salivary glands, breasts, and upper and lower respiratory tract, cervix).[42,43]	No published guidelines. Unclear impact on survival given rare nature of tumor.	No published guidelines. Must distinguish from primary metastasis before diagnosis of PCACC.[43] Consider additional imaging such at US, PET-CT, mammography for workup.	No published guidelines. Authors recommend analogous to high-risk SCC at tumor location with PE including LN examination. Age-appropriate cancer screenings.

(continued on next page)

Table 2
(continued)

Tumor	Treatment	Associations	SLNB	Further Workup	Follow-up
CMT	Excision is TOC (WLE or MMS).[45,46]	None	No published guidelines. Unclear impact on survival given rare nature of tumor.	No published guidelines. Authors recommend complete PE including LN. Consider imaging given propensity for metastasis.[45]	No published guidelines.[a]
PCSC	Excision is TOC (WLE reported).[47]	None	No published guidelines. Likely not needed as no cases of metastasis reported.[47]	No published guidelines. Likely not necessary without high clinical suspicion of metastasis.	No published guidelines.[a]
AA	Excision is TOC (WLE or MMS).[50,60] >50% involvement in LN at time of diagnosis.[51]	May arise from apocrine hyperplasia.[49]	No published guidelines. More than 50% have LN involvement at time of diagnosis.[51] Authors recommend consider SLNB in multidisciplinary approach.	No published guidelines. Consider whole body PET-CT, colonoscopy, mammogram to rule out metastasis. Referral to medical oncology	No published guidelines.[a]
CCC	Excision is TOC (WLE or MMS).[47,52]	None	No published guidelines. Likely not needed as no cases of metastasis reported.[52,53]	No published guidelines. Likely not necessary without high clinical suspicion of metastasis.	No published guidelines.[a]

Abbreviations: AA, apocrine adenocarcinoma; ADPA, aggressive digital papillary adenocarcinoma; CC, cylindrocarcinoma; CCC, cutaneous cribriform carcinoma; CMT, malignant cutaneous mixed tumor; CT, computerized tomography; DRE, digital rectal examination; EMPD, extramammary paget disease; EPC, eccrine porocarcinoma; FNA, fine needle aspiration; GI, gastrointestinal; HAC, hidradenocarcinoma; LN, lymph nodes; MAC, microcystic adnexal carcinoma; MES, malignant eccrine spiradenoma; MMS, Mohs micrographic surgery; MRI, magnetic resonance imaging; PCACC, primary cutaneous adenoid cystic carcinoma; PCMC, primary cutaneous mucinous carcinoma; PCSC, primary cutaneous secretory carcinoma; PE, physical examination; PET-CT, Positron emission tomography – computerized tomography; RT, radiation therapy; SLNB, sentinel lymph node biopsy; TOC, treatment of choice; US, ultrasound; WLE, wide local excision.

[a] Authors recommend analogous to high-risk SCC at tumor location.

Table 3
Key histopathologic characteristics of malignant follicular and sebaceous tumors

Tumor	Figure	Histopathologic Characteristics
TLC	Fig. 10	Neoplasm with lobular, infiltrative growth centered on pilosebaceous unit. Tumor cells are large, polygonal, and clear with glycogen rich cytoplasm. Periphery is often palisaded with occasional pagetoid spread. Trichilemmal keratinization seen. Features similar to trichilemmoma but with cellular atypia.[75]
PC	Fig. 11	Nests of basaloid cells with infrequent eosinophilic ghost "shadow cells".[82] Possible areas of necrosis and mitosis of basaloid cells.[82] Tumor cells surrounded by fibrous desmoplastic stroma.[82]
TBC	Fig. 12	Epithelial keratinocyte hyperplasia with clear cytoplasm.[98] Multiple cords and strands of atypical keratinocytes with deep extension into the dermis.[98] May have extension to adipose and muscle.[99]
SC	Fig. 13	Irregular dermal based unencapsulated aggregates of basaloid and sebaceous cells.[96] "Frothy" appearance of cells due to lipid granules.[96] Variable atypia, with possible extension to vascular, lymphatic, and perineural structures.[96]

Abbreviations: PC, pilomatrix carcinoma; SC, sebaceous carcinoma; TBC, trichoblastic carcinoma; TLC, Trichilemmal carcinoma.

Malignant Follicular Tumors

Trichilemmal carcinoma
Derived from the outer root sheath, Trichilemmal carcinoma (TLC) is most often seen in older patients (mean age 73 years) and generally follows a relatively benign course.[74,75] TLC classically presents in the HNR as a slow-growing papule of nodule with secondary features suggestive of NMSC such as ulceration and telangiectasias.[74,76,77] Excision (WLE or MMS) is TOC, and no guidelines for additional workup exist; however, TLC rarely metastasizes and the prognosis is excellent.[75,76]

Pilomatrix carcinoma
Pilomatrix carcinoma (PC) is derived from the follicular matrix and may arise de novo or via malignant transformation of pilomatrixoma.[78] PC is classically diagnosed in the 6th and 7th decades of life and males are more often affected.[79,80]

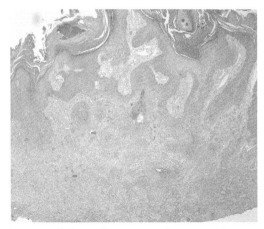

Fig. 10. Trichilemmal carcinoma. (*Courtesy of* Ross M. Levy, MD, Mt Kisco, NY and T Cibull, MD, Evanston, IL.)

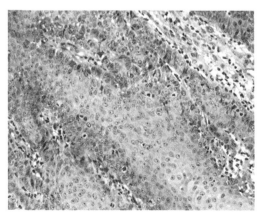

Fig. 11. Pilomatrix carcinoma (10x).

Table 4
Management of malignant follicular and sebaceous tumors

Tumor	Treatment	Associations	SLNB	Imaging	Follow-up
TLC	Excision is TOC (WLE or MMS).[76,100]	No established link with Cowden Disease; however, case reports have postulated this association.[101]	No published guidelines. Likely not needed due to exceedingly rare metastasis.	No published guidelines. Likely not needed due to exceedingly rare metastasis.	No published guidelines.[a]
PC	Excision is TOC (WLE or MMS).[79,82]	May arise from preexisting pilomatrixoma.[102] No established link with conditions involving multiple pilomatrixomas (Gardner syndrome, Rubinstein-Taybi syndrome, Sotos Syndrome, myotonic dystrophy, and Turners syndrome).[80]	No published guidelines. Not performed in most reported cases.[103]	No published guidelines. Not performed in most reported cases.[80]	No published guidelines.[80,a]
TBC	Excision is TOC (WLE or MMS).[84,87]	May arise from preexisting trichoblastoma.[85]	No published guidelines. Not performed in most reported cases.[91]	No published guidelines. Not performed in most reported cases.[91]	No published guidelines.[a]
SC	Excision with MMS is TOC for all SC.[92]	Muir-Torre Syndrome. Solid organ transplant recipients 90 times more likely to develop SC.[93]	Consider for periocular SC stage T2C and above.[92] Not recommended for extraocular SC.[92]	CT or PET-CT considered only in cases of confirmed nodal metastasis.[92]	Every 6 mo for 3 y, then annually.[92]

Abbreviations: CT, computerized tomography; MMS, Mohs micrographic surgery; PC, pilomatrix carcinoma; PET-CT, Positron emission tomography – computerized tomography; SC, sebaceous carcinoma; TBC, trichoblastic carcinoma; TLC, Trichilemmal carcinoma; TOC, treatment of choice; WLE, wide local excision.
[a] Authors recommend analogous to high-risk SCC at tumor location.

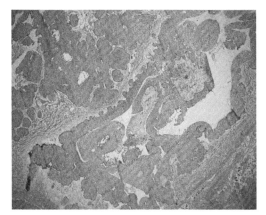

Fig. 12. Trichoblastic carcinoma (4x).

The HNR (especially midface) is the most common location and PC often presents as a cyst-like slow-growing dermal nodule.[80,81] Excision (WLE or MMS) is TOC, and no guidelines for workup exist.[82,83] Metastasis is rare, reported mostly to regional LN, and mortality from PC is likely low.[80]

Trichoblastic carcinoma

Trichoblastic carcinoma (TBC) is derived from the follicular germinal cells and may arise de novo or via malignant transformation of a trichoblastoma.[84,85] TBC most often presents in older patients (mean age of 65 years) in the HNR.[84] Clinical presentation varies widely and includes slow-growing nodules to vegetative tumors.[84] Excision (WLE or MMS) is TOC and is generally curative.[84,86,87] Rare metastasis has been reported, mostly to regional LN, and most cases do not perform SLNB or additional workup at the time of diagnosis.[88–91]

Malignant Sebaceous Tumors

Sebaceous carcinoma

Sebaceous carcinoma (SC) is derived from the adnexal epithelium of sebaceous glands and is most known for its association with Muir-Torre syndrome.[92] Average age at diagnosis is 60 to 70 years with solid organ transplant patients up to 90 times higher risk.[92,93] SC is commonly differentiated as periocular or extraocular, with the HNR the most common extraocular site.[92] Periocular SC occurs in both white and Asian patients; however, extraocular SC almost always arises in white patients.[92] SC often appears as a yellow to pink papule or nodule, but presentation is variable.[94] MMS is the treatment of choice, and SLNB can be considered for periocular cases which have higher rates of nodal metastasis.[92,95] Genetic testing for extraocular SC is recommended for patients with a Mayo Muir-Torre syndrome risk of 2 or greater, but is not routinely recommended for periocular SC.[92] The prognosis of completely excised SC is good, and the most significant predictor of decreased survival is the presence of metastatic disease at the time of diagnosis.[96,97]

SUMMARY

Adnexal and sebaceous neoplasms represent uncommon malignancies with varying predispositions for recurrence and metastasis. As a result of their rare nature, guidelines for management and monitoring are often anecdotal and based on a limited review of case reports. A focused review of literature and expert recommendations on the diagnosis, treatment, prognosis, and follow-up for the management of these tumors are presented.

CLINICS CARE POINTS

- Recurrence rates following Mohs micrographic surgery are often lower than wide local excision for adnexal and sebaceous neoplasms.

- Due to the rarity of many adnexal and sebaceous carcinomas, risk of metastasis and long term prognosis is difficult to establish. Future research in this area can help fill our practice gaps.

DISCLOSURE

The authors have no conflicts of interest to declare.

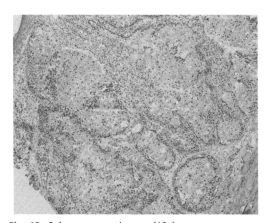

Fig. 13. Sebaceous carcinoma (10x).

REFERENCES

1. Mehregan AH. The origin of the adnexal tumors of the skin: a viewpoint. J Cutan Pathol 1985;12(6): 459–67.
2. Blake PW, Bradford PT, Devesa SS, et al. Cutaneous appendageal carcinoma incidence and survival patterns in the United States: a population-based study. Arch Dermatol 2010;146(6):625–32. https://doi.org/10.1001/archdermatol.2010.105.
3. Avraham JB, Villines D, Maker VK, et al. Survival after resection of cutaneous adnexal carcinomas with eccrine differentiation: risk factors and trends in outcomes. J Surg Oncol 2013;108(1):57–62. https://doi.org/10.1002/jso.23346.
4. Tolkachjov SN. Adnexal Carcinomas Treated With Mohs Micrographic Surgery: A Comprehensive Review. Dermatol Surg 2017;43(10):1199–207. https://doi.org/10.1097/DSS.0000000000001167.
5. Belousova IE, Kazakov DV, Michal M, et al. Vulvar toker cells: the long-awaited missing link: a proposal for an origin-based histogenetic classification of extramammary paget disease. Am J Dermatopathol 2006;28(1):84–6. https://doi.org/10.1097/01.dad.0000194052.65695.f1.
6. Merritt BG, Degesys CA, Brodland DG. Extramammary Paget Disease. Dermatol Clin 2019;37(3): 261–7. https://doi.org/10.1016/j.det.2019.02.002.
7. Morris CR, Hurst EA. Extramammary Paget Disease: A Review of the Literature-Part I: History, Epidemiology, Pathogenesis, Presentation, Histopathology, and Diagnostic Work-up. Dermatol Surg 2020;46(2):151–8. https://doi.org/10.1097/dss.0000000000002064.
8. Fanning J, Lambert HC, Hale TM, et al. Paget's disease of the vulva: prevalence of associated vulvar adenocarcinoma, invasive Paget's disease, and recurrence after surgical excision. Am J Obstet Gynecol 1999;180(1 Pt 1):24–7. https://doi.org/10.1016/s0002-9378(99)70143-2.
9. Kageyama N, Izumi AK. Bilateral scrotal extramammary Paget's disease in a Chinese man. Int J Dermatol 1997;36(9):695–7. https://doi.org/10.1046/j.1365-4362.1997.00044.x.
10. Lee KY, Roh MR, Chung WG, Chung KY. Comparison of Mohs micrographic surgery and wide excision for extramammary Paget's Disease: Korean experience. Dermatol Surg 2009;35(1):34–40. https://doi.org/10.1111/j.1524-4725.2008.34380.x.
11. Morris CR, Hurst EA. Extramammary Paget's Disease: A Review of the Literature Part II: Treatment and Prognosis. Dermatol Surg 2020;46(3):305–11. https://doi.org/10.1097/dss.0000000000002240.
12. Schmitt AR, Long BJ, Weaver AL, et al. Evidence-Based Screening Recommendations for Occult Cancers in the Setting of Newly Diagnosed Extramammary Paget Disease. Mayo Clin Proc 2018; 93(7):877–83. https://doi.org/10.1016/j.mayocp.2018.02.024.
13. Karam A, Dorigo O. Treatment outcomes in a large cohort of patients with invasive Extramammary Paget's disease. Gynecol Oncol 2012;125(2):346–51. https://doi.org/10.1016/j.ygyno.2012.01.032.
14. Goldstein DJ, Barr RJ, Santa Cruz DJ. Microcystic adnexal carcinoma: a distinct clinicopathologic entity. Cancer 1982;50(3):566–72.
15. Amon G, Liszewski W, Maher IA. Epidemiology and Survival of Microcystic Adnexal Carcinoma by Sex in the United States. Dermatol Surg 2021;47(1): 127–9. https://doi.org/10.1097/DSS.0000000000002167.
16. Billingsley EM, Fedok F, Maloney ME. Microcystic adnexal carcinoma. Case report and review of the literature. Arch Otolaryngol Head Neck Surg 1996;122(2):179–82. https://doi.org/10.1001/archotol.1996.01890140065012.
17. Gordon S, Fischer C, Martin A, Rosman IS, Council ML. Microcystic Adnexal Carcinoma: A Review of the Literature. Dermatol Surg 2017;43(8): 1012–6. https://doi.org/10.1097/DSS.0000000000001142.
18. Bier-Laning CM, Hom DB, Gapany M, Manivel JC, Duvall AJ 3rd. Microcystic adnexal carcinoma: management options based on long-term followup. Laryngoscope 1995;105(11):1197–201. https://doi.org/10.1288/00005537-199511000-00011.
19. Behbahani S, Yeh CJ, Pinto JO, et al. Microcystic adnexal carcinoma of the head and neck: Characteristics, treatment, and survival statistics. Dermatol Ther 2021;34(1):e14559. https://doi.org/10.1111/dth.14559.
20. Gauerke S, Driscoll JJ. Hidradenocarcinomas: a brief review and future directions. Arch Pathol Lab Med 2010;134(5):781–5.
21. Cooper PH. Carcinomas of sweat glands. Pathol Annu 1987;22(Pt 1):83–124.
22. Tolkachjov SN, Hocker TL, Hochwalt PC, et al. Mohs micrographic surgery for the treatment of hidradenocarcinoma: the Mayo Clinic experience from 1993 to 2013. Dermatol Surg 2015;41(2):226–31. https://doi.org/10.1097/DSS.0000000000000242.
23. Soni A, Bansal N, Kaushal V, et al. Current management approach to hidradenocarcinoma: a comprehensive review of the literature. Ecancermedicalscience 2015;9:517. https://doi.org/10.3332/ecancer.2015.517.
24. Lim SC, Lee MJ, Lee MS, et al. Giant hidradenocarcinoma: a report of malignant transformation from nodular hidradenoma. Pathol Int 1998;48(10): 818–23. https://doi.org/10.1111/j.1440-1827.1998.tb03843.x.
25. Cohen M, Cassarino DS, Shih HB, et al. Apocrine hidradenocarcinoma of the scalp: a classification

conundrum. Head Neck Pathol 2009;3(1):42–6. https://doi.org/10.1007/s12105-008-0096-8.

26. Brown CW Jr, Dy LC. Eccrine porocarcinoma. Dermatol Ther 2008;21(6):433–8. https://doi.org/10.1111/j.1529-8019.2008.00243.x.

27. Tolkachjov SN, Hocker TL, Camilleri MJ, et al. Treatment of Porocarcinoma With Mohs Micrographic Surgery: The Mayo Clinic Experience. Dermatol Surg 2016;42(6):745–50. https://doi.org/10.1097/DSS.0000000000000763.

28. Snow SN, Reizner GT. Eccrine porocarcinoma of the face. J Am Acad Dermatol 1992;27(2 Pt 2):306–11. https://doi.org/10.1016/0190-9622(92)70187-k.

29. Song SS, Wu Lee W, Hamman MS, et al. Mohs micrographic surgery for eccrine porocarcinoma: an update and review of the literature. Dermatol Surg 2015;41(3):301–6. https://doi.org/10.1097/DSS.0000000000000286.

30. Robson A, Greene J, Ansari N, et al. Eccrine porocarcinoma (malignant eccrine poroma): a clinicopathologic study of 69 cases. Am J Surg Pathol 2001;25(6):710–20. https://doi.org/10.1097/00000478-200106000-00002.

31. Behbahani S, Malerba S, Karanfilian KM, et al. Demographics and outcomes of eccrine porocarcinoma: results from the National Cancer Database. Br J Dermatol 2020;183(1):161–3. https://doi.org/10.1111/bjd.18874.

32. Lennox B, Pearse AG, Richards HG. Mucin-secreting tumours of the skin with special reference to the so-called mixed-salivary tumour of the skin and its relation to hidradenoma. J Pathol Bacteriol 1952;64(4):865–80. https://doi.org/10.1002/path.1700640418.

33. Breiting L, Christensen L, Dahlstrøm K, et al. Primary mucinous carcinoma of the skin: a population-based study. Int J Dermatol 2008;47(3):242–5. https://doi.org/10.1111/j.1365-4632.2008.03558.x.

34. Kamalpour L, Brindise RT, Nodzenski M, et al. Primary cutaneous mucinous carcinoma: a systematic review and meta-analysis of outcomes after surgery. JAMA Dermatol 2014;150(4):380–4. https://doi.org/10.1001/jamadermatol.2013.6006.

35. Reid-Nicholson M, Iyengar P, Friedlander MA, et al. Fine needle aspiration biopsy of primary mucinous carcinoma of the skin: a case report. Acta Cytol 2006;50(3):317–22. https://doi.org/10.1159/000325961.

36. Behbahani S, Pinto JO, Wassef D, et al. Analysis of Head and Neck Primary Cutaneous Mucinous Carcinoma: An Indolent Tumor of the Eccrine Sweat Glands. J Craniofac Surg 2021;32(3):e244–7. https://doi.org/10.1097/scs.0000000000006968.

37. Agni M, Raven ML, Bowen RC, et al. An Update on Endocrine Mucin-producing Sweat Gland Carcinoma: Clinicopathologic Study of 63 Cases and Comparative Analysis. Am J Surg Pathol 2020;44(8):1005–16. https://doi.org/10.1097/pas.0000000000001462.

38. Borik L, Heller P, Shrivastava M, et al. Malignant cylindroma in a patient with Brooke-Spiegler syndrome. Dermatol Pract Concept 2015;5(2):61–5. https://doi.org/10.5826/dpc.0502a09.

39. Dabska M. Malignant transformation of eccrine spiradenoma. Pol Med J 1972;11(2):388–96.

40. Balci MG, Tayfur M, Deger AN, et al. Aggressive papillary adenocarcinoma on atypical localization: A unique case report. Medicine (Baltimore) 2016;95(28):e4110. https://doi.org/10.1097/md.0000000000004110.

41. Hsu HC, Ho CY, Chen CH, et al. Aggressive digital papillary adenocarcinoma: a review. Clin Exp Dermatol 2010;35(2):113–9. https://doi.org/10.1111/j.1365-2230.2009.03490.x.

42. Ferreira S, Conde Fernandes I, Coelho A, et al. Primary cutaneous adenoid cystic carcinoma of the abdomen: a rare entity. Dermatol Online J 2020;26(8). 13030/qt0q979406.

43. Rocas D, Asvesti C, Tsega A, et al. Primary adenoid cystic carcinoma of the skin metastatic to the lymph nodes: immunohistochemical study of a new case and literature review. Am J Dermatopathol 2014;36(3):223–8. https://doi.org/10.1097/DAD.0b013e31829ae1e7.

44. van der Kwast TH, Vuzevski VD, Ramaekers F, et al. Primary cutaneous adenoid cystic carcinoma: case report, immunohistochemistry, and review of the literature. Br J Dermatol 1988;118(4):567–77. https://doi.org/10.1111/j.1365-2133.1988.tb02469.x.

45. Sánchez Herreros C, Belmar Flores P, De Eusebio Murillo E, et al. A case of cutaneous malignant mixed tumor treated with mohs micrographic surgery. Dermatol Surg 2011;37(2):267–70. https://doi.org/10.1111/j.1524-4725.2010.01865.x.

46. Lal K, Morrell TJ, Cunningham M, et al. A Case of a Malignant Cutaneous Mixed Tumor (Chondroid Syringoma) of the Scapula Treated With Staged Margin-Controlled Excision. Am J Dermatopathol 2018;40(9):679–81. https://doi.org/10.1097/dad.0000000000001131.

47. Llamas-Velasco M, Mentzel T, Rütten A. Primary cutaneous secretory carcinoma: A previously overlooked low-grade sweat gland carcinoma. *J Cutan Pathol* Mar 2018;45(3):240–5. https://doi.org/10.1111/cup.13092.

48. Ahn CS, Sangüeza OP. Malignant Sweat Gland Tumors. Hematol Oncol Clin North Am 2019;33(1):53–71. https://doi.org/10.1016/j.hoc.2018.09.002.

49. Miyamoto T, Hagari Y, Inoue S, et al. Axillary apocrine carcinoma with benign apocrine tumours: a case report involving a pathological and

immunohistochemical study and review of the literature. J Clin Pathol 2005;58(7):757–61. https://doi.org/10.1136/jcp.2004.019794.

50. Dhawan SS, Nanda VS, Grekin S, et al. Apocrine adenocarcinoma: case report and review of the literature. J Dermatol Surg Oncol 1990;16(5):468–70. https://doi.org/10.1111/j.1524-4725.1990.tb00066.x.

51. Chamberlain RS, Huber K, White JC, et al. Apocrine gland carcinoma of the axilla: review of the literature and recommendations for treatment. Am J Clin Oncol 1999;22(2):131–5. https://doi.org/10.1097/00000421-199904000-00005.

52. Rütten A, Kutzner H, Mentzel T, et al. Primary cutaneous cribriform apocrine carcinoma: a clinicopathologic and immunohistochemical study of 26 cases of an under-recognized cutaneous adnexal neoplasm. J Am Acad Dermatol 2009;61(4):644–51. https://doi.org/10.1016/j.jaad.2009.03.032.

53. Arps DP, Chan MP, Patel RM, et al. Primary cutaneous cribriform carcinoma: report of six cases with clinicopathologic data and immunohistochemical profile. J Cutan Pathol 2015;42(6):379–87. https://doi.org/10.1111/cup.12469.

54. Durani BK, Kurzen H, Jaeckel A, et al. Malignant transformation of multiple dermal cylindromas. Br J Dermatol 2001;145(4):653–6. https://doi.org/10.1046/j.1365-2133.2001.04460.x.

55. Russ BW, Meffert J, Bernert R. Spiradenocarcinoma of the scalp. Cutis 2002;69(6):455–8.

56. Chen ELA, Nijhawan RI. Aggressive Digital Papillary Adenocarcinoma Initially Misdiagnosed as Basal Cell Carcinoma. Dermatol Surg 2021;47(1):137–9. https://doi.org/10.1097/dss.0000000000002173.

57. Knackstedt RW, Knackstedt TJ, Findley AB, et al. Aggressive digital papillary adenocarcinoma: treatment with Mohs micrographic surgery and an update of the literature. Int J Dermatol 2017;56(10):1061–4. https://doi.org/10.1111/ijd.13712.

58. Naylor E, Sarkar P, Perlis CS, et al. Primary cutaneous adenoid cystic carcinoma. J Am Acad Dermatol 2008;58(4):636–41. https://doi.org/10.1016/j.jaad.2007.12.005.

59. Kazakov DV, Kacerovska D, Hantschke M, et al. Cutaneous mixed tumor, eccrine variant: a clinicopathologic and immunohistochemical study of 50 cases, with emphasis on unusual histopathologic features. Am J Dermatopathol 2011;33(6):557–68. https://doi.org/10.1097/DAD.0b013e318206c1a3.

60. Tolkachjov SN, Brewer JD, Bridges AG. Apocrine Axillary Adenocarcinoma: An Aggressive Adnexal Tumor in Middle-Age Individuals. Dermatol Surg 2018;44(6):876–8. https://doi.org/10.1097/dss.0000000000001430.

61. Wu JD, Changchien CH, Liao KS. Primary cutaneous cribriform apocrine carcinoma: Case report and literature review. Indian J Dermatol Venereol Leprol 2018;84(5):569–72. https://doi.org/10.4103/ijdvl.IJDVL_830_16.

62. Asel M, LeBoeuf NR. Extramammary Paget's Disease. Hematol Oncol Clin North Am 2019;33(1):73–85. https://doi.org/10.1016/j.hoc.2018.09.003.

63. Hatta N, Morita R, Yamada M, et al. Sentinel lymph node biopsy in patients with extramammary Paget's disease. Dermatol Surgt 2004;30(10):1329–34. https://doi.org/10.1111/j.1524-4725.2004.30377.x.

64. Worley B, Owen JL, Barker CA, et al. Evidence-Based Clinical Practice Guidelines for Microcystic Adnexal Carcinoma: Informed by a Systematic Review. JAMA Dermatol 2019;155(9):1059–68. https://doi.org/10.1001/jamadermatol.2019.1251.

65. Belin E, Ezzedine K, Stanislas S, et al. Factors in the surgical management of primary eccrine porocarcinoma: prognostic histological factors can guide the surgical procedure. Br J Dermatol 2011;165(5):985–9. https://doi.org/10.1111/j.1365-2133.2011.10486.x.

66. Shaw M, McKee PH, Lowe D, et al. Malignant eccrine poroma: a study of twenty-seven cases. Br J Dermatol 1982;107(6):675–80. https://doi.org/10.1111/j.1365-2133.1982.tb00527.x.

67. Wick MR, Goellner JR, Wolfe JT 3rd, et al. Adnexal carcinomas of the skin. I. Eccrine carcinomas. Cancer 1985;56(5):1147–62.

68. Adefusika JA, Pimentel JD, Chavan RN, et al. Primary mucinous carcinoma of the skin: the Mayo Clinic experience over the past 2 decades. Dermatol Surg 2015;41(2):201–8. https://doi.org/10.1097/dss.0000000000000198.

69. Kuklani RM, Glavin FL, Bhattacharyya I. Malignant cylindroma of the scalp arising in a setting of multiple cylindromatosis: a case report. Head Neck Pathol 2009;3(4):315–9. https://doi.org/10.1007/s12105-009-0138-x.

70. Lo JS, Peschen M, Snow SN, et al. Malignant cylindroma of the scalp. J Dermatol Surg Oncol 1991;17(11):897–901. https://doi.org/10.1111/j.1524-4725.1991.tb03281.x.

71. Staiger RD, Helmchen B, Papet C, et al. Spiradenocarcinoma: A Comprehensive Data Review. Am J Dermatopathol 2017;39(10):715–25. https://doi.org/10.1097/dad.0000000000000910.

72. Altman CE, Hamill RL, Elston DM. Metastatic aggressive digital papillary adenocarcinoma. Cutis 2003;72(2):145–7.

73. Kempton SJ, Navarrete AD, Salyapongse AN. Aggressive Digital Papillary Adenocarcinoma: Case Report of a Positive Sentinel Lymph Node and Discussion of Utility of Sentinel Lymph Node

Biopsy. Ann Plast Surg 2015;75(1):34–6. https://doi.org/10.1097/sap.0000000000000111.

74. Reis JP, Tellechea O, Cunha MF, et al. Trichilemmal carcinoma: review of 8 cases. J Cutan Pathol 1993; 20(1):44–9. https://doi.org/10.1111/j.1600-0560.1993.tb01248.x.

75. Hamman MS, Brian Jiang SI. Management of trichilemmal carcinoma: an update and comprehensive review of the literature. Dermatol Sur 2014;40(7):711–7. https://doi.org/10.1111/dsu.0000000000000002.

76. Wong TY, Suster S. Tricholemmal carcinoma. A clinicopathologic study of 13 cases. Am J Dermatopatho 1994;16(5):463–73. https://doi.org/10.1097/00000372-199410000-00001.

77. Boscaino A, Terracciano LM, Donofrio V, et al. Tricholemmal carcinoma: a study of seven cases. J Cutan Pathol 1992;19(2):94–9. https://doi.org/10.1111/j.1600-0560.1992.tb01349.x.

78. Lever WF, Griesemer RD. Calcifying epithelioma of Malherbe; report of 15 cases, with comments on its differentiation from calcified epidermal cyst and on its histogenesis. Arch Derm Syphilol 1949;59(5):506–18. https://doi.org/10.1001/archderm.1949.01520300016003.

79. Allaoui M, Hubert E, Michels JJ. Malignant pilomatricoma: two new observations and review of the relevant literature. Turk Patoloji Derg 2014;30(1):66–8. https://doi.org/10.5146/tjpath.2013.01205.

80. Jones C, Twoon M, Ho W, et al. Pilomatrix carcinoma: 12-year experience and review of the literature. J Cutan Pathol 2018;45(1):33–8. https://doi.org/10.1111/cup.13046.

81. Gazic B, Sramek-Zatler S, Repse-Fokter A, et al. Pilomatrix carcinoma of the clitoris. Int J Surg Pathol 2011;19(6):827–30. https://doi.org/10.1177/1066896910397882.

82. Sable D, Snow SN. Pilomatrix carcinoma of the back treated by mohs micrographic surgery. Dermatol Surg 2004;30(8):1174–6. https://doi.org/10.1111/j.1524-4725.2004.30350.x.

83. Xing L, Marzolf SA, Vandergriff T, et al. Facial pilomatrix carcinomas treated with Mohs micrographic surgery. JAAD Case Rep 2018;4(3):253–5. https://doi.org/10.1016/j.jdcr.2018.02.003.

84. Boettler MA, Shahwan KT, Abidi NY, et al. Trichoblastic carcinoma: a comprehensive review of the literature. Arch Dermatol Res 2022;314(5):399–403.

85. Schulz T, Proske S, Hartschuh W, et al. High-grade trichoblastic carcinoma arising in trichoblastoma: a rare adnexal neoplasm often showing metastatic spread. Am J Dermatopathol 2005;27(1):9–16. https://doi.org/10.1097/01.dad.0000142240.93956.cb.

86. Kwock JT, Casady M, Handfield C, et al. A trichogenic tumor with aggressive features

87. Toberer F, Rütten A, Requena L, et al. Eosinophilrich trichoblastic carcinoma with aggressive clinical course in a young man. J Cutan Pathol 2017;44(11):986–90. https://doi.org/10.1111/cup.13031.

88. Battistella M, Mateus C, Lassau N, et al. Sunitinib efficacy in the treatment of metastatic skin adnexal carcinomas: report of two patients with hidradenocarcinoma and trichoblastic carcinoma. J Eur Acad Dermatol Venereol 2010;24(2):199–203. https://doi.org/10.1111/j.1468-3083.2009.03301.x.

89. Regauer S, Beham-Schmid C, Okcu M, et al. Trichoblastic carcinoma ("malignant trichoblastoma") with lymphatic and hematogenous metastases. Mod Pathol 2000;13(6):673–8. https://doi.org/10.1038/modpathol.3880118.

90. Nguyen BD, Seetharam M, Ocal TI. 18F-FDG PET/CT Imaging of Trichoblastic Carcinoma With Nodal Metastasis. Clin Nucl Med 2019;44(7):e423–4. https://doi.org/10.1097/rlu.0000000000002622.

91. Laffay L, Depaepe L, d'Hombres A, et al. Histological features and treatment approach of trichoblastic carcinomas: from a case report to a review of the literature. Tumori 2012;98(2):46e–9e. https://doi.org/10.1700/1088.11948.

92. Owen JL, Kibbi N, Worley B, et al. Sebaceous carcinoma: evidence-based clinical practice guidelines. Lancet Oncol 2019;20(12):e699–714. https://doi.org/10.1016/s1470-2045(19)30673-4.

93. Hoss E, Nelson SA, Sharma A. Sebaceous carcinoma in solid organ transplant recipients. Int J Dermatol 2017;56(7):746–9. https://doi.org/10.1111/ijd.13490.

94. Nelson BR, Hamlet KR, Gillard M, et al. Sebaceous carcinoma. J Am Acad Dermatol 1995;33(1):1–15. https://doi.org/10.1016/0190-9622(95)90001-2. quiz 16-8.

95. Esmaeli B, Nasser QJ, Cruz H, et al. American Joint Committee on Cancer T category for eyelid sebaceous carcinoma correlates with nodal metastasis and survival. Ophthalmology 2012;119(5):1078–82. https://doi.org/10.1016/j.ophtha.2011.11.006.

96. Kyllo RL, Brady KL, Hurst EA. Sebaceous carcinoma: review of the literature. Dermatol Surg 2015;41(1):1–15. https://doi.org/10.1097/dss.0000000000000152.

97. Tryggvason G, Bayon R, Pagedar NA. Epidemiology of sebaceous carcinoma of the head and neck: implications for lymph node management. Head Neck 2012;34(12):1765–8. https://doi.org/10.1002/hed.22009.

98. Garcia A, Nguyen JM, Stetson CL, et al. Facial trichoblastic carcinoma treated with Mohs

initially diagnosed as basal cell carcinoma. Dermatol Online J 2018;24(9).

micrographic surgery: A new indication for Mohs? JAAD Case Rep 2020;6(6):561–2. https://doi.org/10.1016/j.jdcr.2020.02.004.

99. Leeman A, de Cuba EMV, Jaspars LH, et al. A Low-Grade Trichoblastic Carcinoma Treated with Mohs Micrographic Surgery. Case Rep Dermatol 2021; 13(1):129–33. https://doi.org/10.1159/000512871.

100. Tolkachjov SN, Hocker TL, Camilleri MJ, et al. Mohs micrographic surgery in the treatment of trichilemmal carcinoma: the Mayo Clinic experience. J Am Acad Dermatol 2015;72(1):195–6. https://doi.org/10.1016/j.jaad.2014.10.007.

101. Ha JH, Lee C, Lee KS, et al. The molecular pathogenesis of Trichilemmal carcinoma. BMC Cancer 2020;20(1):516.   https://doi.org/10.1186/s12885-020-07009-7.

102. Nishioka M, Tanemura A, Yamanaka T, et al. Pilomatrix carcinoma arising from pilomatricoma after 10-year senescent period: Immunohistochemical analysis. J Dermatol 2010;37(8):735–9. https://doi.org/10.1111/j.1346-8138.2010.00887.x.

103. Herrmann JL, Allan A, Trapp KM, et al. Pilomatrix carcinoma: 13 new cases and review of the literature with emphasis on predictors of metastasis. J Am Acad Dermatol 2014;71(1):38–43.e2.

Cutaneous Mesenchymal Sarcomas

Frances Walocko, MD[a], Rachel E. Christensen, BS[a], Brandon Worley, MD[b],
Murad Alam, MD, MBA, MSCI[a,c,d,e],*

KEYWORDS

- Cutaneous mesenchymal sarcoma • Mohs micrographic surgery • Nonmelanoma skin cancer
- Dermatologic surgery

KEY POINTS

- Cutaneous mesenchymal sarcomas are rare malignancies that lack consensus guidelines on staging, management, and treatment.
- The preferred modality of treatment of locally invasive cutaneous mesenchymal sarcomas is Mohs micrographic surgery or wide local excision.
- Local recurrence is higher, and larger margins are often required for the complete removal of cutaneous mesenchymal sarcomas compared with other forms of nonmelanoma skin cancer.

INTRODUCTION

Cutaneous mesenchymal sarcomas develop from the soft tissue of the dermis and subcutis. Given the overall rarity of these cutaneous malignancies, limited consensus guidelines exist on staging and management. This article provides an overview on evaluation, diagnosis, staging, and management of the most reported cutaneous mesenchymal sarcomas, including dermatofibrosarcoma protuberans (DFSP), atypical fibroxanthoma (AFX), pleomorphic dermal sarcoma (PDS), cutaneous angiosarcoma, myofibrosarcoma, and leiomyosarcoma.

DISCUSSION

Dermatofibrosarcoma Protuberans

DFSP is a soft tissue tumor that involves the dermis, subcutis, and rarely the muscle or fascia. Incidence rate ranges from 0.8 to 5 cases per million persons per year.[1–3] The tumor typically presents as an indurated, slow-growing plaque that can be violaceous, pink, or hyperpigmented (**Fig. 1**A). The most common location is the trunk (50%), followed by the extremities (35%) and head/neck (15%).[2,4–6] DFSP most commonly presents in patients aged from 20 to 50 years.[2] A chromosomal translocation between chromosomes 17 and 22 (t(17:22)) presents in a significant number of DFSP cases and is thought to play a key role in tumor pathogenesis.[7]

Diagnosis should be performed with a biopsy to the deep subcutaneous tissue. On histopathologic evaluation, spindled tumor cells are arranged in a "storiform" architecture with infiltration from the dermis into underlying tissue (**Fig. 1**B).[8] Immunohistochemistry can aid in diagnosis. CD34 is commonly positive (**Fig. 1**C), whereas Factor 13a is negative.[2,9] DFSP with fibrosarcomatous change (FS-DSFP) on histology are thought to be associated with a more aggressive clinical course

[a] Department of Dermatology, Feinberg School of Medicine, Northwestern University, 676 North Saint Clair Street, 1600, Chicago, IL 60611, USA; [b] Florida Dermatology and Skin Cancer Centers, 421 Linden Lane, Lake Wales, Lake Wales, FL 33853, USA; [c] Department of Surgery, Feinberg School of Medicine, Northwestern University, 676 North Saint Clair Street, 1600, Chicago, IL 60611, USA; [d] Department of Otolaryngology, Feinberg School of Medicine, Northwestern University, 676 North Saint Clair Street, 1600, Chicago, IL 60611, USA; [e] Department of Medical Social Sciences, Feinberg School of Medicine, Northwestern University, 676 North Saint Clair Street, 1600, Chicago, IL 60611, USA
* Corresponding author. Department of Dermatology, Feinberg School of Medicine, Northwestern University, 676 North Saint Clair Street, 1600, Chicago, IL 60611.
E-mail address: m-alam@northwestern.edu

Dermatol Clin 41 (2023) 133–140
https://doi.org/10.1016/j.det.2022.07.011

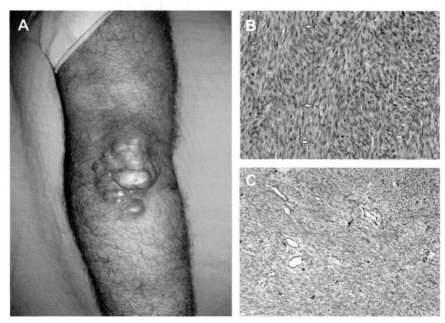

Fig. 1. Dermatofibrosarcoma protuberans. (*A*) Indurated skin-colored plaque on upper extremity. (*B*) Spindled tumor cells with mitoses (*arrows*) arranged in elongated fascicles (H&E). (*C*) CD34 expression by tumor cells. (*From* [*A*] Brooks J, Ramsey ML. Dermatofibrosarcoma Protuberans. In: StatPearls. Treasure Island (FL): StatPearls Publishing; 2022. Licensed under CC BY 4.0; and [*B*] Chen Y, Shi YZ, Feng XH, Wang XT, He XL, Zhao M. Novel TNC-PDGFD fusion in fibrosarcomatous dermatofibrosarcoma protuberans: a case report. Diagn Pathol. 2021 Jul 13;16(1):63. Licensed under CC BY 4.0.)

with increased potential for metastatic spread but research is conflicting.[10] Fibrosarcomatous change occurs when spindle cells are seen intersecting at angles, forming a "herringbone" pattern.[11] The National Comprehensive Cancer Network (NCCN) recommends that FS-DFSP be treated similar to visceral sarcomas; management is not covered by their guidelines for DFSP.[12,13]

No staging system is specific for DFSP; however, larger diameter tumors tend to be more infiltrative and have been associated with a higher potential for metastasis. Whether these metastases resulted from missed FS-DFSP is unclear. Sentinel lymph node biopsy (SLNB) or regional node dissection is currently not recommended because there is no known benefit and node-positive disease is rare. MRI may be useful in larger or recurrent tumors to evaluate for infiltrative disease.[14] Treatment should follow the NCCN guidelines as summarized here.[12,13] Local disease is treated with surgical resection with a goal of complete extirpation to minimize recurrence. Mohs micrographic surgery (MMS) or complete circumferential peripheral and deep margin assessment are preferred to prevent the escape of any infiltrative strands that could be missed by the traditional bread loaf processing. However, when wide local excision (WLE) is chosen, margin

sizes of 2 to 4 cm are required to reduce the chance of recurrence.[12] Radiation may be used as an adjuvant therapy after surgery or considered in cases where surgery is contraindicated.[12,15] Therapeutics that target platelet-derived growth factor receptor, such as imatinib, may be considered in advanced or metastatic disease.[16]

Local recurrence can surpass 60%, even with clear surgical margins. However, recent reviews have shown recurrence rates at 7% to 9% with WLE and 1% to 1.5% with MMS.[2,17,18] Recurrences tend to occur within 3 years of excision.[2] Distant metastasis is rare (<5%), with the most common location being the lung.[19]

Atypical Fibroxanthoma/Pleomorphic Dermal Sarcoma

AFX and PDS are both rare, fibrohistiocytic tumors of mesenchymal origin.[20] AFX is typically located within the dermis, whereas PDS often presents within deeper subcutaneous spread and can invade into fascia and deeper tissue (**Fig 2A**).[20] PDS is considered a more aggressive tumor with increased morbidity and mortality compared with AFX. It is currently unclear if AFX and PDS exist on a clinicopathologic spectrum or are distinct entities. Both cutaneous tumors clinically present

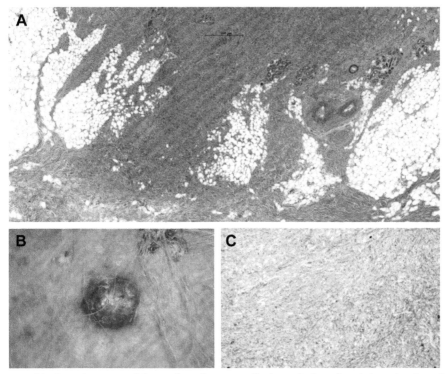

Fig. 2. Pleomorphic dermal sarcoma. (*A*) Invasion of tumor cells through the subcutis into the deep fascia (H&E, magnification 30×). (*B*) Exophytic, violaceous nodule located on the scalp. (*C*) CD10 expression by tumor cells. (*From* [*A, B*] Bowe CM, Godhania B, Whittaker M, Walsh S. Pleomorphic dermal sarcoma: a clinical and histological review of 49 cases. Br J Oral Maxillofac Surg. 2021 May;59(4):460-465; and [*C*] Klebanov N, Hoang MP, Reddy BY. Pleomorphic Dermal Sarcoma of the Scalp. Cureus. 2018 Jul 13;10(7):e2979. Licensed under CC BY 4.0.)

with exophytic, ulcerated, violaceous to erythematous nodules (**Fig. 2**B). The most common location is the head or neck in an elderly patient.[20,21]

Biopsy to the deep subcutaneous tissue should be performed for diagnosis. Histologic features of AFX include haphazardly arranged pleomorphic, atypical-appearing spindle cells that extend into the reticular dermis or superficial subcutaneous fat.[20] PDS has similar histologic features but with deeper subcutaneous invasion. Tumor necrosis, perineural invasion, and/or lymphovascular invasion may be seen. CD10 and procollagen-1 positivity can help distinguish AFX and PDS from other histologic mimickers, such as spindle cell melanoma or squamous cell carcinoma (**Fig. 2**C).[20,22] However, CD10 may be negative in AFX, leading to diagnostic challenges. CD99 may help distinguish AFX from PDS because it shows moderate to strong and diffuse staining in AFX in contrast with weaker and focal staining in PDS; larger studies are needed demonstrating these staining patterns.[23]

No consensus guidelines exist for staging (including SLNB) or treatment. Imaging, such as MRI, may be helpful for PDS given the deeper

invasion and increased metastatic potential.[21] WLE was historically the standard of care for both AFX and PDS with an average margin of at least 2 cm. Clinical tumor width size is proportional to the margins needed to clear most tumors of that size.[24] MMS is the preferred surgical modality for AFX; studies are limited for the treatment of PDS with MMS. Radiation may be used for the treatment of poor surgical candidates.

AFX recurrence rates when treated with MMS and WLE are 2.7% and 9.4%, respectively.[18,25] Recurrence typically occurs within 2 years.[21] The metastasis rate ranges from 1% to 5%.[18,21] It is possible that some aggressive AFX tumors could have been misclassified in studies and were in fact PDS. PDS has an overall higher local recurrence and metastatic rate at 20% to 28% and 10% to 42%, respectively.[26,27] Risk factors for metastasis include tumor site (trunk or extremities), tumor size (larger than 2 cm), invasion beyond subcutaneous fat, and lymphovascular invasion.[28]

Overall, AFX is an indolent but locally invasive tumor with 20-year survival rate of greater than 97%.[29,30] PDS has a 61.9% 5-year disease-specific survival.[31] Risk factors for overall mortality mirror those that predispose a patient to metastasis. Older age (>60) patients have poorer survival compared with those in a younger cohort.[28]

Cutaneous Angiosarcoma

Cutaneous angiosarcoma is a rare, aggressive vascular tumor (incidence rate of 2.25 per 100,000).[32] It most commonly arises as an erythematous or violaceous plaque on the head or neck in elderly, Caucasian patients (**Fig. 3**A).[33] Delays in diagnosis may occur as angiosarcoma can mimic an ecchymosis or hematoma.[34] There are several tumor subtypes: classic angiosarcoma of the head and neck, angiosarcoma associated with lymphedema (Stewart-Treves syndrome), angiosarcoma arising in sites of previous irradiation, and epithelioid angiosarcoma.[34]

Histologic features include irregular vascular channels with atypical spindle cells. Tumors with poor-differentiation may seem as sheets of spindled-shaped or epithelioid-shaped cells with increased mitotic activity (**Fig.** 3B).[34] Positive staining for CD31 and CD34 can help confirm the diagnosis (**Fig.** 3C).[34] S-100, smooth muscle actin, and desmin are typically negative.[34]

No consensus guidelines exist for staging or management. SLNB is currently not recommended given lack of data. MRI may help delineate tumor extension in larger lesions.[34] Surgical removal with WLE is considered the standard of care but recurrence rates are high. MMS is not recommended in these tumors as noncontiguous spread is common, making reliable margin control with narrow margins infeasible.[18] Adjuvant radiation is often recommended because it improves local disease control after WLE.[33] Taxane-based chemotherapy may be considered for distant disease but the benefit on overall survival is unclear.[33] Targeted therapies against vascular endothelial growth factor, tropomyosin receptor kinase, and mitogen-activated protein kinase are under investigation but data are limited.[35] A multidisciplinary approach is key given the high recurrence and metastases rate.[34]

Local recurrence rates with WLE with and without radiation or chemotherapy range from 43% to 100%.[33,36,37] Recurrence rates following MMS are unknown. Metastatic rates range from 36% to 49%.[33] Five-year disease-specific survival ranges between 12% and 60%.[32,33] Older age, tumor size (>5 cm), presence of satellite cutaneous lesions, and tumor location (scalp) are associated with poor prognosis.[32,33]

Myofibrosarcoma

Myofibrosarcoma is a rare sarcoma comprising myofibroblasts. They most often occur in the deep soft tissue but can also be found in subcutaneous tissue, submucosa, or bone.[38] The typical presentation is an indurated papule or nodule but they can be clinically indistinct to identify them by morphology alone.[34,39] A biopsy is required for diagnosis. An estimated one-third of cases are observed on the head and neck, although cases have been reported on the upper extremities and trunk.[40]

The tumor presents on histopathology as unencapsulated sheets of long, uniform spindle cells in fascicular or storiform patterns (**Fig.** 4A).[38] Abnormal mitotic figures may be seen but necrosis is rarely observed.[40] Positive staining for smooth muscle actin (**Fig.** 4B), desmin, calponin, vimentin, and factor XIIIA may help confirm the

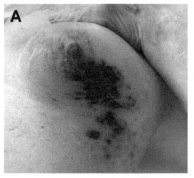
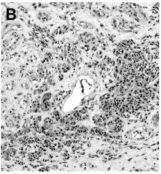
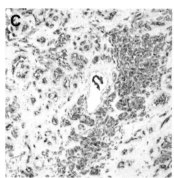

Fig. 3. Cutaneous angiosarcoma. (*A*) Erythematous plaque arising on the left breast following irradiation. (*B*) Sheets of atypical spindle cells (H&E, magnification 20×). (*C*) CD31 expression by tumor cells. (*From* [*A*] Abbenante D, Malossa M, Raone B. Radiation-Induced Cutaneous Angiosarcoma of the Breast. Am J Med. 2020;133(10):1156-1157; and [*B, C*] Verdura V, Di Pace B, Concilio M, Guastafierro A, Fiorillo G, Alfano L, Nicoletti GF, Savastano C, Cascone AM, Rubino C. A new case of radiation-induced breast angiosarcoma. Int J Surg Case Rep. 2019;60:152-155. Licensed under CC BY 4.0.)

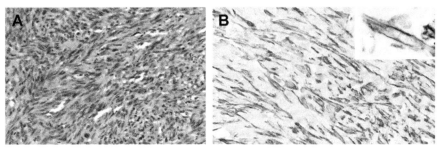

Fig. 4. Myofibrosarcoma. (A) Spindle cells arranged in fascicular pattern. (B) Positive stain for smooth-muscle actin with peripheral enhancement (top corner). (*From* Fisher C. Myofibrosarcoma. Virchows Arch. 2004 Sep;445(3):215-23.)

diagnosis.[34,40] H-caldesmon (protein expressed in smooth and nonsmooth muscle cells) negativity can help differentiate myofibrosarcoma from leiomyosarcoma.[40]

No consensus guidelines exist for staging, SLNB, or management. Myofibrosarcoma is most often treated by WLE. Patients may benefit from adjunctive radiotherapy or chemotherapy but data on best practices are lacking.[39,41]

Myofibrosarcomas are characterized by aggressive spread to adjacent structures with local recurrence rates between 18% and 54%.[38,39,41] Metastasis is rare but several cases of spread to the lungs have been reported.[38,39,42] Data are lacking on survival rates given the rarity of this tumor.

Leiomyosarcoma

Leiomyosarcomas are malignant tumors originating from smooth muscle cells. They represent 0.04% of all tumors and 2% to 3% of all soft tissue sarcomas.[43,44] Leiomyosarcomas are categorized as cutaneous or subcutaneous. Cutaneous leiomyosarcomas, also referred to as superficial or dermal leiomyosarcomas, most often present on hair-bearing surfaces of the body as a solitary, slowly growing, firm pink nodule (Fig. 5A).[45,46] Subcutaneous leiomyosarcomas present as a deeper, well-defined nodule.[44,47] Both cutaneous and subcutaneous leiomyosarcomas most frequently affect patients between 50 and 80 years of age.[44]

Diagnosis requires biopsy to the deep subcutaneous tissue.[46] On histopathology, tumors contain fascicles of spindle cells with hyperchromatic, blunt-ended nuclei (Fig. 5B).[39,46,47] Varied cellularity can be present with some tumors demonstrating a nodular pattern with high cellularity, nuclear atypia, and necrosis, whereas others have a diffuse pattern with low cellularity, well-differentiated cells, and no necrosis.[46,47] Tumors stain positive for vimentin, smooth muscle actin (Fig. 5C), H-caldesmon, and calponin in most cases.[39,48]

No consensus guidelines exist for staging or management specifically for leiomyosarcoma. SLNB is unclear in its utility. Initial management is with WLE using 2 to 5 cm margins; however, no consensus exists for most appropriate margin size.[40] Adjuvant radiotherapy has been documented in some treatment approaches, although

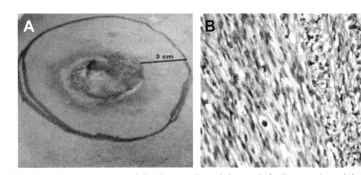
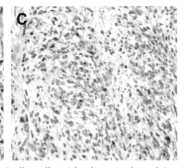

Fig. 5. Leiomyosarcoma. (A) Ulcerated nodule on left iliac region. (B) Spindle cells with elongated nuclei arranged in a fascicular pattern with abnormal mitoses and areas of necrosis (H&E). (C) Expression of smooth muscle actin by tumor cells. (*From* Antakle M, Alshaghel MM, Ghannam G, Al-Ibraheem M, Shehade L, Agha S, Etr A. Primary cutaneous Leiomyosarcoma on the left iliac region: A rare case report from Syria. Ann Med Surg (Lond). 2021 Oct 30;71:102992. Licensed under CC BY 4.0.)

Table 1
Management of cutaneous mesenchymal sarcomas

Tumor	Local Disease	Locally Advanced, Margin Positive or Metastatic Disease
Dermatofibrosarcoma protuberans	Based on NCCN guidelines:[12] MMS or CCDMA are preferred. Consider radiation for positive surgical margins	Imatinib Chemotherapy Radiation
Atypical fibroxanthoma	MMS or CCPDMA is preferred	Radiation
Pleomorphic dermal sarcoma	No consensus. MMS or CCPDMA may have advantages over WLE	Radiation
Cutaneous angiosarcoma	WLE ± radiation. MMS or CCPDMA discouraged	Radiation Chemotherapy
Myofibrosarcoma	WLE. Margin control techniques can be tissue sparing	Radiation Chemotherapy
Leiomyosarcoma Cutaneous Subcutaneous	No consensus guidelines: MMS, CCPDMA or WLE WLE ± radiation	Radiation Radiation

Abbreviations: CCPDMA, complete circumferential and deep margin assessment; MMS, Mohs micrographic surgery; NCCN, National Comprehensive Cancer Network; WLE, wide local excision.

evidence-based recommendations for its use are lacking.[43]

Limited data exist on recurrence, prognosis, and survival. Overall, local recurrence rates for cutaneous leiomyosarcoma range from 18% to 35% and metastasis rates range from 12% to 14%.[49] Subcutaneous leiomyosarcoma carries an increased risk of recurrence and metastasis, with regional recurrence reported in 28% to 61% of cases and metastasis in 51% to 62% of cases.[49] Metastatic spread occurs most commonly to the lung.[42,49] Five-year overall survival is estimated at 98% for cutaneous leiomyosarcoma and 88% for subcutaneous leiomyosarcoma. Tumor size of 5 cm or greater, fascial involvement, and high histologic grade may be associated with decreased survival.[50–52]

SUMMARY

Cutaneous mesenchymal sarcomas are rare entities with limited guidelines on diagnosis, staging, and management. A summary of management is provided to assist clinicians when encountering these tumors (**Table 1**). Higher rates of local recurrence with surgical excision are experienced compared with more common forms of nonmelanoma skin cancer. In addition, patients with cutaneous angiosarcoma, PDS, and subcutaneous leiomyosarcoma are at higher risk of metastatic disease. Collection of tumor characteristics and treatment outcomes within large databases may help further standardize the management of these rare carcinomas.

CLINICS CARE POINTS

- Cutaneous mesenchymal sarcomas are a diverse group of neoplasms that require individualized care and, sometimes, multidisciplinary consultation because there is a lack of evidence-based guidelines.

- With the exception of angiosarcoma, margin control with complete circumferential and peripheral deep margin assessment allows for tissue sparing while reducing the chance of recurrence.

- Immunohistochemistry is often helpful to confirm the diagnosis and rule out mimickers.

- Metastasis rates vary within the group of tumors. The lungs are a favorite distant site for spread.

DISCLOSURE

The authors have no conflicts of interest to disclose.

REFERENCES

1. Criscione VD, Weinstock MA. Descriptive epidemiology of dermatofibrosarcoma protuberans in the United States, 1973 to 2002. J Am Acad Dermatol 2007;56(6):968–73.

2. Bogucki B, Neuhaus I, Hurst EA. Dermatofibrosarcoma protuberans: a review of the literature. Dermatol Surg 2012;38(4):537–51.

3. Tolkachjov SN, Schmitt AR, Muzic JG, et al. Incidence and Clinical Features of Rare Cutaneous Malignancies in Olmsted County, Minnesota, 2000 to 2010. Dermatol Surg 2017;43(1):116–24.

4. Bowne WB, Antonescu CR, Leung DH, et al. Dermatofibrosarcoma protuberans: A clinicopathologic analysis of patients treated and followed at a single institution. Cancer 2000;88(12):2711–20.

5. Chang CK, Jacobs IA, Salti GI. Outcomes of surgery for dermatofibrosarcoma protuberans. Eur J Surg Oncol 2004;30(3):341–5.

6. Gloster HM. Dermatofibrosarcoma protuberans. J Am Acad Dermatol 1996;35(3 Pt 1):355–74.

7. Pedeutour F, Simon MP, Minoletti F, et al. Ring 22 chromosomes in dermatofibrosarcoma protuberans are low-level amplifiers of chromosome 17 and 22 sequences. Cancer Res 1995;55(11):2400–3.

8. Hao X, Billings SD, Wu F, et al. Dermatofibrosarcoma Protuberans: Update on the Diagnosis and Treatment. J Clin Med 2020;9(6):1752.

9. Kim HJ, Lee JY, Kim SH, et al. Stromelysin-3 expression in the differential diagnosis of dermatofibroma and dermatofibrosarcoma protuberans: comparison with factor XIIIa and CD34. Br J Dermatol 2007;157(2):319–24.

10. Liang CA, Jambusaria-Pahlajani A, Karia PS, et al. A systematic review of outcome data for dermatofibrosarcoma protuberans with and without fibrosarcomatous change. J Am Acad Dermatol 2014;71(4):781–6.

11. Wrotnowski U, Cooper PH, Shmookler BM. Fibrosarcomatous change in dermatofibrosarcoma protuberans. Am J Surg Pathol 1988;12(4):287–93.

12. Miller SJ, Alam M, Andersen JS, et al. Dermatofibrosarcoma protuberans. J Natl Compr Canc Netw 2012;10(3):312–8.

13. National Comprehensive Cancer Network. Dermatofibrosarcoma protuberans. Available at: NCCN.org. Accessed January 18, 2022.

14. Thornton SL, Reid J, Papay FA, et al. Childhood dermatofibrosarcoma protuberans: role of preoperative imaging. J Am Acad Dermatol 2005;53(1):76–83.

15. Chen YT, Tu WT, Lee WR, et al. The efficacy of adjuvant radiotherapy in dermatofibrosarcoma protuberans: a systemic review and meta-analysis. J Eur Acad Dermatol Venereol 2016;30(7):1107–14.

16. Navarrete-Dechent C, Mori S, Barker CA, et al. Imatinib Treatment for Locally Advanced or Metastatic Dermatofibrosarcoma Protuberans: A Systematic Review. JAMA Dermatol 2019;155(3):361–9.

17. Foroozan M, Sei JF, Amini M, et al. Efficacy of Mohs micrographic surgery for the treatment of dermatofibrosarcoma protuberans: systematic review. Arch Dermatol 2012;148(9):1055–63.

18. Rosenfeld DJ, Cappel MA, Tolkachjov SN. Cutaneous mesenchymal tumors treated with Mohs micrographic surgery: a comprehensive review. Int J Dermatol 2021;60(11):1334–42.

19. Rutgers EJ, Kroon BB, Albus-Lutter CE, et al. Dermatofibrosarcoma protuberans: treatment and prognosis. Eur J Surg Oncol 1992;18(3):241–8.

20. Soleymani T, Aasi SZ, Novoa R, et al. Atypical Fibroxanthoma and Pleomorphic Dermal Sarcoma: Updates on Classification and Management. Dermatol Clin 2019;37(3):253–9.

21. Phelan PS, Rosman IS, Council ML. Atypical Fibroxanthoma: The Washington University Experience. Dermatol Surg 2019;45(12):1450–8.

22. de Feraudy S, Mar N, McCalmont TH. Evaluation of CD10 and procollagen 1 expression in atypical fibroxanthoma and dermatofibroma. Am J Surg Pathol 2008;32(8):1111–22.

23. Hartel PH, Jackson J, Ducatman BS, et al. CD99 immunoreactivity in atypical fibroxanthoma and pleomorphic malignant fibrous histiocytoma: a useful diagnostic marker. J Cutan Pathol 2006;33(Suppl 2):24–8.

24. Jibbe A, Worley B, Miller CH, et al. Surgical excision margins for fibrohistiocytic tumors, including atypical fibroxanthoma and undifferentiated pleomorphic sarcoma: A probability model based on a systematic review. J Am Acad Dermatol 2021. S0190-9622(21)02519-02526.

25. Tolkachjov SN, Kelley BF, Alahdab F, et al. Atypical fibroxanthoma: Systematic review and meta-analysis of treatment with Mohs micrographic surgery or excision. J Am Acad Dermatol 2018;79(5):929–34.e6.

26. Miller K, Goodlad JR, Brenn T. Pleomorphic dermal sarcoma: adverse histologic features predict aggressive behavior and allow distinction from atypical fibroxanthoma. Am J Surg Pathol 2012;36(9):1317–26.

27. Tardío JC, Pinedo F, Aramburu JA, et al. Pleomorphic dermal sarcoma: a more aggressive neoplasm than previously estimated. J Cutan Pathol 2016;43(2):101–12.

28. Winchester D, Lehman J, Tello T, et al. Undifferentiated pleomorphic sarcoma: Factors predictive of adverse outcomes. J Am Acad Dermatol 2018;79(5):853–9.

29. Koch M, Freundl AJ, Agaimy A, et al. Atypical Fibroxanthoma - Histological Diagnosis, Immunohistochemical Markers and Concepts of Therapy. Anticancer Res 2015;35(11):5717–35.

30. Sandhu N, Sauvageau AP, Groman A, et al. Cutaneous Leiomyosarcoma: A SEER Database Analysis. Dermatol Surg 2020;46(2):159–64.

31. Ibanez MA, Rismiller K, Knackstedt T. Prognostic factors, treatment, and survival in cutaneous pleomorphic sarcoma. J Am Acad Dermatol 2020;83(2):388–96.

32. Conic RRZ, Damiani G, Frigerio A, et al. Incidence and outcomes of cutaneous angiosarcoma: A SEER population-based study. J Am Acad Dermatol 2020;83(3):809–16.

33. Guadagnolo BA, Zagars GK, Araujo D, et al. Outcomes after definitive treatment for cutaneous angiosarcoma of the face and scalp. Head Neck 2011;33(5):661–7.

34. Hollmig ST, Sachdev R, Cockerell CJ, et al. Spindle cell neoplasms encountered in dermatologic surgery: a review. Dermatol Surg 2012;38(6):825–50.

35. Wagner MJ, Lyons YA, Siedel JH, et al. Combined VEGFR and MAPK pathway inhibition in angiosarcoma. Sci Rep 2021;11(1):9362.

36. Maddox JC, Evans HL. Angiosarcoma of skin and soft tissue: a study of forty-four cases. Cancer 1981;48(8):1907–21.

37. Pawlik TM, Paulino AF, McGinn CJ, et al. Cutaneous angiosarcoma of the scalp: a multidisciplinary approach. Cancer 2003;98(8):1716–26.

38. Montgomery E, Goldblum JR, Fisher C. Myofibrosarcoma: a clinicopathologic study. Am J Surg Pathol 2001;25(2):219–28.

39. Mentzel T, Dry S, Katenkamp D, et al. Low-grade myofibroblastic sarcoma: analysis of 18 cases in the spectrum of myofibroblastic tumors. Am J Surg Pathol 1998;22(10):1228–38.

40. Fisher C. Myofibrosarcoma. Virchows Arch 2004; 445(3):215–23.

41. Keller C, Gibbs CN, Kelly SM, et al. Low-grade myofibrosarcoma of the head and neck: importance of surgical therapy. J Pediatr Hematol Oncol 2004; 26(2):119–20.

42. Watanabe K, Ogura G, Tajino T, et al. Myofibrosarcoma of the bone: a clinicopathologic study. Am J Surg Pathol 2001;25(12):1501–7.

43. Wong GN, Webb A, Gyorki D, et al. Cutaneous leiomyosarcoma: dermal and subcutaneous. Australas J Dermatol 2020;61(3):243–9.

44. Rodríguez-Lomba E, Molina-López I, Parra-Blanco V, et al. Clinical and Histopathologic Findings of Cutaneous Leiomyosarcoma: Correlation with Prognosis in 12 Patients. Actas dermo-sifiliograficas 2018;109(2):140–7.

45. Ciurea ME, Georgescu C v, Radu CC, et al. Cutaneous leiomyosarcoma - Case report. J Med Life 2014;7(2):270–3.

46. Chalfant V, Schriber T, Sabri A, et al. Primary Cutaneous Leiomyosarcoma of the Lower Extremity: A Case Report and Literature Review. Cureus 2021; 13(4):e14282.

47. Soares Queirós C, Filipe P, Soares de Almeida L. Cutaneous leiomyosarcoma: a 20-year retrospective study and review of the literature. An Bras Dermatol 2021;96(3):278–83.

48. González-Sixto B, de la Torre C, Pardavila R, et al. Leiomyosarcoma arising from scrofuloderma scar. Clin Exp Dermatol 2008;33(6):776–8.

49. Kaddu S, Beham A, Cerroni L, et al. Cutaneous leiomyosarcoma. Am J Surg Pathol 1997;21(9):979–87.

50. Murphy-Chutorian B, Routt E, Vinelli G, et al. A Systematic Review of the Treatment of Superficial Leiomyosarcoma With Mohs Micrographic Surgery. Dermatol Surg 2019;45(12):1437–41.

51. Winchester DS, Hocker TL, Brewer JD, et al. Leiomyosarcoma of the skin: clinical, histopathologic, and prognostic factors that influence outcomes. J Am Acad Dermatol 2014;71(5):919–25.

52. Jensen ML, Jensen OM, Michalski W, et al. Intradermal and subcutaneous leiomyosarcoma: a clinicopathological and immunohistochemical study of 41 cases. J Cutan Pathol 1996;23(5):458–63.

Cutaneous Oncology in the Immunosuppressed

Leo L. Wang, MD, PhD[a,1], Stephanie K. Lin, BA[b,1], Carolyn M. Stull, MD[a],
Thuzar M. Shin, MD, PhD[a], H. William Higgins, MD, MBE[a], Cerrene N. Giordano, MD[a],
Stacy L. McMurray, MD[a], Jeremy R. Etzkorn, MD[a], Christopher J. Miller, MD[a],
Joanna L. Walker, MD[a,*]

KEYWORDS

- Immunosuppression • Organ transplant recipients • Keratinocyte carcinoma • Melanoma
- Merkel cell carcinoma • Kaposi sarcoma • Chronic lymphocytic leukemia • HIV

KEY POINTS

- The risk of developing skin cancers increases with higher doses, longer duration, and certain types of immunosuppression; therefore, proactive management of immunosuppressants can reduce skin cancer risk.
- Managing advanced skin cancers in immunosuppressed patients often requires interdisciplinary teams to weigh the risks and benefits of surgery, radiation, or systemic therapy.
- Close surveillance and early detection can prevent immunosuppressed patients from developing advanced skin cancers.

INTRODUCTION

Compared with the general population, patients with immunodeficiencies and lymphoproliferative disorders have an increased risk for frequent and aggressive skin cancers (**Table 1**). Immunosuppression reduces immune-mediated tumor surveillance, increases activation of oncogenic viruses (ie, human papillomavirus [HPV], Merkel cell polyomavirus [MCPyV]), and promotes oncogenesis.[1] This review covers the management of skin cancers (excluding cutaneous lymphomas) in acquired and iatrogenic immunodeficiencies.

SKIN CANCER IN ACQUIRED IMMUNODEFICIENCIES
Chronic Lymphocytic Leukemia

Chronic lymphocytic leukemia (CLL), the most common type of adult-onset leukemia, is associated with increased risk for developing keratinocyte carcinoma (KC, an inclusive term for both basal cell carcinoma [BCC] and squamous cell carcinoma [SCC]) and other skin cancers (**Table 2**). CLL lymphocytes downregulate CD40 ligand expression on activating T cells, impairing antigen presentation and tumor surveillance, thus creating an immunosuppressed milieu where tumors may behave more aggressively.[2] KCs have higher rates of subclinical spread, and peritumoral lymphocytic infiltrates make histologic assessment more challenging[3]; this leads to 7 to 14 times higher local recurrence following Mohs micrographic surgery (MMS) compared with controls.[4] In CLL patients with SCC, mortality is as high from SCC as from CLL.[5] In addition, overall survival (OS) and disease-specific survival (DSS) are worse for melanoma, Merkel cell carcinoma (MCC), and SCC when concomitant CLL is present.[2–4]

[a] Department of Dermatology, Perelman Center for Advanced Medicine, University of Pennsylvania, 1st Floor South Pavilion, 3400 Civic Center Boulevard, Philadelphia, PA 19104, USA; [b] Donald and Barbara Zucker School of Medicine at Hofstra/Northwell, 500 Hofstra Boulevard, Hempstead, NY 11549, USA
[1] Co-first author.
* Corresponding author.
E-mail address: joanna.walker@pennmedicine.upenn.edu

Dermatol Clin 41 (2023) 141–162
https://doi.org/10.1016/j.det.2022.07.012

Table 1
Immunosuppressive conditions associated with increased skin cancer risk

Lymphoproliferative Disorder	Genetic and Acquired Immunodeficiencies	Iatrogenic Immunodeficiencies
• Chronic lymphocytic leukemia (CLL) • Hodgkin lymphoma • Non-Hodgkin lymphoma • Multiple myeloma	• Human immunodeficiency virus (HIV)/AIDS • Primary immune deficiency diseases • Rheumatologic and autoimmune diseases (medication and/or immune dysregulation risk)	• Solid organ transplant • Hematopoietic stem cell transplant • Rheumatologic and autoimmune diseases Immunosuppressive medications in solid organ transplant recipients • Calcineurin inhibitors (cyclosporine, tacrolimus) • mTOR inhibitors (sirolimus, everolimus) • Azathioprine Immunosuppressive/modulating medications in rheumatologic and autoimmune disease • Corticosteroids • Methotrexate • Anti-TNF therapy

Abbreviation: TNF, tumor necrosis factor.

Human Immunodeficiency Virus

Human immunodeficiency virus (HIV) infection is associated with increased risk of several cutaneous malignancies and requires specific management considerations (**Table 3**).[6–9] Among individuals with HIV, lower CD4 count (<200 cells/mm^3) and higher viral load (≥10,000 copies/mm^3) are strongly associated with risk of SCC in particular (**Fig. 1**).[7] Notably, patients with HIV are at increased risk of anogenital SCC, often related to high-risk HPV strains.[6] HPV vaccination is recommended for all HIV-positive individuals younger than 26 years, regardless of CD4 count, and may be beneficial beyond this age range for high-risk individuals including men who have sex with men.[8] The most common cutaneous malignancy in HIV-infected individuals is Kaposi sarcoma (KS), although incidence has decreased significantly following widespread use of combination antiretroviral therapy (cART).[7]

SKIN CANCER IN ORGAN TRANSPLANT RECIPIENTS

Immunosuppression to prevent rejection of transplanted organs increases malignancy risk. Skin cancer accounts for nearly 50% of all malignancies in organ transplant recipients (OTRs) and is the most common cause of cancer-related death in this population (**Table 4**). Skin cancers have a higher risk to metastasize in OTRs. For example, SCC metastasizes at a rate of 8% in OTRs compared with less than 5% in the general population (**Fig. 2**).[10]

KCs comprise most of the skin cancers (>90%) in OTRs.[11] Although BCC is more common in the immunocompetent population, SCC is more common in OTRs.[10,12–16]

Pretransplant Approach

Risk stratification
Before transplant, dermatology consultation is crucial to determine skin cancer risk (**Table 5**).[16] Pretransplant skin cancer increases risk of other solid organ cancers, death, graft rejection, and lymphoproliferative disorders.[17] High-risk patients should have prompt treatment of premalignant and malignant skin lesions, education on strict photoprotection, and interdisciplinary discussion regarding modification of immunosuppressive regimens and chemoprophylaxis.

Management of pretransplant skin cancer
Pretransplant skin cancers may affect eligibility for solid organ transplant (SOT). Consensus guidelines recommend delaying transplantation for 2 to 3 years following the diagnosis of a high-risk SCC (defined as size >2 cm on trunk/extremities or >1 cm on face, recurrent, immunosuppressed, site of prior radiation/scar, depth >2 mm, perineural/perivascular involvement). For patients with a history of melanoma, pretransplant imaging is advised for stage IIA or higher disease, and SOT should be delayed for more than or equal to 1 year for stage IA, IB, and IIA; 1 to 2 years for stage IIIA; and 2 to 4 years for stages IIB, IIC, and IIIB.[18] Nodal disease of any skin cancer requires delay of transplantation.

Table 2
Chronic lymphocytic leukemia disease-specific risk and management considerations

Associated Risk By Tumor Type	Diagnosis and Staging WorkUp	Localized Disease Management	Advanced Disease Management	Surveillance
BCC • 2x ↑ risk • ↑ subclinical tumoral spread • ↑ local recurrence SCC • 5-8x ↑ risk • ↑ subclinical tumoral spread • ↑ local recurrence • ↑ nodal and distant metastasis • ↑ death from disease Melanoma • 2-7x ↑ risk • → OS • → DS MCC • 8x ↑ risk • → OS • → DSS KS • 3x ↑ risk	• ↓ threshold for biopsy of suspicious lesions • Obtain adequate sampling to assess high-risk histologic features such as depth and differentiation • ↓ threshold for radiologic and histologic assessment of enlarged lymph nodes • Consider 18F-FDG PET/CT as part of baseline workup in high-risk patients • FDG uptake often more intense in nodal metastases compared with CLL/SLL nodes	• Consider MMS or excision with complete circumferential and deep margin assessment given ↑ subclinical tumoral spread • Immunohistochemistry may enhance margin assessment in presence of peritumoral lymphocytic infiltrate	• Multidisciplinary team • No CLL-specific contraindication to standard therapies such as RT or ICIs	• Education on photoprotection • self-skin examination • Full body skin and regional lymph node examination by dermatologist at least yearly • ↑ frequency of surveillance in high-risk patients

Abbreviations: DSS, disease-specific survival; FDG-PET/CT, fluorodeoxyglucose-positron emission tomography/computed tomography; ICIs, immune checkpoint inhibitors; KS, Kaposi sarcoma; MCC, Merkel cell carcinoma; MMS, Mohs micrographic surgery; OS, overall survival; RT, radiation therapy; SLL, small lymphocytic leukemia.

Table 3
Human immunodeficiency virus disease-specific risk and management considerations

Associated Risk by Tumor Type	Diagnosis and Staging WorkUp	Localized Disease Management	Advanced Disease Management	Surveillance
BCC • 2x ↑ risk SCC • 5x ↑ risk • ↑ risk HPV-associated anogenital SCC Melanoma • 2x ↑ risk • ↓ OS • ↓ DSS MCC • 13x ↑ risk • ↓ OS • ↓ DSS	• Test for HIV in patients presenting with skin cancer without typical risk factors • Test for HIV in patients presenting with HPV-associated anogenital SCC • ↓ threshold to stage with imaging	• Consider MMS or excision with complete circumferential and deep margin assessment ± immunohistochemistry for tumor identification • Consider testing SCC tumors of the anogenital, nail, or perioral regions for high-risk HPV strains	• Multidisciplinary team • No HIV-specific contraindication to standard therapies such as RT and ICIs	• Frequent skin cancer surveillance including genital examination • Optimize HIV treatment to keep viral load undetectable and CD4 count normal • Offer HPV vaccine if not previously vaccinated
KS • ↑ risk with ↓ CD4 count	• Test for HIV in patients presenting with KS • Baseline CBC with differential, CMP, FOBT, CXR • Additional imaging if symptoms raise concern for visceral involvement	• Treatment of HIV per infectious disease experts • Initiation of cART alone may induce regression of early stage tumors • Intralesional vinblastine • RT • Alitretinoin 0.1% gel	• Avoid systemic corticosteroids • Chemotherapy • Consider ICIs	• Frequent skin cancer surveillance including oral and genital examination • Monitor for KS-IRIS following initiation of cART

Abbreviations: cART, combination antiretroviral therapy; CBC, complete blood count; CMP, complete metabolic panel; CXR, chest radiograph; FOBT, fecal occult blood test; ICIs, immune checkpoint inhibitors; IRIS, immune reconstitution inflammatory syndrome; RT, radiation therapy.

African Americans at low risk, but education is important to avoid delayed skin cancer detection.[16]

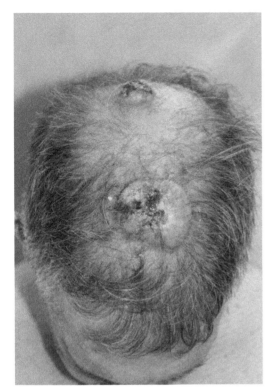

Fig. 1. Multiple aggressive SCCs in an HIV-positive patient.

Distant metastatic disease is a contraindication to transplantation.[19]

Transplant immunosuppression is associated with worse melanoma outcomes.[20,21] Intermediate and deeply invasive melanomas (Breslow depth >1.5) are associated with especially poor prognosis in OTRs.[21] However, limited data suggest that patients with a history of pretransplant melanoma rarely develop recurrence or die from melanoma after transplant and should therefore remain eligible for transplant.[21]

Posttransplant Approach

Transplant recipients should be counseled to practice strict sun avoidance and protection and perform monthly self-skin examinations. Careful sun protection decreases risk of actinic keratosis (AK) and SCC in OTRs by nearly 3-fold.[22,23] The SUNTRAC score is a multivariate model developed to stratify skin cancer risk and guide dermatologic screening recommendations (Fig. 3).[16,24] From this model, anyone with a prior skin cancer is screened within 1 to 2 years. Male patients with heart and lung transplants or patients older than 50 years require screening within 6 months. All other demographics should be screened within 5 years. No consensus has been reached in

Approach to Immunosuppressant Regimen Adjustment

In patients with life-threatening skin cancer or a high burden of primary skin cancers, reducing or changing immunosuppressive therapy may be warranted (Table 6). These decisions must balance the risk of skin cancer progression and graft survival, as well as the patient's age, prior rejection history, human leukocyte antigen match, medication levels, allograft type, and time after transplantation.[11,25]

Replacing calcineurin-based regimens (cyclosporine, tacrolimus) with mTOR-based therapies (sirolimus, everolimus) reduces skin cancer risk by 56%.[26] However, mTOR inhibitors are associated with higher rates of infection and death; therefore, multidisciplinary teams must weigh risks and benefits.[27] Among cell-cycle inhibitors, replacing azathioprine with mycophenolate mofetil reduces skin cancer risk.[28]

In addition to modifying immunosuppressants, OTRs must beware of other medications that increase skin cancer risk (Table 7).[29–32] For example, voriconazole, which is used to treat or prevent invasive aspergillosis, increases risk of SCC by 73%, and this risk increases by 3% with each month of use.[33] Physicians caring for lung transplant recipients should avoid or limit voriconazole and emphasize strict photoprotection when voriconazole is used. Photosensitizing medications should be minimized and therapeutic phototherapy avoided.

Systemic Chemoprophylaxis

In patients who develop multiple skin cancers per year, chemoprophylaxis with acitretin or isotretinoin should be considered (Fig. 4). Specific indications for oral retinoids are development of 5 to 10 SCCs or 1 to 2 high-risk SCCs per year, although this may vary in individual circumstances.[19]

Oral nicotinamide demonstrates modest reduction in KCs in immunocompetent individuals, although studies are underpowered to detect efficacy in OTRs.[15,34] Nicotinamide and retinoid therapy may be used concomitantly. These medications should be implemented with appropriate clinical and laboratory monitoring in collaboration with the transplant team. Retinoid and nicotinamide discontinuation may cause a "rebound effect" in which patients quickly develop multiple SCCs; therefore, treatment should be continued long-term.[11,35] Finally, systemic

Table 4
Organ transplant recipient disease-specific risk and management considerations

Associated Risk By Tumor Type	Diagnosis and Staging WorkUp	Localized Disease Management	Advanced Disease Management	Surveillance
BCC • 10x ↑ risk SCC • 60–250x ↑ risk • ↑recurrence • ↓ OS • ↓ DSS Melanoma • 2–5x ↑ risk MCC • 10–24x ↑ risk KS • 84x ↑ risk Soft tissue sarcomas • 4x ↑ risk Adnexal tumors • 2.7x ↑ risk HPV-associated nonkeratinocytic tumors • 1–10x ↑ risk Overall • ↑risk with ↑ degree of immunosuppression • ↑risk with ↑ length of immunosuppression • ↑risk with certain medication classes (see Table 6)	• Obtain adequate sampling to assess high-risk histologic features such as depth and differentiation • ↓ threshold to obtain imaging studies for staging and baseline in high-risk tumors	• Excision with complete circumferential and deep margin assessment (such as MMS) for tumors with high-risk features (see Tables 8 and 10) • Immunohistochemistry staining to enhance detection of deeply invasive, recurrent, infiltrative, single-cell, perineural, or lymphovascular spread • Avoid tissue transfer or large reconstruction until negative margins confirmed	• Multidisciplinary team • Consider salvage RT with uncertain or unresectable positive margins • Consider adjuvant RT for large-caliber/multifocal perineural invasion (SCC, BCC) • ICIs relatively contraindicated	• Skin cancer surveillance based on SUNTRAC algorithm, including genital examination • More frequent skin and lymph node examinations for high-risk tumors • Imaging surveillance for high-risk tumors • Consider decreasing or changing immunosuppressant regimen • 49x ↑ risk of subsequent KC after first KC development

Abbreviations: ICIs, immune checkpoint inhibitors; RT radiation therapy.

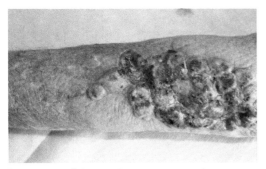

Fig. 2. SCC with in-transit metastases on the upper extremity in an OTR.

capecitabine has been used for high-volume SCCs in the OTR.[36]

KERATINOCYTE CARCINOMA
Overview

KCs, particularly SCC, are the most common malignancy in the immunosuppressed.[1]

Risk Stratification and Staging

To guide treatment, KCs should be stratified based on their risk for local recurrence, metastases, or DSS. The National Comprehensive Cancer Network (NCCN) publishes categories to determine risk for local recurrence and metastasis, and staging systems estimate prognosis. High-risk SCC and BCC are defined by the NCCN guidelines along with recommendation for complete margin-controlled surgery in the setting of immunosuppression (**Tables 8** and **9**).[14,15,37]

Multiple staging systems exist for cutaneous SCC. The American Joint Committee on Cancer

8th edition (AJCC-8) Staging System applies to cutaneous SCC of the head and neck; the Brigham and Women's Hospital (BWH) system and International Union Against Cancer (UICC) system apply to cutaneous SCC of any location (**Table 10**).[38–41] Staging remains challenging due to the numerous systems, nonuniform high-risk criteria, and the reliance on pathologic criteria that may not be available before surgical treatment.

Staging for BCC is also based on AJCC-8 and newly developed BWH BCC tumor categorization (**Table 11**).[42]

Approach to Low-Risk Disease

Immunosuppressed patients have higher rates of AK progression, lower rates of regression, and multiple AKs can obscure early invasive SCC lesions. Therefore, AKs should be proactively managed and treated. Discrete AKs are commonly treated with liquid nitrogen cryotherapy, although alternatives include curettage and topical drugs.[35] Small SCC in situ (SCCIS) in low-risk sites may be treated with standard surgical excision, shave excision, electrodessication and curettage (ED&C), or topical 5-fluorouracil (5-FU). In terminal hair-bearing sites (eg, scalp or beard), high-risk anatomic sites, or lesions greater than 0.6 cm, surgery with MMS provides reduced risk of recurrence and tissue sparing.[14,35]

For SCC without NCCN high-risk features other than immunosuppression, prompt surgical excision with at least 4 to 6 mm margins or MMS is recommended.[14] MMS is associated with lower recurrence than local resection for all skin cancers including SCC and BCC.[43] MMS is appropriate for

---

Table 5
History and physical examination factors associated with posttransplantation skin cancer risk

Genetic	Medical History	Exposures	Physical Examination
• Increased age • Male gender • Lighter Fitzpatrick skin type and eye color • Family history of skin cancer • Inheritable disorders (basal cell nevus syndrome, xeroderma pigmentosum, oculocutaneous albinism, etc.)	• Personal history of skin cancer • Dermatologic disease (psoriasis, eczema, etc.) • Rheumatologic/auto-immune condition • PUVA treatment • Immunosuppressing/photosensitizing medications • HHV-8 seropositivity	• Low-latitude geography • Recreational UV exposure • Occupational UV exposure • Severe sunburns • Indoor tanning • Carcinogen exposure (ionizing radiation, tobacco, arsenic)	• Skin cancer • Premalignant AKs • Lentigines • Multiple melanocytic nevi/atypical nevi • Disseminated porokeratoses • Other examination findings of actinic damage

Abbreviations: AKs, actinic keratoses; HHV-8, human herpesvirus-8; PUVA, psoralen and ultraviolet A radiation therapy; UV, ultraviolet.

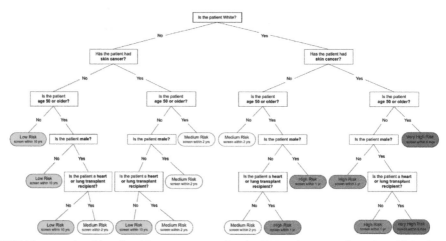

Fig. 3. SUNTRAC score algorithm for skin cancer screening in SOTRs. (*From* Jambusaria-Pahlajani A, Crow LD, Lowenstein S, Garrett GL, Melcher ML, Chan AW, Boscardin J, Arron ST. Predicting skin cancer in organ transplant recipients: development of the SUNTRAC screening tool using data from a multicenter cohort study. Transpl Int. 2019 Dec;32(12):1259-1267.)

most SCCs in the immunocompromised patient (**Table 12**).[14,43]

The standard of care for low-risk BCC is excision with 4 mm margins, although wider margins may be necessary in immunosuppressed.[43] ED&C can also be considered, particularly for less than 1 cm primary low-risk BCCs on the trunk and extremities.[37] MMS provides improved cure rate and tissue conservation (see **Table 12**).[43] Watchful waiting may be appropriate for patients with limited life expectancy and asymptomatic nodular or superficial BCCs in low-risk anatomic sites.[44]

Approach to High-Burden Disease

The simultaneous presence of adjacent SCCs and AKs may require "field" therapy (**Fig. 5**).[35] Biopsy of any lesions with potential dermal invasion is important to assess depth of invasion and high-risk features. For invasive SCC, surgery is indicated. For hypertrophic AKs and early SCCIS, numerous lesions may be treated with curettage with or without topical field therapy.[19] Topical 5-

FU and cyclical photodynamic therapy are effective for AKs without hyperkeratosis.[11] Other treatments including topical 5-FU combined with calcipotriol, diclofenac, imiquimod, tirbanibulin, chemical peels, and carbon-dioxide laser may also be considered.[11,45]

Approach to High-Risk and Locally Advanced Disease

Early multidisciplinary involvement is essential for high-risk SCC in immunocompromised patients, given the significantly higher rate of SCC recurrence, metastasis, and disease-specific death.[46] The goal in high-risk SCC is complete tumor removal for highest cure rate and improved outcomes, preferably with MMS, as it enables 100% microscopic margin assessment.[11,14,43] When MMS is not accessible or feasible, surgical excision with at least 6 to 10 mm margins with intraoperative or postoperative margin examination is acceptable.[14] Reconstruction with tissue rearrangement should be delayed until negative margins are histologically confirmed.

Table 6		
Comparative risk for skin cancer development among commonly used transplant medications		
High Risk[a]	Moderate Risk[a]	Low Risk[a]
• Azathioprine • Calcineurin inhibitors (cyclosporine > tacrolimus) • Voriconazole	• Mycophenolate mofetil	• mTOR inhibitors (sirolimus, everolimus)

Seek expert interdisciplinary advice for individual patient care.
[a] Rough estimate of risk based on available data.

Table 7
Medications associated with increased risk of skin cancer (immune-related, photosensitizing, and other/unknown mechanisms)

Medication[a]	Risk
Cyclosporine	6x in OTR
Azathioprine	1.5x in OTR
Voriconazole	1.7x in OTR
Hydrochlorothiazide	4x
Oral steroids	2.3x
Hydroxyurea	2.2x
PDE-5 inhibitors	2.2x
BRAF inhibitors	1.3x
JAK inhibitors[b]	2x
TNF inhibitors[b]	1.3x
Methotrexate[b]	1.6x
Tacrolimus Mycophenolate Photosensitizing 　medications 　(antibiotic, 　antiepileptic, 　diuretic) Abatacept Thiopurine	Not well quantified

Abbreviations: JAK, Janus kinase; PDE, phosphodiesterase; TNF, tumor necrosis factor.

[a] List is not exhaustive; most of the available data show association rather than causation between medication and skin cancer risk.

[b] Association with skin cancer risk is uncertain due to conflicting outcomes in current research.

Table 13 provides strategies for managing high-risk SCC in the immunocompromised patient based on NCCN guidelines (see **Table 8**).[14] For high-risk SCC, (eg, BWH T2b/T3, AJCC T3, or T2 with multiple high-risk features), preoperative imaging should be considered to guide surgical approach and treatment plan.[47] Although sentinel lymph node biopsy (SLNB) is more sensitive than imaging studies to detect subclinical metastases, there is insufficient evidence to identify which patients may benefit from an SLNB and whether it alters disease management/outcomes at this time.[14,48]

Radiation therapy

Primary radiation therapy (RT) is reserved for patients who are not surgical candidates, but it is significantly less effective in high-risk tumors, with local recurrence for higher T-stage SCC exceeding 25.9%.[49] More often, RT is used as an adjuvant therapy following definitive surgical treatment when there are high-risk features (eg, perineural involvement). Alternatively, salvage RT may be used following an incomplete/uncertain resection when further surgery is unlikely to be successful or has great risk of morbidity.[48] Despite bimodal therapy with surgery and adjuvant RT, immunosuppressed patients experience inferior outcomes for recurrence and progression-free survival (PFS), and proactive surveillance is advised.[50]

Systemic therapy for squamous cell carcinoma

Systemic therapy is indicated for patients who are ineligible for curative excision or RT or who have

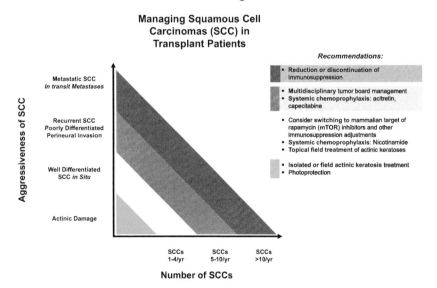

Fig. 4. Recommendations on SCC management. (*Adapted from* Mittal A, Colegio OR. Skin Cancers in Organ Transplant Recipients. Am J Transplant. 2017 Oct;17(10):2509-2530.)

Table 8
National Comprehensive Cancer Network squamous cell carcinoma risk stratification and treatment recommendation

	Low Risk	High Risk	Very High Risk
Location	• Trunk, extremities ≤ 2 cm	• Trunk, extremities >2–4 cm • Head, neck, hands, feet, pretibial, and anogenital (any size)	• > 4 cm, any location
Features	• Well-defined borders • Primary lesion • Well or moderately differentiated • ≤ 6 mm and no invasion beyond subcutaneous fat	• Poorly defined borders • Recurrent lesion • Immunosuppression • Site of prior radiation therapy or chronic inflammation • Rapidly growing • Neurologic symptom • Acantholytic, adenosquamous, metaplastic subtypes	• Poor differentiation • Desmoplastic SCC • > 6 mm or invasion beyond subcutaneous fat • Tumor cells within nerve sheath of nerve lying deeper than dermis or measuring ≥0.1 mm • Lymphatic or vascular involvement

Treatment	• ED&C, excluding terminal hair-bearing areas
	• Standard excision with 4–6 mm clinical margins and post-op margin assessment
	• MMS or other peripheral and deep en face margin assessment
	• RT for nonsurgical candidates
		• MMS or other peripheral and deep en face margin assessment
		• Standard excision with wider surgical margins and postoperative margin assessment
		• For nonsurgical candidates
		  ○ RT ± systemic therapy
		  ○ Systemic therapy if curative RT not feasible	

Abbreviations: ED&C, electrodesiccation and curettage; RT, radiation therapy.

Table 9
National Comprehensive Cancer Network basal cell carcinoma risk stratification and treatment recommendation

	Low Risk	High Risk
Location	• Trunk, extremities < 2 cm	• Trunk, extremities ≥2 cm • Cheeks, forehead, scalp, neck, and pretibial (any size) • Head, neck, hands, feet, pretibial, and anogenital (any size)
Features	• Well-defined borders • Primary lesion • Well or moderately differentiated • ≤ 6 mm and no invasion beyond sub-cutaneous fat	• Poorly defined borders • Recurrent lesion • Immunosuppression • Site of prior RT • Aggressive growth pattern (mixed infiltrative, micronodular, morphea-form, basosquamous, sclerosing, or carcinosarcomatous)

Treatment	• ED&C, excluding terminal hair-bearing areas
	• Standard excision with 4 mm clinical margins and post-op margin assessment
	• MMS or other peripheral and deep en face margin assessment
	• RT for nonsurgical candidates
		• MMS or other peripheral and deep en face margin assessment
		• Standard excision with wider surgical margins and postoperative margin assessment
		• For nonsurgical candidates
		  ○ RT
		  ○ Systemic therapy if curative RT not feasible

Abbreviations: ED&C, electrodesiccation and curettage; RT, radiation therapy.

Table 10
AJCC 8 versus BWH versus UICC squamous cell carcinoma staging systems

AJCC 8th Edition for Head and Neck SCC		BWH		UICC	
T1	<2 cm in greatest diameter	T1	0 High-risk factors	T1	≤2 cm in greatest diameter
T2	≥2 cm, but <4 cm in greatest diameter	T2a	1 High-risk factor	T2	>2 cm in greatest diameter
		T2b	2–3 High-risk factors		
T3	Tumor ≥4 cm in greatest diameter or minor bone invasion or perineural invasion[a] or deep invasion[b]	T3	≥4 High-risk factors or bone invasion	T3	Tumor with invasion of deep structures (eg, muscle, cartilage, bone, orbit)
T4a	Tumor with gross cortical bone and/or marrow invasion	BWH High-Risk Factors • Tumor diameter ≥2 cm • Poorly differentiated histology		T4	Tumor with invasion of axial skeleton or direct perineural invasion of skull base
T4b	Tumor with skull bone invasion and/or skull base foramen involvement	• Perineural invasion of nerve ≥0.1 mm in caliber • Tumor invasion beyond subcutaneous fat			

Abbreviations: AJCC, American Joint Committee on Cancer; BWH, Brigham and Women's Hospital; UICC, International Union Against Cancer.

[a] Perineural invasion defined as tumor cells in the nerve sheath of a nerve deeper than the dermis or measuring ≥0.1 mm in caliber or presenting with clinical or radiographic involvement of named nerves without skull base invasion.
[b] Deep invasion beyond subcutaneous fat or >6 mm.

Data from Amin MB, Greene FL, Edge SB, et al. The Eighth Edition AJCC Cancer Staging Manual: Continuing to build a bridge from a population-based to a more "personalized" approach to cancer staging. *CA Cancer J Clin.* 2017;67(2):93-99. Sobin LH, Gospodarowicz MK, Wittekind C. *TNM classification of malignant tumours.* John Wiley & Sons; 2011. Jambusaria-Pahlajani A, Kanetsky PA, Karia PS, et al. Evaluation of AJCC tumor staging for cutaneous squamous cell carcinoma and a proposed alternative tumor staging system. *JAMA Dermatol.* 2013;149(4):402-410.

metastatic, recurrent, or refractory disease **(Table 14).**[37,48,51–60]

Cemiplimab and pembrolizumab, programmed cell death protein 1 (PD-1) inhibitors within the category of immune checkpoint inhibitor (ICI) therapy, have a 35% to 50% objective response rate in locally advanced unresectable and metastatic SCC.[51,52] Notably, safety and efficacy have not

Table 11
AJCC 8 versus BWH basal cell carcinoma staging systems

AJCC 8th Edition for Head and Neck BCC		Brigham and Women's Hospital (BWH)	
T1	<2 cm in greatest diameter	T1	Tumor diameter of < 2 cm or tumor diameter of ≥ 2 cm with 0–1 risk factors
T2	≥2 cm, but <4 cm in greatest diameter	T2	Tumor diameter of ≥ 2 cm with 2–3 risk factors
T3	Tumor ≥4 cm in greatest diameter or minor bone invasion or perineural invasion or deep invasion	BWH High-Risk Factors • Tumor diameter ≥ 4 cm • Head or neck location • Depth beyond fat	
T4a	Tumor with gross cortical bone and/or marrow invasion		
T4b	Tumor with skull bone invasion and/or skull base foramen involvement		

Abbreviations: AJCC, American Joint Committee on Cancer; BWH, Brigham and Women's Hospital.

Adapted from Morgan FC, Ruiz ES, Karia PS, Besaw RJ, Neel VA, Schmults CD. Brigham and Women's Hospital tumor classification system for basal cell carcinoma identifies patients with risk of metastasis and death. J Am Acad Dermatol. 2021 Sep;85(3):582-587.

Table 12
Mohs appropriate use criteria for immunocompromised patients

	Immunocompromised Patients		
	Appropriate	Uncertain	Inappropriate
Area H: mask areas of the face, genitalia, hands, feet, nail units, ankles, nipple/areola			
SCC	Primary or recurrent: aggressive, nonaggressive, KA-type SCC, in situ SCC		AK with focal SCC in situ
BCC	Primary or recurrent: aggressive, nodular, superficial		
Area M: cheeks, forehead, scalp, neck, jawline, pretibial surface			
SCC	Primary or recurrent: aggressive, nonaggressive, KA-type SCC, in situ SCC		AK with focal SCC in situ
BCC	Primary or recurrent: aggressive, nodular, superficial		
Area L: trunk and extremities			
SCC	Primary • Aggressive • Nonaggressive > 1.1 cm • In situ SCC > 1.1 cm • KA-type SCC ≥ 0.6 cm Recurrent: • Aggressive • KA-type SCC • Nonaggressive	Primary • Nonaggressive ≤ 1 cm • SCC in situ 0.6-1 cm • KA-type SCC ≤ 0.5 cm Recurrent • SCC in situ/Bowen	Primary • Primary SCC in situ < 0.5 cm • AK with focal SCC in situ Recurrent • AK with focal SCC in situ
BCC	Primary • Aggressive ≥0.6 cm • Nodular ≥ 1.1 cm Recurrent: • Aggressive • Nodular	Primary • Aggressive ≤ 0.5 cm • Nodular 0.6–1 cm • Superficial ≥ 1.1 cm	Primary • Nodular ≤ 0.5 cm • Superficial ≤ 1 cm Recurrent • Superficial

Abbreviations: AK, actinic keratosis; H, high-risk; KA, keratoacanthoma; L, low-risk; M, medium-risk.

Adapted from Ad Hoc Task Force, Connolly SM, Baker DR, Coldiron BM, Fazio MJ, Storrs PA, Vidimos AT, Zalla MJ, Brewer JD, Smith Begolka W; Ratings Panel, Berger TG, Bigby M, Bolognia JL, Brodland DG, Collins S, Cronin TA Jr, Dahl MV, Grant-Kels JM, Hanke CW, Hruza GJ, James WD, Lober CW, McBurney EI, Norton SA, Roenigk RK, Wheeland RG, Wisco OJ. AAD/ACMS/ASDSA/ASMS 2012 appropriate use criteria for Mohs micrographic surgery: a report of the American Academy of Dermatology, American College of Mohs Surgery, American Society for Dermatologic Surgery Association, and the American Society for Mohs Surgery. J Am Acad Dermatol. 2012 Oct;67(4):531-50.

been well established in OTRs and other immuno-suppressed patients due to their exclusion from clinical trials. Although ICI is better tolerated than other classes of cancer drugs, the immune-mediated adverse events from ICIs can be life-threatening and long-lasting. However, PD-1 in-hibitor OS and PFS is superior to epidermal growth factor receptor (EGFR) inhibitors and platinum-based chemotherapy based on indirect comparisons.[56]

ICIs have immune-stimulating effects that may mediate allograft rejection in OTRs and therefore are relatively contraindicated in this population. ICIs' benefits must be weighed against the often-catastrophic risks of organ rejection, and other treatment modalities are favored.[61] Generally, kid-ney OTRs have an option of dialysis should their organ fail, but this still carries significant risk and morbidity. For other transplanted organs, graft fail-ure is considered lethal. A review of 39 OTRs with advanced SCC demonstrated 100% overall response rate to ICIs, but 41% experienced allo-graft rejection with 33% graft failure.

Traditional cytotoxic chemotherapy is used in patients with metastatic SCC but has limited response rates and poor tolerance by elderly pa-tients. Platin-based therapy alone or combination with 5-FU is the most common drug used.[48]

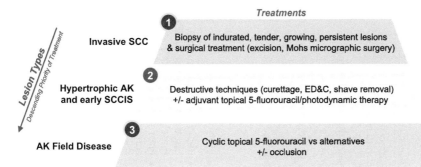

Fig. 5. Management of field cancerization. AK, actinic keratosis; ED&C, electrodesiccation and curettage; SCC, squamous cell carcinoma; SCCIS, squamous cell carcinoma in situ.

Chemotherapy combined with radiotherapy is also used for advanced SCC; however, the only randomized controlled trial investigating chemoradiation demonstrated that addition of carboplatin to radiotherapy was not superior to radiotherapy alone.[57]

EGFR inhibitors, such as cetuximab and panitumumab, are targeted therapies used for unresectable cutaneous SCC.[53] Although data in OTRs are very limited, a report of fatal alveolar damage in 2 lung transplant patients cautions use in lung transplant recipients.[54] EGFR inhibitors are better

tolerated than standard cytotoxic chemotherapy, but their effect is typically short-lived.[48]

Systemic therapy for basal cell carcinoma
Oral small molecule inhibitors of the hedgehog signaling pathway, vismodegib and sonidegib, treat metastatic and unresectable locally advanced BCC.[37] Data for the immunosuppressed population are very limited, but vismodegib appears safe and efficacious in case reports of OTRs.[62] Development of drug resistance to smoothened inhibitors is typical, and tolerability

Table 13	
Approach to high-risk localized squamous cell carcinoma	
1. Multidisciplinary Tumor Board	• Obtain interdisciplinary collaborations • Reference current NCCN guidelines • Enroll in clinical trial where available
2. Staging Workup	Imaging (general strengths of imaging modality) • CT (cortical bone or lymph node involvement) • MR (soft tissue and/or perineural visualization, brain evaluation) • PET/CT (increased sensitivity, evaluation for distant disease) • Ultrasound (regional lymph node evaluation) SLNB • Consider in select cases • Insufficient evidence to recommend for or against
3. Treatment	*1st line:* complete surgical tumor extirpation • May require multispecialty surgical team • Delay reconstruction with tissue rearrangement until histologic confirmation of negative margins *2nd line:* RT and/or systemic therapy

4. Adjuvant Therapy	• Consider RT
	  ○ Adjuvant RT: very high-risk cases, extensive perineural involvement
	  ○ Salvage RT: margin status close/uncertain
	• Consider adjuvant chemoradiation in select cases

5. Surveillance	• Complete skin and lymph node examination at least every 3 months for 2–5 years • Consider imaging studies to supplement examination and ROS

Abbreviations: CT, computed tomography; MR, magnetic resonance; PET, positron emission tomography; ROS, review of systems; RT, radiation therapy; SLNB, sentinel lymph node biopsy.

Table 14
Systemic therapy in keratinocyte carcinoma for immunocompromised[a]

Drug Class	ICIs	Targeted Therapy (SCC)	Chemotherapy (Cytotoxic)	Targeted Therapy (BCC)
Examples	Cemiplimab Pembrolizumab	Cetuximab Panitumumab	Cisplatin Carboplatin Capecitabine (5-FU)	Vismodegib Sonidegib
MOA	PD-1 inhibitor	EGFR inhibitor	DNA synthesis inhibitors	Smoothened inhibitor
FDA approval for CSCC	Yes	No	No	N/A
FDA approval for BCC	Yes	No	No	Yes
Objective response rates	35-50%	28-31%	17-54%	8-60%
Durability of response	+++	+	++	+
Tolerability	+++	++	+	++
Key features	• Durable response • Immune-mediated adverse events • Safe in HIV and lymphoproliferative disorders	• Rapid response possible, but drug resistance typical • Can be used in immunocompromised	• Low response rates • Radio-sensitizing chemo may be beneficial in the setting of chemoradiation[b] • Can be used in immunocompromised	• Rapid response possible, but drug resistance typical (median 7.6 months) • Poor tolerability due to common side effects • Can be used in immunocompromised
Key contraindications	• OTR (risk of graft rejection) • Autoimmune disease	• Lung transplant (risk of alveolar damage)	• Poor performance status • Poor renal function	• Pregnancy (severe birth defects)

Abbreviations: CSCC, cutaneous squamous cell carcinoma; DNA, deoxyribonucleic acid; EGFR, epidermal growth factor receptor; FDA, US Food and Drug Administration; HIV, human immunodeficiency virus; ICI, immune checkpoint inhibitor; MOA, mechanism of action; N/A, not applicable; PD-1, programmed cell death protein 1.

[a] Summary based on limited available evidence.

[b] Carboplatin radiotherapy did not improve outcomes compared with radiotherapy monotherapy.[57]

Table 15
NCCN *melanoma* sentinel lymph node biopsy and margin recommendations for immunosuppressed and immunocompetent

Tumor Stage	Workup	Margins for Conventional Wide Local Excision[a]
Melanoma in situ	History and physical examination	0.5–1.0 cm[b]
T1a <0.8 mm thick without ulceration	History and physical examination	1.0 cm[b]
T1b <1 mm thick with ulceration 0.8–1.0 mm thick without ulceration	Consider SLNB	1.0 cm[b]
T2 1.1–2.0 mm thick without (T2a) or with (T2b) ulceration	Offer SLNB	1.0-2.0 cm
T3 2.1–4.0 mm thick without (T3a) or with (T3b) ulceration	Offer SLNB	2.0 cm
T4 >4.0 mm thick without (T4a) or with (T4b) ulceration	Offer SLNB	2.0 cm

[a] Excision depth to the superficial fascia; avoid extensive undermining, delay tissue rearrangement or large reconstruction until final pathology for staging and margin status is complete.
[b] MMS with immunostains for comprehensive margin assessment decreases rates of reexcision for positive margin and recurrence for anatomically constrained areas (head, neck, hands/feet, pretibial, genitalia).

is poor over a longer duration of treatment. Cemiplimab is approved for locally advanced and metastatic BCC that has failed treatment with smoothened inhibitor therapy.[55] As indicated earlier, cemiplimab use in OTRs is discouraged, but it can be used in lymphoproliferative and other acquired immunodeficiencies.

MELANOMA
Overview

Although the risk for melanoma in the immunosuppressed is lower than for other types of skin cancer, the prevalence is at least double, and OS and DSS are decreased compared with the general population[10,20] (see **Tables 2–4**). In the OTR, median time to diagnosis ranges from 1.5 to 2.5 years following transplantation. The risk of stage III and IV melanoma is highest within 4 years of transplantation, whereas the risk of in situ and localized melanoma remains consistently elevated over time.[20] Alterations in immunosuppression should be guided by the patient's transplant team, accounting for factors including melanoma stage, type of allograft, and alternative options in the event of graft failure.[25]

Stage 0–II Melanoma

Immunosuppressed patients who develop in situ or localized invasive melanoma should be managed in accordance with NCCN guidelines,

including with SLNB for T1b or higher tumor category (**Table 15**).[63] Newly approved adjuvant immunotherapy for high-risk stage II disease is discouraged in the OTR but may be considered for other immunosuppressed conditions, despite exclusion of this population from clinical trials.[64]

Stage III–IV Melanoma

NCCN guidelines specify appropriate staging workup including baseline imaging in advanced disease. Multidisciplinary collaboration to assess risks and benefits of therapeutic intervention is recommended, particularly for the immunosuppressed patient.

Local nonsurgical therapy for melanoma

Intralesional talimogene laherparepvec (T-VEC), an oncolytic modified herpes simplex virus, is an emerging option for in-transit metastases. T-VEC is approved for treatment of melanoma with unresectable cutaneous, subcutaneous, and nodal lesions and can be administered in a clinical setting. Case reports have described complete remission following administration of T-VEC in OTRs with locally advanced melanoma.[65,66] Although T-VEC is an immunogenic therapy, no cases were complicated by graft failure or rejection; however, caution is advised, given lack of safety data for the OTR population. In addition, it is unknown if efficacy is decreased in the

Table 16
Merkel cell carcinoma–specific risk and management considerations in immunocompromised

Associated Risk	Staging	Localized Disease Management	Advanced Disease Management	Surveillance
Overall • 13–24x ↑ risk among immunosuppressed[a] • ↓ OS • ↓ DSS [a]Immunosuppressed more likely to be seronegative for MCPyV antibodies including: • OTR • HIV/AIDs • Lympho-proliferative • Other immune suppressing medications; azathioprine and cyclosporine associated with highest risk	• FDG-PET/CT at baseline • SLNB • MCPyV antibodies within 3 months of diagnosis • Immunocompromised more likely to be seronegative for MCPyV antibodies	• Surgery (MMS or standard excision) • Primary tissue closure preferred to avoid delay in initiation of adjuvant RT • Adjuvant RT indicated for all MCC cases in the immunosuppressed	• Reduce/eliminate immunosuppression; avoid azathioprine and cyclosporine when possible • ICIs for nontransplant population • ICIs relatively contraindicated in OTR • Consider standard chemotherapy in OTR	• Complete skin and lymph node examination every 3–6 mo for 3 years, then every 6–12 mo • Consider more frequent follow-up in high-risk population[67] • Consider routine imaging to detect occult disease • Track MCPyV oncoprotein antibodies in baseline seropositive cases

Abbreviation: FDG-PET/CT, fluorodeoxyglucose-positron emission tomography/computed tomography.

Table 17
Kaposi sarcoma–specific risk and management considerations

Associated Risk	Staging	Localized Disease Management[a]	Advanced Disease Management	Surveillance
Overall • ↑ risk among Mediterranean, Jewish, Arabic, Caribbean, African descent due to higher HHV-8 prevalence Epidemic • ↑ risk with ↓ CD4 count Iatrogenic • 208x ↑ risk in OTRs	• Examine skin, mucosa, and lymph nodes; assess for lower extremity edema • ↓threshold for biopsy of suspicious lesions • Consider ID consultation to assess for opportunistic infections • CBC with differential, CMP, HIV testing • FOBT to assess for GI involvement • CXR to assess for pulmonary involvement • Additional imaging if symptoms raise concern for visceral involvement	• Initiation of cART alone may induce regression of early stage tumors • Wide local excision • Cryosurgery • Intralesional vinblastine • Radiation therapy • Alitretinoin 0.1% gel • Imiquimod 5% cream • Observation	• Reduce/eliminate immunosuppression or switch to sirolimus when clinically acceptable • Avoid systemic corticosteroids • Chemotherapy: doxorubicin, paclitaxel • Consider ICIs (relatively contraindicated in OTR)	• Monitor for KS-IRIS following initiation of cART • Treatment does not prevent recurrence • Frequent skin, mucosa, and lymph node examination • Periodic lab monitoring • Routine imaging not recommended, unless signs or symptoms concerning for visceral involvement arises

Abbreviations: CBC, complete blood count; CMP, complete metabolic panel; CXR, chest radiograph; FOBT, fecal occult blood test; GI, gastrointestinal; ID, infectious disease; IRIS, immune reconstitution inflammatory syndrome.

[a] Based on limited data.

immunosuppressed owing to potentially decreased immunogenic response to treatment.

Systemic therapy for melanoma

In patients with V600-activating BRAF mutations, treatment with combination BRAF/MEK inhibitors improves outcomes, including survival for advanced stage melanoma.[64] Although the mechanism of these drugs poses no theoretical harm to OTRs, minimal data exist for targeted melanoma treatment in the immunosuppressed, and further evaluation of this approach is needed.[66]

As discussed in the setting of advanced SCC treatment, the use of ICIs for treatment of melanoma in the OTR is associated with significant risk for graft rejection. Based on reviews of ICI use in OTRs that include 77 melanoma patients total, graft rejection occurs in approximately 40%. Of those who experience rejection, end-stage organ failure and death secondary to graft rejection occur in 71% and 14%, respectively.[58] Subanalysis indicates that higher efficacy against disease also correlates with increased risk for graft failure. Pembrolizumab has been associated with the highest rate of remission (20%), in addition to the highest rate of death secondary to graft rejection (30%). In contrast, no patients who received ipilimumab died from graft rejection; however, 70% experienced progression or death secondary to disease. Nivolumab was associated with a 50% partial response rate, and no cases of remission or death due to graft rejection were reported.[61] Use of ICIs in OTRs should be considered with caution, and patients should be thoroughly counseled regarding associated risks.

MERKEL CELL CARCINOMA
Overview

The relationship between MCC and immunosuppression is well documented, theoretically relating to the virally mediated pathogenesis of MCC.[67] Incidence of MCC is increased in patients with hematologic malignancies, HIV, and organ transplantation, and approximately 10% of patients with MCC are immunocompromised.[68]

MCC is a highly aggressive tumor; nearly one-third of patients present at primary diagnosis with stage III disease, and more than one-third of patients die from MCC-related causes. Outcomes, including OS, DSS, and PFS, are reduced in OTRs compared with immunocompetent patients with MCC.[13,67,68]

Management

The approach to workup and management of MCC in the immunosuppressed should be discussed in a multidisciplinary setting (Table 16). Immunosuppressive therapy should be modified or reduced when possible. The combination maintenance regimen of cyclosporine and azathioprine has been associated with the highest MCC risk, whereas tacrolimus and mycophenolate mofetil have been associated with lower MCC incidence.[13]

All patients with MCC should receive a complete skin and lymph node (LN) examination, baseline imaging, ideally with fluorodeoxyglucose-PET/computed tomography, and SLNB.[69] In addition to imaging and nodal assessment, quantitation of serum MCPyV capsid and oncoprotein antibodies assists in prognostication and surveillance. Patients who are seronegative for capsid antibodies at baseline are at higher risk for recurrence, and in seropositive patients, increasing oncoprotein titers are an early indicator of progression. Owing to their immunocompromised status, OTRs may be less likely to be seropositive at baseline than immunocompetent patients.[70]

Localized MCC in the immunosuppressed without evidence of nodal involvement on imaging or SLNB should be managed with surgical excision and adjuvant RT according to current NCCN guidelines.[69]

Although evidence supports the use of ICIs for metastatic MCC, these agents are avoided in OTRs due to concerns regarding safety and risk of graft rejection.[71] Systemic chemotherapy may be considered as a second-line therapy in select patients.

KAPOSI SARCOMA
Overview

Two of the four epidemiological subtypes of KS, epidemic/AIDS-related KS and iatrogenic/transplant-related KS, are associated with immunosuppression (Table 17).

Epidemic KS is considered an AIDS-defining illness, and the risk of development is inversely related to CD4 count. Initiation of cART alone may induce regression of early stage tumors.[72] Following initiation of cART, a subset of patients may experience KS immune reconstitution inflammatory syndrome (KS-IRIS) characterized by clinical worsening. Although KS-IRIS can be self-limited, addition of chemotherapy is necessary in some cases. As in other types of KS, corticosteroids may cause exacerbation and should be avoided. Focal cutaneous KS can be observed or treated with locally directed therapy.[12,72–76] Chemotherapy is the mainstay of treatment of advanced AIDS-related KS; however, ICIs may be an emerging alternative.[72]

Iatrogenic/transplant-related KS is diagnosed 1 year after transplantation on average, and the mean age at diagnosis is 40 years. Approximately 90% of iatrogenic KS presents with cutaneous and/or mucosal lesions, whereas 10% of cases present with purely visceral disease.[12] Visceral involvement is more common in patients with heart or liver transplants compared with kidney transplants.[12]

Presentation

Iatrogenic KS often presents with angiomatous lesions on the lower extremities that may cause lymphedema. However, mucosal surfaces including the conjunctiva and oropharynx may also be affected. Visceral disease has a predilection for the LNs, gastrointestinal tract, and lungs and is associated with worse prognosis.[12]

Incidence of KS is highest in geographic regions with increased prevalence of the human herpesvirus-8 (HHV-8).[12] Because most cases of posttransplant KS occur as a result of HHV-8 reactivation, individuals who are seropositive for HHV-8 before transplantation are more susceptible. Of note, several cases of donor-derived KS have been reported, and pretransplant screening of donors and recipients at high risk for HHV-8 infection has been proposed.[74]

Management

The diagnosis of KS should be established histologically with immunohistochemistry. Because certain opportunistic infections including bacillary angiomatosis, blastomycosis, and cryptococcus may resemble KS in immunocompromised individuals, consultation with an infectious disease specialist may be prudent. Once the diagnosis of KS has been confirmed, initial workup should include comprehensive physical examination along with baseline labs (see **Table 17**).

In patients with iatrogenic KS, lesions often spontaneously regress following cessation of immunosuppression.[72,76] Glucocorticoids have been associated with KS progression and should be avoided, whereas sirolimus may inhibit KS progression. In a study of 15 kidney transplant recipients who developed KS and were switched from cyclosporine to sirolimus, all KS lesions resolved and graft function remained viable.[75] Of note, a recent study in OTRs reported significantly reduced incidence of KS with initiation of prophylactic valacyclovir; however, further studies are needed to explore the effectiveness of this approach.[76]

For patients with limited cutaneous disease, a variety of therapeutic approaches have been used with variable success (see **Table 17**). Because individual KS lesions are often distinct clones as opposed to metastases, treatment of existing lesions does not prevent recurrence of new ones. In the setting of advanced cutaneous, mucosal or visceral disease, use of systemic chemotherapy may be considered. Doxorubicin and paclitaxel are considered first-line therapies in immunocompetent patients, but potential benefits should be weighed carefully against potential side effects in OTRs.[12,72]

No established guidelines exist for surveillance in patients with KS, but frequent skin, mucosal, and LN examinations along with periodic laboratory monitoring are advised.

SUMMARY

Patients with immunosuppression have an increased risk for skin cancer and worse outcomes. Prevention, early diagnosis, and proactive management of localized cancer should be optimized. Immunosuppressed patients with advanced skin cancer may not be eligible for the same systemic therapies as immunocompetent patients. Outcomes improve with early identification of risk factors, early detection, effective local therapies, and new targeted therapies.

CLINICS CARE POINTS

- Organ transplant recipients are at high risk for all skin cancers, and particularly cutaneous squamous cell carcinomas. Early dermatology involvement with risk stratification and appropriate skin cancer screening improves outcomes.

- Among organ transplant recipients who are at high risk for skin cancer, consider alternatives to cyclosporine, azathioprine, and voriconazole, which are highly associated with increased skin cancer risk.

- In immunocompromised patients, surgical excision with complete circumferential peripheral and deep margin assessment is the standard of care for most forms of localized skin cancer

- A multidisciplinary approach is needed to weigh the risks and benefits of surgery, radiation, or systemic therapy for locally advanced or metastatic disease.

CONFLICTS OF INTEREST/FUNDING DISCLOSURES

None.

REFERENCES

1. Brin L, Zubair AS, Brewer JD. Optimal management of skin cancer in immunosuppressed patients. Am J Clin Dermatol 2014;15(4):339–56.

2. Brewer JD, Habermann TM, Shanafelt TD. Lymphoma-associated skin cancer: incidence, natural history, and clinical management. Int J Dermatol 2014;53(3):267–74.

3. Mehrany K, Byrd DR, Roenigk RK, et al. Lymphocytic infiltrates and subclinical epithelial tumor extension in patients with chronic leukemia and solid-organ transplantation. Dermatol Surg 2003; 29(2):129–34.

4. Mehrany K, Weenig RH, Pittelkow MR, et al. High recurrence rates of squamous cell carcinoma after Mohs' surgery in patients with chronic lymphocytic leukemia. Dermatol Surg 2005;31(1):38–42 [discussion: 42].

5. Velez NF, Karia PS, Vartanov AR, et al. Association of advanced leukemic stage and skin cancer tumor stage with poor skin cancer outcomes in patients with chronic lymphocytic leukemia. JAMA Dermatol 2014;150(3):280–7.

6. Reusser NM, Downing C, Guidry J, et al. HPV Carcinomas in Immunocompromised Patients. J Clin Med 2015;4(2):260–81.

7. Asgari MM, Ray GT, Quesenberry CP Jr, et al. Association of Multiple Primary Skin Cancers With Human Immunodeficiency Virus Infection, CD4 Count, and Viral Load. JAMA Dermatol 2017;153(9):892–6.

8. Deshmukh AA, Chhatwal J, Chiao EY, et al. Long-term outcomes of adding HPV vaccine to the anal intraepithelial neoplasia treatment regimen in hiv-positive men who have sex with men. Clin Infect Dis 2015;61(10):1527–35.

9. Yarchoan R, Uldrick TS. HIV-associated cancers and related diseases. N Engl J Med 2018;378(11):1029–41.

10. O'Reilly Zwald F, Brown M. Skin cancer in solid organ transplant recipients: advances in therapy and management: part I. Epidemiology of skin cancer in solid organ transplant recipients. J Am Acad Dermatol 2011;65(2):253–61.

11. O'Reilly Zwald F, Brown M. Skin cancer in solid organ transplant recipients: advances in therapy and management: part II. Management of skin cancer in solid organ transplant recipients. J Am Acad Dermatol 2011;65(2):263–79.

12. Euvrard S, Kanitakis J, Claudy A. Skin cancers after organ transplantation. N Engl J Med 2003;348(17):1681–91.

13. Clarke CA, Robbins HA, Tatalovich Z, et al. Risk of merkel cell carcinoma after solid organ transplantation. J Natl Cancer Inst 2015;107(2).

14. National Comprehensive Cancer N. Squamous cell skin cancer (Version 2.2021. Available at: https://www.nccn.org/professionals/physician_gls/pdf/squamous.pdf. Accessed November 10, 2021.

15. National Comprehensive Cancer N. Basal cell skin cancer (Version 2.2021. Available at: https://www.nccn.org/professionals/physician_gls/pdf/nmsc.pdf. Accessed November 10, 2021.

16. Crow LD, Jambusaria-Pahlajani A, Chung CL, et al. Initial skin cancer screening for solid organ transplant recipients in the United States: Delphi method development of expert consensus guidelines. Transpl Int 2019;32(12):1268–76.

17. Kang W, Sampaio MS, Huang E, et al. Association of pretransplant skin cancer with posttransplant malignancy, graft failure and death in kidney transplant recipients. Transplantation 2017;101(6):1303–9.

18. Al-Adra DP, Hammel L, Roberts J, et al. Preexisting melanoma and hematological malignancies, prognosis, and timing to solid organ transplantation: A consensus expert opinion statement. Am J Transplant 2021;21(2):475–83.

19. Massey PR, Schmults CD, Li SJ, et al. Consensus-based recommendations on the prevention of squamous cell carcinoma in solid organ transplant recipients: a delphi consensus statement. JAMA Dermatol 2021;157(10):1219–26.

20. Robbins HA, Clarke CA, Arron ST, et al. Melanoma risk and survival among organ transplant recipients. J Invest Dermatol 2015;135(11):2657–65.

21. Brewer JD, Christenson LJ, Weaver AL, et al. Malignant melanoma in solid transplant recipients: collection of database cases and comparison with surveillance, epidemiology, and end results data for outcome analysis. Arch Dermatol 2011;147(7):790–6.

22. Ulrich C, Jurgensen JS, Degen A, et al. Prevention of non-melanoma skin cancer in organ transplant patients by regular use of a sunscreen: a 24 months, prospective, case-control study. Br J Dermatol 2009;161(Suppl 3):78–84.

23. Acuna SA, Huang JW, Scott AL, et al. Cancer screening recommendations for solid organ transplant recipients: a systematic review of clinical practice guidelines. Am J Transpl 2017;17(1):103–14.

24. Jambusaria-Pahlajani A, Crow LD, Lowenstein S, et al. Predicting skin cancer in organ transplant recipients: development of the SUNTRAC screening tool using data from a multicenter cohort study. Transpl Int 2019;32(12):1259–67.

25. Otley CC, Berg D, Ulrich C, et al. Reduction of immunosuppression for transplant-associated skin cancer: expert consensus survey. Br J Dermatol 2006;154(3):395–400.

26. Dantal J, Morelon E, Rostaing L, et al. Sirolimus for secondary prevention of skin cancer in kidney transplant recipients: 5-year results. J Clin Oncol 2018;36(25):2612–20.

27. Knoll GA, Kokolo MB, Mallick R, et al. Effect of sirolimus on malignancy and survival after kidney transplantation: systematic review and meta-analysis of individual patient data. BMJ 2014;349:g6679.

28. Coghill AE, Johnson LG, Berg D, et al. Immunosuppressive medications and squamous cell skin carcinoma: nested case-control study within the skin cancer after organ transplant (SCOT) cohort. Am J Transpl 2016;16(2):565–73.

29. Scott FI, Mamtani R, Brensinger CM, et al. Risk of nonmelanoma skin cancer associated with the use of immunosuppressant and biologic agents in patients with a history of autoimmune disease and nonmelanoma skin cancer. JAMA Dermatol 2016; 152(2):164–72.

30. Karagas MR, Cushing GL Jr, Greenberg ER, et al. Non-melanoma skin cancers and glucocorticoid therapy. Br J Cancer 2001;85(5):683–6.

31. Barbui T, Ghirardi A, Masciulli A, et al. Second cancer in Philadelphia negative myeloproliferative neoplasms (MPN-K). A nested case-control study. Leukemia 2019;33(8):1996–2005.

32. Johnson NM, Prickett KA, Phillips MA. Systemic medications linked to an increased risk for skin malignancy. Cutis 2019;104(4):E32–6.

33. D'Arcy ME, Pfeiffer RM, Rivera DR, et al. Voriconazole and the risk of keratinocyte carcinomas among lung transplant recipients in the United States. JAMA Dermatol 2020;156(7):772–9.

34. Tee LY, Sultana R, Tam SYC, et al. Chemoprevention of keratinocyte carcinoma and actinic keratosis in solid-organ transplant recipients: Systematic review and meta-analyses. J Am Acad Dermatol 2021; 84(2):528–30.

35. Mittal A, Colegio OR. Skin Cancers in Organ Transplant Recipients. Am J Transpl 2017;17(10): 2509–30.

36. Breithaupt AD, Beynet D, Soriano T. Capecitabine for squamous cell carcinoma reduction in solid organ transplant recipients. JAAD Case Rep 2015; 1(6):S16–8.

37. Totonchy M, Leffell D. Emerging concepts and recent advances in basal cell carcinoma. F1000Res 2017;6:2085.

38. Ruiz ES, Karia PS, Besaw R, et al. Performance of the american joint committee on cancer staging manual, 8th edition vs the brigham and women's hospital tumor classification system for cutaneous squamous cell carcinoma. JAMA Dermatol 2019; 155(7):819–25.

39. Amin MB, Greene FL, Edge SB, et al. The eighth edition AJCC cancer staging manual: continuing to build a bridge from a population-based to a more "personalized" approach to cancer staging. CA Cancer J Clin 2017;67(2):93–9.

40. Jambusaria-Pahlajani A, Kanetsky PA, Karia PS, et al. Evaluation of AJCC tumor staging for cutaneous squamous cell carcinoma and a proposed alternative tumor staging system. JAMA Dermatol 2013;149(4):402–10.

41. Sobin LH, Gospodarowicz MK, Wittekind C. TNM classification of malignant tumours. Oxford, UK: John Wiley & Sons; 2011.

42. Morgan FC, Ruiz ES, Karia PS, et al. Brigham and Women's Hospital tumor classification system for basal cell carcinoma identifies patients with risk of metastasis and death. J Am Acad Dermatol 2021; 85(3):582–7.

43. American Academy of D, American College of Mohs S, American Society for Dermatologic Surgery A, et al. AAD/ACMS/ASDSA/ASMS 2012 appropriate use criteria for Mohs micrographic surgery: a report of the American Academy of Dermatology, American College of Mohs Surgery, American Society for Dermatologic Surgery Association, and the American Society for Mohs Surgery. Dermatol Surg 2012;38(10):1582–603.

44. van Winden MEC, Hetterschijt CRM, Bronkhorst EM, et al. Evaluation of watchful waiting and tumor behavior in patients with basal cell carcinoma: an observational cohort study of 280 basal cell carcinomas in 89 patients. JAMA Dermatol 2021; 157(10):1174–81.

45. Rosenberg AR, Tabacchi M, Ngo KH, et al. Skin cancer precursor immunotherapy for squamous cell carcinoma prevention. JCI Insight 2019;4(6):e125476.

46. McLaughlin EJ, Miller L, Shin TM, et al. Rate of regional nodal metastases of cutaneous squamous cell carcinoma in the immunosuppressed patient. Am J Otolaryngol 2017;38(3):325–8.

47. Ruiz ES, Karia PS, Morgan FC, et al. The positive impact of radiologic imaging on high-stage cutaneous squamous cell carcinoma management. J Am Acad Dermatol 2017;76(2):217–25.

48. Claveau J, Archambault J, Ernst DS, et al. Multidisciplinary management of locally advanced and metastatic cutaneous squamous cell carcinoma. Curr Oncol 2020;27(4):e399–407.

49. Krausz AE, Ji-Xu A, Smile T, et al. A Systematic review of primary, adjuvant, and salvage radiation therapy for cutaneous squamous cell carcinoma. Dermatol Surg 2021;47(5):587–92.

50. Manyam BV, Garsa AA, Chin RI, et al. A multi-institutional comparison of outcomes of immunosuppressed and immunocompetent patients treated with surgery and radiation therapy for cutaneous squamous cell carcinoma of the head and neck. Cancer 2017;123(11):2054–60.

51. Hughes BGM, Munoz-Couselo E, Mortier L, et al. Pembrolizumab for locally advanced and recurrent/metastatic cutaneous squamous cell carcinoma (KEYNOTE-629 study): an open-label, nonrandomized, multicenter, phase II trial. Ann Oncol 2021; 32(10):1276–85.

52. Migden MR, Rischin D, Schmults CD, et al. PD-1 blockade with cemiplimab in advanced cutaneous squamous-cell carcinoma. N Engl J Med 2018; 379(4):341–51.

53. Maubec E, Petrow P, Scheer-Senyarich I, et al. Phase II study of cetuximab as first-line single-drug therapy in patients with unresectable squamous cell carcinoma of the skin. J Clin Oncol 2011;29(25):3419–26.

54. Leard LE, Cho BK, Jones KD, et al. Fatal diffuse alveolar damage in two lung transplant patients treated with cetuximab. J Heart Lung Transpl 2007; 26(12):1340–4.

55. Stratigos AJ, Sekulic A, Peris K, et al. Cemiplimab in locally advanced basal cell carcinoma after hedgehog inhibitor therapy: an open-label, multi-centre, single-arm, phase 2 trial. Lancet Oncol 2021;22(6): 848–57.

56. Keeping S, Xu Y, Chen CI, et al. Comparative efficacy of cemiplimab versus other systemic treatments for advanced cutaneous squamous cell carcinoma. Future Oncol 2021;17(5):611–27.

57. Porceddu SV, Bressel M, Poulsen MG, et al. Postoperative concurrent chemoradiotherapy versus postoperative radiotherapy in high-risk cutaneous squamous cell carcinoma of the head and neck: the randomized phase III TROG 05.01 trial. J Clin Oncol 2018;36(13):1275–83.

58. d'Izarny-Gargas T, Durrbach A, Zaidan M. Efficacy and tolerance of immune checkpoint inhibitors in transplant patients with cancer: A systematic review. Am J Transpl 2020;20(9):2457–65.

59. Cook MR, Kim C. Safety and efficacy of immune checkpoint inhibitor therapy in patients with HIV infection and advanced-stage cancer: a systematic review. JAMA Oncol 2019;5(7):1049–54.

60. Leiter U, Loquai C, Reinhardt L, et al. Immune checkpoint inhibition therapy for advanced skin cancer in patients with concomitant hematological malignancy: a retrospective multicenter DeCOG study of 84 patients. J Immunother Cancer 2020;8(2).

61. Fisher J, Zeitouni N, Fan W, et al. Immune checkpoint inhibitor therapy in solid organ transplant recipients: a patient-centered systematic review. J Am Acad Dermatol 2020;82(6):1490–500.

62. Cusack CA, Nijhawan R, Miller B, et al. Vismodegib for locally advanced basal cell carcinoma in a heart transplant patient. JAMA Dermatol 2015;151(1): 70–2.

63. Rzepecki AK, Hwang CD, Etzkorn JR, et al. The rule of 10s versus the rule of 2s: High complication rates after conventional excision with postoperative margin assessment of specialty site versus trunk

and proximal extremity melanomas. J Am Acad Dermatol 2021;85(2):442–52.

64. Flaherty KT, Infante JR, Daud A, et al. Combined BRAF and MEK inhibition in melanoma with BRAF V600 mutations. N Engl J Med 2012;367(18): 1694–703.

65. Ressler J, Silmbrod R, Stepan A, et al. Talimogene laherparepvec (T-VEC) in advanced melanoma: complete response in a heart and kidney transplant patient. A case report. Br J Dermatol 2019;181(1): 186–9.

66. Tripathi SV, Morris CR, Alhamad T, et al. Metastatic melanoma after solid organ transplantation: An interdisciplinary, institution-based review of management with systemic and targeted therapies. J Am Acad Dermatol 2018;78(1):184–5.

67. Paulson KG, Iyer JG, Blom A, et al. Systemic immune suppression predicts diminished Merkel cell carcinoma-specific survival independent of stage. J Invest Dermatol 2013;133(3):642–6.

68. Engels EA, Frisch M, Goedert JJ, et al. Merkel cell carcinoma and HIV infection. Lancet 2002; 359(9305):497–8.

69. National Comprehensive Cancer N. Merkel Cell Carcinoma (Version 2.2021. Available at: https://www.nccn.org/professionals/physician_gls/pdf/mcc.pdf. Accessed November 10, 2021.

70. Paulson KG, Lewis CW, Redman MW, et al. Viral oncoprotein antibodies as a marker for recurrence of Merkel cell carcinoma: A prospective validation study. Cancer 2017;123(8):1464–74.

71. Nghiem P, Bhatia S, Lipson EJ, et al. Durable Tumor Regression and Overall Survival in Patients With Advanced Merkel Cell Carcinoma Receiving Pembrolizumab as First-Line Therapy. J Clin Oncol 2019;37(9):693–702.

72. Cesarman E, Damania B, Krown SE, et al. Kaposi sarcoma. Nat Rev Dis Primers 2019;5(1):9.

73. Frances C, Mouquet C, Marcelin AG, et al. Outcome of kidney transplant recipients with previous human herpesvirus-8 infection. Transplantation 2000;69(9): 1776–9.

74. Regamey N, Tamm M, Wernli M, et al. Transmission of human herpesvirus 8 infection from renal-transplant donors to recipients. N Engl J Med 1998;339(19):1358–63.

75. Stallone G, Schena A, Infante B, et al. Sirolimus for Kaposi's sarcoma in renal-transplant recipients. N Engl J Med 2005;352(13):1317–23.

76. Donia AF, Fouda MA, Ghoneim ME, et al. The previously common post-kidney transplant Kaposi sarcoma has become non-existent for a decade: an Egyptian experience. J Cancer Res Clin Oncol 2021;147(5):1493–8.

Approaches to Tumors of the Nail Unit and Genitalia

Kishan M. Shah, MD[1], Kevin Y. Shi, MD, PhD[1], Rajiv I. Nijhawan, MD, Divya Srivastava, MD*

KEYWORDS

- Nail unit tumors • Penile cancer • Vulvar cancer • Outcomes • Dermatology • Surgical specialties
- Mohs micrographic surgery

INTRODUCTION

The nail unit and genitalia represent rare locations where malignant tumors may arise. Human papillomavirus has emerged as a causative agent of the development of the most common malignancies in these sites. Tissue preservation with surgery is of utmost importance, and tissue-sparing approaches are increasingly emphasized in the dermatology, urology, and gynecology literature. In addition to its tissue-sparing nature, Mohs micrographic surgery (MMS) allows the complete evaluation of histologic margins to ensure tumor extirpation and may be the ideal treatment modality. The authors herein present approaches for the evaluation and treatment of malignant tumors of the nail unit and genitalia.

APPROACH TO TUMORS OF THE NAIL

Treatment of nail unit tumors requires a thorough understanding of the unique anatomy and histology of the entire nail apparatus. The most common nail malignancy is squamous cell carcinoma (nSCC) followed by melanoma and more rarely basal cell carcinoma (nBCC). In the last decade, there has been much progress in establishing optimal treatments for malignant nail tumors, particularly SCC and melanoma. There are special considerations for nail surgery involving approach to anesthesia, surgical preparation, and instrumentation.

Anatomy

The nail unit is composed of the nail matrix, proximal nail fold and eponychium, lateral nail folds, nail bed, nail plate, and hyponychium. The nail matrix is composed of onychocytes, melanocytes, Langerhans cells, and Merkel cells.[1] The distal aspect of the matrix can be visualized as the lunula. The proximal and distal aspects of the matrix comprise the dorsal and ventral aspects of the nail plate, respectively.[2] This knowledge assists in surgical planning and patient counseling for location of neoplasms and risk of permanent nail dystrophy. The remaining matrix is covered by the proximal nail fold. The matrix itself extends laterally past the proximal nail fold, particularly in the case of the great toe, in which the matrix may be found as far as halfway into the lateral nail fold.[2] The extensor tendon inserts ~1.4 mm proximal to the nail matrix and is at risk for injury during en bloc resection.

The nail bed extends from the lunula to the hyponychium and contains a rich vascular supply. Longitudinal parallel ridges that interlock between the nail plate and nail bed create a strongly adherent seal between these 2 structures.[1] Approximately 3 mm thickness separates the nail bed epithelium from the underlying periosteum, with a dense connective tissue network encompassing the underlying neurovascular bundle.[1]

The innervation of the digits includes paired volar and dorsal nerves that course along the lateral aspect of the digits. Although anatomic variations exist, generally the second through fourth digits are innervated by palmar digital nerves, and the first and fifth fingers are innervated by dorsal nerves.[2] Three anastomosing arterial arcades, the superficial, proximal, and distal, provide the main blood supply to the nail unit.[2]

Conflicts of Interest: None declared.
Department of Dermatology, University of Texas Southwestern Medical Center, 5939 Harry Hines Boulevard, 4th Floor Suite 100, Dallas, TX 75390, USA
[1] These authors contributed equally to this work.
* Corresponding author.
E-mail address: divya.srivastava@utsouthwestern.edu

Dermatol Clin 41 (2023) 163–174
https://doi.org/10.1016/j.det.2022.07.016

Malignant Nail Neoplasms

Squamous cell carcinoma

nSCC is the most common nail unit malignancy, although it remains rare.[3] It is a slow-growing, low-grade malignancy most commonly diagnosed in middle-aged and older individuals and in men.[4] Presenting signs include onycholysis, hyperkeratosis, verrucous mass, ulceration, paronychia, and granulation tissue (**Fig. 1**). Subungual hyperkeratosis with erythronychia or melanonychia is a clue to matrical involvement. Clinical appearance may mimic benign entities, such as verruca vulgaris, subungual exostosis, onychomycosis, onychomatricoma, infectious paronychia, and trauma. Because of the varying clinical appearance and lack of pain in the majority of tumors, diagnosis is often delayed for an average of 2 years.[4–7] Despite delays in diagnosis, 1 study demonstrated no correlation between time to biopsy and rate of recurrence or invasive disease.[4]

The authors recommend a low threshold for biopsying suspicious lesions. A deep shave for nail bed and nail fold lesions and a nail matrix shave biopsy for matrical lesions are recommended.[4]

Fingers are more commonly affected than toes, which may reflect a role of UV radiation and human papilloma virus (HPV) in the pathogenesis.[8,9] HPV infection, in particular, serotype 16, has been strongly linked to development of nSCC.[10] There are estimations that HPV infections are acquired through genitodigital transmission, as nearly one-third of patients report a personal history of HPV-associated genital disease or a sexual partner with such a history.[3] Other risk factors include radiation, tobacco use, and chronic inflammation.[1,11]

Although lower rates of metastasis are reported for nSCC, there is potential for bony involvement given the proximity of the nail apparatus to the periosteum and distal phalanx.[4] There are 3 types of bone involvement that are seen with nSCC.[12] The most common occurrence is when SCC in situ grows downward from the nail bed rete ridges and abuts the periosteum but does not invade the dermis. The second occurrence involves invasive nSCC that microscopically invades the periosteum and superficial bone. Last, the bone can be grossly involved as evidenced by pitting or bone loss and is typically noted on radiograph. In the last case, partial amputation may be required.

There are no clear guidelines for obtaining preoperative imaging for nSCC. Perioperative imaging may be inconclusive, as inflammation and periosteal compression can obscure the ability to reliably identify true bony invasion.[13] Keratoacanthomas can cause bone resorption, and mass effect may appear as a lytic lesion on radiograph.[14–16] Imaging is more likely obtained for painful tumors. Some investigators argue that histologic examination of the resection specimen is a better evaluation of bone tissue involvement than radiograph, which may help avoid digit amputation.[13] Thus, it is not the authors' standard practice to obtain preoperative imaging. However, should histopathology during resection reveal bone involvement, it must be addressed as described in later discussion.[11,12]

Several treatment modalities exist for nSCC, including MMS, wide local excision, amputation, destruction, and topical therapy.[4,11] A recent systemic review highlighted that complete surgical resection is first-line therapy for nSCC. MMS is optimal for superior cure rates, tissue preservation, which can lead to better function and wound healing, and verification of clear margins in real time. Often much of the nail unit can be spared, and MMS for nSCC does not require en bloc resection. If MMS is not available, wide local excision with complete peripheral and deep margin control should be performed. In cases of bony involvement, amputation can be considered. If there is only microscopic disease, the authors use a nail nipper or bone rongeur to remove the superficial bone and either process it as a frozen section or as a permanent section, thereby avoiding amputation if possible. Repair options following surgical removal include full-thickness skin grafts, secondary intention, and split-thickness skin grafts.[4]

Topical therapies, such as imiquimod or 5-fluorouracil, are not optimal for first-line treatment of nSCC owing to challenges in completely treating the sulci of the nail folds. Imiquimod may have a benefit as adjuvant field therapy in patients with HPV-related nSCC.[1] Radiation is an option for patients with multiple affected digits or if surgery is contraindicated. However, radiation exposure

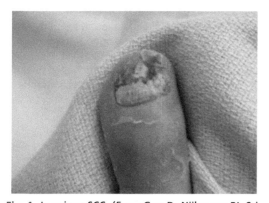

Fig. 1. Invasive nSCC. (*From* Gou D, Nijhawan RI, Srivastava D. Mohs Micrographic Surgery as the Standard of Care for Nail Unit Squamous Cell Carcinoma. Dermatol Surg. 2020 Jun;46(6):725-732.)

has also been reported as a causative agent in the formation of nSCC.[1] Overall recurrence rates for modalities other than surgical resection is 3-fold higher.[17]

Postresection recurrences are hypothesized, in part, to be driven by persistent HPV field effect.[4,6] There is a paucity of data in adjuvant treatments and the role of HPV vaccination in the role of treatment and prevention.

Nail unit melanoma

Nail unit melanoma is a rare variant of acral lentiginous melanoma.[18–21] It is more common in darker-skinned and Asian patients.[18–20,22] Delays in diagnosis are due to the asymptomatic nature of the lesions and common presentation with other benign causes, such as onychomycosis and trauma. There are challenges with histologic diagnosis as well, given features overlap with other benign melanocytic lesions.[10,21,23,24] The ABCDE rule for melanoma of the nail unit is useful in evaluating melanonychia, as well as Hutchinson sign, in which pigment extends on the proximal nail matrix or nail folds.[1] These include age in the fifth to seventh decade of life, African, Asian, or Native American ethnicity, brown or black pigment greater than 3 mm in width, change in the nail or failure to improve with treatment, which digit is involved, most pertinently the thumb or great toe, and extension of the pigment to the lateral or proximal nail fold.[1]

Surgical treatment options range from digital amputation, en bloc nail unit resection, and MMS.[11,25–28] It is necessary to balance maintaining digit function with prioritizing an optimal oncologic cure. Treatment has evolved toward digit-sparing surgery, as outcomes (recurrence and metastasis) are equivalent to proximal or distal amputation.[27,29,30] For invasive melanoma, treatment recommendations are based on depth of invasion. A recent meta-analysis analyzed 5 studies reporting on 109 patients with in situ or minimally invasive (<0.5 mm) melanoma of the nail bed demonstrated no difference in recurrence between those who had "functional" surgery (en bloc nail excisions or MMS) versus digit amputation.[31] For deeper melanomas, amputation and sentinel lymph node (LN) biopsy are indicated.

MMS has been used for melanoma in situ as well as invasive melanoma using melanoma antigen recognized by T cells-1 (MART-1) immunostains.[22] The authors' approach is to resect the entire nail unit, including nail bed, hyponychium, proximal nail fold, and matrix, plus a minimum of 5 mm from the margin of clinically evident tumor, marked as demonstrated in **Fig. 2**. The excision is extended 8 to 10 mm proximally and 4 to 6 mm

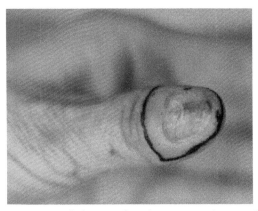

Fig. 2. Surgical planning for adequate margin control of clinical lesion. (*From* Matsumoto A, Strickland N, Nijhawan RI, Srivastava D. Nail Unit Melanoma In Situ Treated With Mohs Micrographic Surgery. Dermatol Surg. 2021 Jan 1;47(1):98-103.)

laterally from the proximal nail fold to ensure excision of the lateral horns of the nail matrix, which is the most common site for recurrence.[25] The depth of excision is the deepest extent of subcutaneous tissue and to periosteum under the nail apparatus (**Fig. 3**). Jellinek and Bauer[29] suggest incising the lateral nail fold and then extending distally to the phalangeal tuft at the level of the periosteum. The proximal dissection to the level of the extensor tendon is performed using blunt-tipped scissors with "tips down" to prevent injury to the overlying matrix.[29]

The authors do not perform nail avulsion before removal of the Mohs layer to minimize shearing of the nail bed epithelium and allow complete histologic examination of the epithelium.[32,33] Removal of the nail unit is their preferred method for decreasing risk of recurrence and growth of nail spicules, which can cause postoperative sequalae.[34] Tissue is processed with standard Mohs technique and stained with hematoxylin and eosin (H&E) and MART-1 immunostaining. Positive margins identified on the frozen section are further resected with an additional 3-mm margin and processed with the standard Mohs technique. After the tissue is cleared by MMS, the excised specimen is thawed and sent in for permanent sections with H&E for standard bread-loaf sectioning to evaluate depth for accurate staging.[33]

MMS remains an excellent treatment modality for melanoma in situ (MIS) of the nail unit, providing a noninferior recurrence rate demonstrated across multiple studies and excellent functional outcomes.[33] MMS for nail unit melanoma requires extensive training and understanding of nail anatomy, nail histology, and MART-1 stains. En bloc resection can also achieve excellent results while

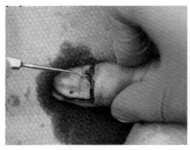 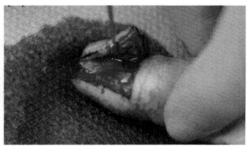

Fig. 3. After initial incisions around the phalanx, the nail unit is dissected immediately above the periosteum. (*From* Matsumoto A, Strickland N, Nijhawan RI, Srivastava D. Nail Unit Melanoma In Situ Treated With Mohs Micrographic Surgery. Dermatol Surg. 2021 Jan 1;47(1):98-103.)

preserving the digit. Knackstedt and Jellinek[21] reported high satisfaction rates of 87% after digit-sparing surgery for nail unit MIS. There was minimal impact on quality of life or disability. In contrast, distal or proximal amputation of the thumb is associated with 50% and 100% impairment of the digit.

Basal cell carcinoma
BCC of the nail unit is the least commonly encountered malignant tumor of the nail.[1] These tumors may present within the nail bed, or along the nail-fold. Chronic erythema and scaling are the 2 most common findings, whereas the typical features of translucency, telangiectasias, and ulceration are less frequent.[1] Although local destruction with topical medications and curettage has been used for treatment, MMS remains the most appropriate modality for treatment.[1]

Aggressive papillary digital adenocarcinoma
Aggressive digital papillary adenocarcinoma (ADPA) is a rare adenocarcinoma of the sweat glands that can be treated by MMS.[35] ADPA can mimic benign conditions, such as ganglion cysts, pyogenic granulomas, paronychia, and giant cell tumor of the tendon sheath. Definite treatment is not well established, as there are high rates of local recurrent and distant metastases reported.[36] Although some advise amputation as definitive treatment owing to the aggressive nature of the tumor, MMS represents an enticing treatment that significantly decreases morbidity.

Special Considerations

Anesthesia and surgical preparation
A successful nail procedure requires adequate anesthesia. Lidocaine is the most widely available and used by the authors. Other options include bupivacaine and ropivacaine.[37] The onset of action of each anesthetic is inversely proportional to its duration. **Table 1** delineates onset and duration of action for each anesthetic. Although

longer-acting anesthetics provide postoperative pain minimizations, they may mask possible complications, including compartment syndrome, infection, and ischemia.[37] Ropivacaine is associated with vasoconstrictive properties without epinephrine and less postprocedure pain.[38]

It is safe to use epinephrine in the anesthetic. Previous concerns regarding risk of necrosis from vasoconstriction have been disproven in the absence of other contraindications (ie, vasospastic disease).[39] It is important to be cautious with the volume of anesthetic injected. Lidocaine 1% with epinephrine 1:100,000 can safely be used for 1 mL per side of the digit for the digital block and 1 to 2 mL for the wing block. The maximum volume that should be injected is 5 mL; however, much lower volumes can achieve adequate anesthesia.[37] The benefits of epinephrine include prolonged anesthesia, postoperative analgesia, and decreased bleeding.[37] The usual techniques for decreasing pain during injection, including buffering, warming, slow injection, using the gate theory of pain, and "talkesthesia," may all help improve comfort.[37]

Injection techniques include infiltrative anesthesia, in the form of wing block and/or digital nerve blocks. Wing blocks use anesthesia at the proximal nail fold initially, and additional anesthesia is placed in the lateral nail fold and then the digital tip. Fluid injection acts as a tamponade

Table 1		
Various anesthetics, their onset, and duration of action		
Anesthetic	Onset of Action (min)	Duration of Action with Epinephrine (h)
Lidocaine	<1	1–6.5
Bupivacaine	2–5	4–8
Ropivacaine	1–15	Up to 20

that aids in hemostasis.[37] The traditional digital block requires 2 needle punctures, one on each side of the digit, to anesthetize the paired dorsal and volar digital nerves. These punctures may be made at either the metacarpophalangeal/metatarsophalangeal joint or slightly more proximally. The authors prefer injection at the distal interphalangeal to achieve more rapid anesthesia with less volume.[40] After injection, onset of action can range from 3 to 20 minutes.[37] Patients may soak their digits in chlorhexidine to soften the nail plate while waiting. The distal digit must be tested before initiation of the procedure. Anesthesia is injected as the needle is pulled back, diffusing laterally to affect the digital nerves.[37] The authors perform a digital block followed by a wing block after 5 to 10 minutes.

Before surgery, the affected digit can be soaked in a chlorhexidine saline mixture to soften the plate. This can be done while the digital block is taking effect. The surgical field should be prepared with chlorhexidine or povidone-iodine and draped. Some advocate for sterile preparation, and others have similar outcomes with clean preparation. Hemostasis can be achieved using a tourniquet. A Penrose drain can be used as a tourniquet. A sterile glove with the affected tip cut away can be placed on the patient's hand, and the tip can be rolled back to create compression. It is critical to remove the tourniquet within 10 to 15 minutes to avoid digital ischemia. A clear visual field can also be obtained if the surgical assistant applies pressure to the sides of the digit to tamponade the vessels.

Nail instruments
Dermatologic surgeons can benefit from specialized instruments for nail surgery (**Fig. 4**). The Freer septum elevator has a thin curved blade that can be used to separate the nail plate from the nail bed and matrix. The English nail splitter consists of 1 sharp cutting edge and 1 flat surface. The dual-action nail nippers are used to excise thick nails. The authors also use this instrument to remove soft tissue remnants, periosteum, and superficial bone, as needed. A bone rongeur can also be used for removing bone.

Complications
Patients can experience prolonged pain after nail surgery. It is important to counsel them appropriately. Pain management can be achieved with alternating ibuprofen and acetaminophen. Some patients may require a short course of opioids. In patients undergoing en bloc resection, it is important to counsel on total lack of nail regrowth. For partial resections, as in the case of nSCC, the location of the nSCC will dictate whether the

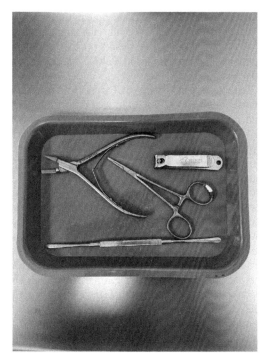

Fig. 4. Nail instruments.

patient develops nail dystrophy from nail matrix involvement. If lateral horns of the matrix remain postresection, painful spicules can develop and should be removed along with the residual matrix. For patients undergoing second intention healing or flap/graft repair, it is important to counsel them to use the digit and move the joints regularly to prevent formation of a thick scar.

In summary, it is critical to understand nail anatomy and physiology in order to perform effective nail surgery for malignant neoplasms. As excellent outcomes can be achieved with digit-sparing surgery, dermatologic surgeons need to gain training and expertise in nail surgery to optimize digit function.

APPROACH TO TUMORS OF THE GENITALIA
Malignant Neoplasms of the Penis and Scrotum

Penile cancer accounts for less than 1% of all cancers in men, with SCC accounting for ~95% of cases.[41,42] Invasive SCC can arise de novo or evolve from a precursor, penile intraepithelial neoplasm (PeIN). Infection from HPV-16, -18, and other high-risk subtypes accounts for 30% to 50% of cases. Concurrent lichen sclerosis is seen in up to 33% of invasive SCC and is the most important factor for HPV-independent tumorigenesis.[41] PeIN can present as Bowenoid papulosis, Bowen disease, or erythroplasia of

Queyrat (EQ). EQ undergoes malignant transformation in 10% to 30% of cases. Histologic grading of PeIN (grades 1–3) is based on the extent of epithelial involvement, with PeIN 3 featuring full-thickness atypia.[41]

The majority of invasive SCCs are located on the glans, followed by the prepuce, corona sulcus, and, rarely, the shaft.[41] Regional metastases occur in 15% to 25% of patients.[43] The American Joint Committee on Cancer (AJCC) 8th edition and Union for International Cancer Control TNM staging system offer prognostic information for penile carcinomas.[43] Because of lower rates of regional metastasis, T1a and lower staged tumors do not require routine LN dissection. In comparison, T1b stage (presence of either lymphovascular invasion, perineural invasion, or high histologic grade) is associated with greater than 25% of regional metastasis and requires superficial inguinal LN dissection or dynamic sentinel lymph node biopsy (SLNB). Deep invasion into the corpus spongiosum and beyond is associated with 36% to 56% nodal involvement and worse disease-specific survival.

For PeIN, topical 5-fluorouracil 5% and imiquimod 5% creams have an overall complete response rate of 57%.[44] Destruction with cryotherapy, with or without imiquimod, has also been described.[45] The outcomes of these conservative modalities based on the severity of PeIN are not well defined. If a nonsurgical modality is chosen, a punch or incisional biopsy should be performed to rule out SCC, because 20% of PeIN may harbor invasive disease.[41]

National Comprehensive Cancer Network (NCCN) guidelines recommend organ-sparing approaches for the surgical treatment of Tis (ie, PeIN), Ta, or T1 SCC.[46] A local recurrence rate (LRR) of 6.4% was reported for wide local excision (WLE) compared with 3% to 10% for penectomy, and margin control was imperative as narrow clearance of less than 1 mm had nearly 6 times the risk for recurrence.[47] Circumcision with a margin of 5 mm offers excellent outcomes for SCC confined to the prepuce. Laser ablation, WLE, glans resurfacing, glansectomy, and radiation are effective treatments.[48]

MMS for penile carcinomas has shown favorable outcomes (LRR, 1.2%–32%).[49–53] In the largest series to date, a single recurrence was seen for 22 invasive SCC and 63 squamous cell carcinoma in situ (SCCis) after a median follow-up of 2.36 years.[50] In addition, patients reported high degrees of satisfaction for cosmetic outcomes and preservation of organ functionality after MMS.[49,51] HPV field effect or technique-related differences may account for the range of LRR.[49] These case series included some AJCC stage T1b or greater tumors, which did not significantly differ in outcomes compared with lower-stage tumors.[49,52] Therefore, MMS may still offer excellent local disease control for deep and large tumors in combination with appropriate nodal staging. An evolving application of MMS is for carcinoma with urethral involvement. Urethral invasion is not a reliable prognostic factor and is not associated with T stage. In fact, involvement of the distal urethra can occur in Tis meatal tumors. In practice, 2 series described the use of MMS for urethral invasion without any cases of recurrence.[49,54]

Other rare malignancies of the penis include melanoma, extramammary Paget disease (EMPD), and BCC.[42] MMS of EMPD has demonstrated superior outcomes to WLE in both male and female patients and are discussed further later. Although historically associated with occupational exposures in chimney sweeps, scrotal cancers are exceedingly rare, with SCC, EMPD, and BCC as the most commonly reported tumors.[55,56] Despite their rarity, MMS has been shown to be effective for treating scrotal SCC, EMPD, and BCC.[55]

Operative Considerations

Local anesthesia with 1% lidocaine with epinephrine can be safely used.[49] A dorsal penile block (infiltration of 0.4 mL of 1% lidocaine without epinephrine at the 2 and 10 o'clock positions deep to the pubic symphysis) or a ring block at the base of the shaft can also be performed.[57] Of note, the dorsal penile nerves do not supply the frenulum.

Preoperative MRI with artificial erection is the method of choice for assessing deep invasion and urethral involvement, with cystoscopy as an adjunct procedure.[43,54] Standard procedure for MMS also applies for penile tumors.[58] The lesion can first be debulked to define the extent of tumor, and then a margin of ∼2 mm can be taken into the clinically health tissue (**Fig. 5**).[49] For carcinoma in situ, a depth to the Buck fascia for the shaft and superficial corpus spongiosum for the glans may be appropriate (see **Fig. 5**A, C). As discussed previously, deep invasion of the corpus spongiosum and cavernosum is not an indication for aborting surgery based on the experience of the surgeon. If urethral involvement is detected on microscopic examination, some investigators perform ventral meatotomy and urethrotomy to allow access to planar gross tissue containing the urethra.[49] Analogous to actinic damage, if significant field cancerization from low-grade PeIN is seen on frozen section, a postoperative course of imiquimod

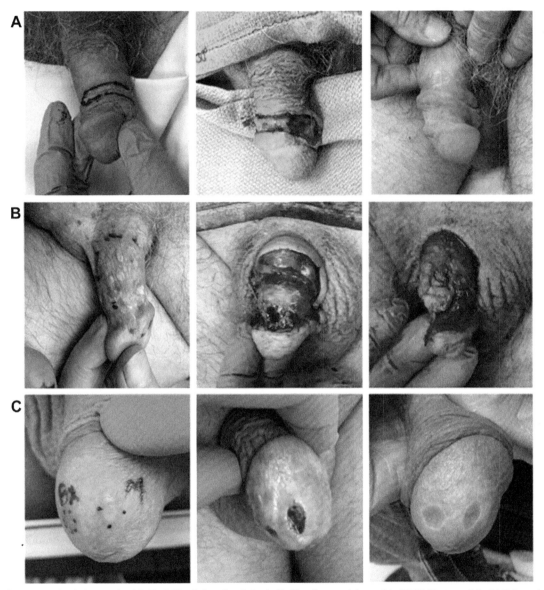

Fig. 5. MMS of the penis. (A) Tis SCC of the distal shaft (*left*), after excision with MMS (2 stages) (*middle*), and healing by secondary intention (*right*). (B) Extensive Tis/T1a SCC involving the dorsolateral shaft, corona, and glans (*left*), after MMS stage 1 (*middle*), and stage 2 (*right*). (C) Tis SCC (marked "M") isolated to the glans (*left*), after excision with MMS (1 stage) (*middle*), and healing by secondary intention (*right*).

should be considered. Hemostasis for superficial defects can be accomplished with electrodessication. A temporary tourniquet can be applied to the base of the shaft if significant hemorrhage is encountered.[59] Catheterization may be implemented postexcision for defects involving the meatus/urethra to prevent tissue stenosis before reconstruction. Healing by secondary intention can yield excellent cosmetic and functional outcomes for both mucosal or cutaneous defects and even those that involve the distal urethra (see **Fig. 5**A, C).[49,51] Primary closures of small shaft defects may be easily performed as an outpatient, but reconstruction of extensive defects involving the glans, deep erectile tissue, or proximal urethra requires additional specialty referral. For surgery without incision of the urethra, perioperative antibiotic is not indicated.

Malignant Neoplasms of the External Female Genitalia

Vulvar cancer comprises 4% of all gynecologic malignancies with SCC representing 90% of cases.[60,61] Vulvar intraepithelial neoplasms (VIN) are the malignant precursor of SCC; the most common sites are the labia majora and minora. Low-grade intraepithelial lesion is associated with HPV-6, -11, and other high-risk subtypes and is equivalent to condyloma accuminata. High-grade intraepithelial lesion (HSIL, previously VIN 2 or 3) is usually associated with HPV-16, -18, and -31. Approximately 9% of HSIL will progress to SCC; 20% may harbor invasive, and up to 25% will recur after treatment.[60,62–64] HPV-independent, differentiated VIN (dVIN) develop in older patients with chronic inflammatory dermatoses, with a risk for malignant transformation of 50% over 10 years.

Based on the AJCC and The International Federation of Gynecology and Obstetrics TNM staging system, T1a/IA tumors (localized to the vulva/perineum, <2 cm in diameter, and <1 mm of stromal invasion) have less than 1% concurrent nodal metastasis. Tumors T1b or greater demonstrate greater than 8% nodal involvement, and lymphadenectomy or SLNB should be performed at the time excision.[65,66] Incisional or punch biopsies should be performed for diagnosis as the depth of invasion is used to guide treatment planning.

For HSIL, surgical excision, ablative laser, or topical imiquimod 5% cream offers similar cure rates.[62,67] Ablative laser or imiquimod may be advantageous for multifocal lesions and those that involve the clitoris, urethra, anus, or introitus to minimize loss of function and anatomical distortion from surgical scarring. Nonsurgical approaches should be avoided in hair-bearing sites owing to potential follicular extension of tumor, and imiquimod should be avoided in pregnancy.[67]

Surgical margins of 0.5 to 1 cm are recommended for WLE of HSIL or dVIN.[67,68] NCCN guidelines recommend a margin of at least 1 cm for T1a SCC. LRR and disease-specific death are similar for WLE and vulvectomy. If narrow margins are necessary based on anatomical constraints, a referral to gynecologic surgery is appropriate, and adjuvant radiation may be indicated. Although there is no current recommendation for the use of MMS for HSIL or SCC, it should be considered owing to its tissue-sparing nature and ability to examine all tissue margins.[69–71] In the largest case series to date, no recurrence was seen after MMS for 16 carcinoma in situ and 3 SCC.[71]

Genital melanoma represents 2% of all melanomas in women and is the second most common vulvar malignancy.[72] The labia majora and clitoris are the most common sites. Current literature recommends that vulvar melanoma and precursor lesions should be treated similarly to its cutaneous counterpart. T1a tumors can be treated with WLE with 1-cm margins, which appears as effective as radical vulvectomy for disease-specific survival.[73] For melanoma in situ, MMS should be strongly considered given its tissue-sparing nature, as a narrow initial margin of 2 to 3 mm can be taken compared with 5 to 10 mm for WLE.[74] Numerous studies have shown minimal LRR after MMS and superiority over WLE, and a recent case highlighted its successful application to the vulva.[74–76]

Primary EMPD is an adenocarcinoma of keratinocytic precursor or apocrine duct cells.[77] The vulva is the most common site for EMPD. The tumor is typically confined to the epidermis, but invasive disease of the dermis complicated by metastasis has been reported. Other rare tumors include BCC and dermatofibroma protuberance.

Because of its penchant for subclinical extension, WLE of EMPD (even with a margin of 3–5 cm) has historically resulted in recurrence rates of 30% to 60%. For MMS, compiled data from both female and male patients showed LRR of 12.2% for both primary and recurrent tumors.[77] Hendi and colleagues[78] reported that a margin of 5 cm was required to clear 97% of tumors. Therefore, MMS can help to identify where extra margins are needed while potentially sparing vital local structures. The use of intraoperative cytokeratin-7 immunostaining further improved LRR to 3.3% for 61 tumors over average follow-up of 43.5 months.[79]

Operative Consideration

Presurgical counseling is imperative regarding the possible effect of surgery on sexual or urinary function, and any psychosocial concern should be addressed. Local anesthesia with 1% lidocaine with epinephrine is usually adequate. The patient should be situated in a lithotomy position whenever possible with feet placed in stirrups to facilitate access and decrease tension on wound edges during reconstruction. A head lamp can be worn to aid in the visualization of the field.

WLE should be performed in an elliptical manner oriented anterior-posteriorly. Lesions involving the mucosal surface can be oriented in a curvilinear fashion along anatomical contours. For vulvar SCC, guidelines recommend that the excision should be carried to the deep subcutaneous fascia to facilitate accurate staging. Standard MMS procedure applies to the vulva.[58] Immediate reconstruction of small to medium defects can be accomplished with primary closure or local random pattern flaps (Fig. 6). Healing by secondary intention of shallow defects can also be

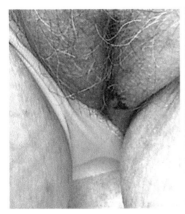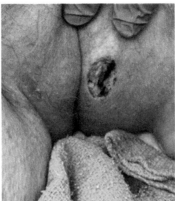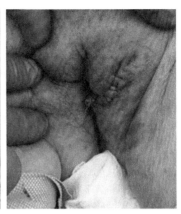

Fig. 6. MMS of the vulva. Nodular basal cell carcinoma of the left labia majus (*left*), post-MMS defect (*middle*), and repair by primary closure (*right*).

considered. For exceptionally large tumors, mostly encountered for EMPD, a modified MMS procedure can be used to selectively assess margin control at the periphery of the lesion, whereas the center island of tumor can be excised in the deep subcutaneous plane.[78–80] Preoperative scouting shave biopsies can also be used to aid first-stage planning.[79] Similarly observed in sun-damaged skin, increased density of basilar melanocytes due to background vulvar lentiginosis may complicate frozen-section interpretation of MIS.[75] The routine use of MART-1 staining during MMS can help to discriminate MIS-specific features, such as contiguous or nesting melanocytes, pagetoid spread, and/or adnexal involvement, whereas biopsy of the surrounding skin can also serve as a negative control.[74] Postexcision, sanitary napkin or adult diaper may be provided to prevent soiling of garments. Although postsurgical infection rates may be as high as 58%, gynecologic guidelines consider vulvar surgery to be a clean-contaminated procedure and do not make definitive recommendations for perioperative antibiotics.[81]

CLINICS CARE POINTS

- Knowledge of nail anatomy and anesthesia techniques are vital components of successful tumor extirpation

- Squamous cell carcinoma of the nail unit is often driven by HPV infections, and can result in bony invasion

- Digit sparing surgery with en bloc resection or Mohs micrographic surgery for melanoma of the nail unit results in significant

functional improvement with noninferior recurrence rates

- HPV-related squamous cell carcinoma is the most common cancer of the external genitalia

- Surgical and non-surgical treatments of genital cancers need to minimize long-term functional and cosmetic morbidities

- Mohs micrographic surgery is an effective and emerging tissue-sparing treatment of genital cancers

REFERENCES

1. Jellinek NJ. Primary malignant tumors of the nail unit. Adv Dermatol 2005;21:33–64.
2. Richert B, Rich P. Nail surgery. In: Bolognia JL, Schaffer JV, Cerroni L, editors. Dermatology. Philadelphia: Elsevier; 2018. p. 2531–40.
3. Richert B, Lecerf P, Caucanas M, et al. Nail tumors. Clin Dermatol 2013;31(5):602–17.
4. Gou D, Nijhawan RI, Srivastava D. Mohs micrographic surgery as the standard of care for nail unit squamous cell carcinoma. Dermatol Surg 2020;46(6):725–32.
5. Lecerf P, Richert B, Theunis A, et al. A retrospective study of squamous cell carcinoma of the nail unit diagnosed in a Belgian general hospital over a 15-year period. J Am Acad Dermatol 2013;69(2):253–61.
6. Gormley RH, Groft CM, Miller CJ, et al. Digital squamous cell carcinoma and association with diverse high-risk human papillomavirus types. J Am Acad Dermatol 2011;64(5):981–5.
7. Clark MA, Filitis D, Samie FH, et al. Evaluating the utility of routine imaging in squamous cell carcinoma of the nail unit. Dermatol Surg 2020;46(11):1375–81.

8. Ormerod E, de Berker D. Nail unit squamous cell carcinoma in people with immunosuppression. Br J Dermatol 2015;173(3):701–12.

9. Riddel C, Rashid R, Thomas V. Ungual and periungual human papillomavirus-associated squamous cell carcinoma: a review. J Am Acad Dermatol 2011;64(6):1147–53.

10. Baltz JO, Jellinek NJ. Nail surgery: six essential techniques. Dermatol Clin 2021;39(2):305–18.

11. Lambertini M, Piraccini BM, Fanti PA, et al. Mohs micrographic surgery for nail unit tumours: an update and a critical review of the literature. J Eur Acad Dermatol Venereol 2018;32(10):1638–44.

12. Jariwala N, Jellinek NJ, Srivastava DS, et al. Commentary on "treatment options and outcomes for squamous cell carcinoma of the nail unit: a systematic review". Dermatol Surg 2022;48(3):274–5.

13. Dika E, Fanti PA, Patrizi A, et al. Mohs surgery for squamous cell carcinoma of the nail unit: 10 years of experience. Dermatol Surg 2015;41(9):1015–9.

14. Sinha A, Marsh R, Langtry J. Spontaneous regression of subungual keratoacanthoma with reossification of underlying distal lytic phalynx. Clin Exp Dermatol 2005;30(1):20–2.

15. Cramer SF. Subungual keratoacanthoma. A benign bone-eroding neoplasm of the distal phalanx. Am J Clin Pathol 1981;75(3):425–9.

16. Choi JH, Shin DH, Shin DS, et al. Subungual keratoacanthoma: ultrasound and magnetic resonance imaging findings. Skeletal Radiol 2007;36(8): 769–72.

17. Ning AY, Levoska MA, Zheng DX, et al. Treatment Options and Outcomes for Squamous Cell Carcinoma of the Nail Unit: A Systematic Review. Dermatol Surg 2021;48(3):267–73.

18. Chang JW. Acral melanoma: a unique disease in Asia. JAMA Dermatol 2013;149(11):1272–3.

19. Duarte AF, Correia O, Barros AM, et al. Nail matrix melanoma in situ: conservative surgical management. Dermatology 2010;220(2):173–5.

20. Jung HJ, Kweon SS, Lee JB, et al. A clinicopathologic analysis of 177 acral melanomas in Koreans: relevance of spreading pattern and physical stress. JAMA Dermatol 2013;149(11):1281–8.

21. Knackstedt T, Jellinek NJ. Limitations and challenges of nail unit dermoscopy in longitudinal melanonychia. J Am Acad Dermatol 2017;76(2):e71–2.

22. Brodland DG. The treatment of nail apparatus melanoma with Mohs micrographic surgery. Dermatol Surg 2001;27(3):269–73.

23. Albertini JG, Elston DM, Libow LF, et al. Mohs micrographic surgery for melanoma: a case series, a comparative study of immunostains, an informative case report, and a unique mapping technique. Dermatol Surg 2002;28(8):656–65.

24. High WA, Quirey RA, Guilen DR, et al. Presentation, histopathologic findings, and clinical outcomes in 7 cases of melanoma in situ of the nail unit. Arch Dermatol 2004;140(9):1102–6.

25. Reilly DJ, Aksakal G, Gilmour RF, et al. Subungual melanoma: management in the modern era. J Plast Reconstr Aesthet Surg 2017;70(12):1746–52.

26. Banfield CC, Dawber RP, Walker NP, et al. Mohs micrographic surgery for the treatment of in situ nail apparatus melanoma: a case report. J Am Acad Dermatol 1999;40(1):98–9.

27. Cochran AM, Buchanan PJ, Bueno RA Jr, et al. Subungual melanoma: a review of current treatment. Plast Reconstr Surg 2014;134(2):259–73.

28. Park KG, Blessing K, Kernohan NM. Surgical aspects of subungual malignant melanomas. The Scottish Melanoma Group. Ann Surg 1992;216(6): 692–5.

29. Jellinek NJ, Bauer JH. En bloc excision of the nail. Dermatol Surg 2010;36(9):1445–50.

30. Sureda N, Phan A, Poulalhon N, et al. Conservative surgical management of subungual (matrix derived) melanoma: report of seven cases and literature review. Br J Dermatol 2011;165(4):852–8.

31. Jo G, Cho SI, Choi S, et al. Functional surgery versus amputation for in situ or minimally invasive nail melanoma: a meta-analysis. J Am Acad Dermatol 2019;81(4):917–22.

32. Jellinek NJ, Cordova KB. Frozen sections for nail surgery: avulsion is unnecessary. Dermatol Surg 2013;39(2):312–4.

33. Matsumoto A, Strickland N, Nijhawan RI, et al. Nail Unit Melanoma In Situ Treated With Mohs Micrographic Surgery. Dermatol Surg 2021;47(1):98–103.

34. Terushkin V, Brodland DG, Sharon DJ, et al. Digit-Sparing Mohs Surgery for Melanoma. Dermatol Surg 2016;42(1):83–93.

35. Knackstedt RW, Knackstedt TJ, Findley AB, et al. Aggressive digital papillary adenocarcinoma: treatment with Mohs micrographic surgery and an update of the literature. Int J Dermatol 2017;56(10): 1061–4.

36. Duke WH, Sherrod TT, Lupton GP. Aggressive digital papillary adenocarcinoma (aggressive digital papillary adenoma and adenocarcinoma revisited). Am J Surg Pathol 2000;24(6):775–84.

37. Jellinek NJ, Velez NF. Nail surgery: best way to obtain effective anesthesia. Dermatol Clin 2015; 33(2):265–71.

38. Di Chiacchio N, Ocampo-Garza J, Villarreal-Villarreal CD, et al. Post-nail procedure analgesia: a randomized control pilot study. J Am Acad Dermatol 2019;81(3):860–2.

39. Harness NG. Digital block anesthesia. J Hand Surg Am 2009;34(1):142–5.

40. Jariwala NN, Dasilva DR, Sobanko JF, et al. Modified distal digital block for nail unit surgery. J Am Acad Dermatol 2021;. https://doi-org.foyer.swmed.edu/10.1016/j.jaad.2021.10.056.

41. Thomas A, Necchi A, Muneer A, et al. Penile cancer. Nat Rev Dis Primers 2021;7(1):11.

42. Brady KL, Mercurio MG, Brown MD. Malignant tumors of the penis. Dermatol Surg 2013;39(4):527–47.

43. Khalil MI, Kamel MH, Dhillon J, et al. What you need to know: updates in penile cancer staging. World J Urol 2021;39(5):1413–9.

44. Manjunath A, Brenton T, Wylie S, et al. Topical Therapy for non-invasive penile cancer (Tis)-updated results and toxicity. Transl Androl Urol 2017;6(5):803–8.

45. Shaw KS, Nguyen GH, Lacouture M, et al. Combination of imiquimod with cryotherapy in the treatment of penile intraepithelial neoplasia. JAAD Case Rep 2017;3(6):546–9.

46. Clark PE, Spiess PE, Agarwal N, et al. Penile cancer: clinical practice guidelines in oncology. J Natl Compr Canc Netw 2013;11(5):594–615.

47. Sri D, Sujenthiran A, Lam W, et al. A study into the association between local recurrence rates and surgical resection margins in organ-sparing surgery for penile squamous cell cancer. BJU Int 2018;122(4):576–82.

48. Babbar P, Yerram N, Crane A, et al. Penile-sparing modalities in the management of low-stage penile cancer. Urol Ann 2018;10(1):1–6.

49. Machan M, Brodland D, Zitelli J. Penile Squamous Cell Carcinoma: Penis-Preserving Treatment With Mohs Micrographic Surgery. Dermatol Surg 2016;42(8):936–44.

50. Lukowiak TM, Perz AM, Aizman L, et al. Mohs micrographic surgery for male genital tumors: Local recurrence rates and patient-reported outcomes. J Am Acad Dermatol 2021;84(4):1030–6.

51. Mohs FE, Snow SN, Larson PO. Mohs micrographic surgery for penile tumors. Urol Clin North Am 1992;19(2):291–304.

52. Brown MD, Zachary CB, Grekin' RC, et al. Penile tumors: their management by Mohs micrographic surgery. J Dermatol Surg Oncol 1987;13(11):1163–7.

53. Shindel AW, Mann MW, Lev RY, et al. Mohs micrographic surgery for penile cancer: management and long-term followup. J Urol 2007;178(5):1980–5.

54. Erlendsson AM, Wilson BN, Bellia P, et al. Mohs micrographic surgery for penile carcinoma with urethral invasion: A multidisciplinary approach. J Am Acad Dermatol 2020;83(6):1803–5.

55. Roberson D, Chelluri R, Skokan AJ, et al. Outcomes of Mohs microgrpahic resection for cutaneous malignancy involving the scrotum. Urol Oncol 2021;39(8):501.e11–6.

56. Wright JL, Morgan TM, Lin DW. Primary scrotal cancer: disease characteristics and increasing incidence. Urology 2008;72(5):1139–43.

57. McPhee AS, McKay AC. StatPearls Publishing Copyright © 2021. Treasure Island (FL: StatPearls Publishing LLC; 2021.

58. Chen ELA, Srivastava D, Nijhawan RI. Semin Plast Surg 2018;32(2):60–8.

59. Parsons BA, Kalejaiye O, Mohammed M, et al. The penile tourniquet. Asian J Androl 2013;15(3):364–7.

60. Thuijs NB, van Beurden M, Bruggink AH, et al. Vulvar intraepithelial neoplasia: Incidence and long-term risk of vulvar squamous cell carcinoma. Int J Cancer 2021;148(1):90–8.

61. Siegel RL, Miller KD, Fuchs HE, et al. Cancer Statistics, 2021. CA Cancer J Clin 2021;71(1):7–33.

62. Lawrie TA, Nordin A, Chakrabarti M, et al. Medical and surgical interventions for the treatment of usual-type vulval intraepithelial neoplasia. Cochrane Database Syst Rev 2016;2016(1):Cd011837.

63. van Seters M, van Beurden M, de Craen AJ. Is the assumed natural history of vulvar intraepithelial neoplasia III based on enough evidence? A systematic review of 3322 published patients. Gynecol Oncol 2005;97(2):645–51.

64. Modesitt SC, Waters AB, Walton L, et al. Vulvar intraepithelial neoplasia III: occult cancer and the impact of margin status on recurrence. Obstet Gynecol 1998;92(6):962–6.

65. Olawaiye AB, Cuello MA, Rogers LJ. Cancer of the vulva: 2021 update. Int J Gynaecol Obstet 2021;155(Suppl 1):7–18.

66. Hacker NF, Berek JS, Lagasse LD, et al. Individualization of treatment for stage I squamous cell vulvar carcinoma. Obstet Gynecol 1984;63(2):155–62.

67. Committee Opinion No. 675 Summary: Management of Vulvar Intraepithelial Neoplasia. Obstet Gynecol 2016;128(4):937–8.

68. DeSimone CP, Crisp MP, Ueland FR, et al. Concordance of gross surgical and final fixed margins in vulvar intraepithelial neoplasia 3 and vulvar cancer. J Reprod Med 2006;51(8):617–20.

69. Boaz A, Joseph A. Letter: Mohs micrographic surgery for the treatment of vulvar Bowen's disease. Dermatol Surg 2007;33(3):388–9.

70. Dudley C, Kircik LH, Bullen R, et al. Vulvar squamous cell carcinoma metastatic to the skin. Dermatol Surg 1998;24(8):889–92.

71. Spiker AM, Hankinson AC, Petrick MG, et al. Single Institution Review of Mohs Surgery for Vulvar Neoplasms. Dermatol Surg 2019;45(12):1698–700.

72. Tan A, Bieber AK, Stein JA, et al. Diagnosis and management of vulvar cancer: a review. J Am Acad Dermatol 2019;81(6):1387–96.

73. Suwandinata FS, Bohle RM, Omwandho CA, et al. Management of vulvar melanoma and review of the literature. Eur J Gynaecol Oncol 2007;28(3):220–4.

74. Beaulieu D, Fathi R, Srivastava D, et al. Current perspectives on Mohs micrographic surgery for melanoma. Clin Cosmet Investig Dermatol 2018;11:309–20.

75. Grewal SK, Leboit PE, Saylor DK. Mohs for vulvar melanoma in situ. Dermatol Surg 2021;47(5):695–6.

76. Nosrati A, Berliner JG, Goel S, et al. Outcomes of melanoma in situ treated with Mohs micrographic surgery compared with wide local excision. JAMA Dermatol 2017;153(5):436–41.

77. Bae JM, Choi YY, Kim H, et al. Mohs micrographic surgery for extramammary Paget disease: a pooled analysis of individual patient data. J Am Acad Dermatol 2013;68(4):632–7.

78. Hendi A, Brodland DG, Zitelli JA. Extramammary Paget's disease: surgical treatment with Mohs micrographic surgery. J Am Acad Dermatol 2004;51(5):767–73.

79. Damavandy AA, Terushkin V, Zitelli JA, et al. Intraoperative Immunostaining for Cytokeratin-7 During Mohs Micrographic Surgery Demonstrates Low Local Recurrence Rates in Extramammary Paget's Disease. Dermatol Surg 2018;44(3):354–64.

80. Chang MS, Mulvaney PM, Danesh MJ, et al. Modified peripheral and central Mohs micrographic surgery for improved margin control in extramammary Paget disease. JAAD Case Rep 2021;7:71–3.

81. ACOG practice bulletin no. 195: prevention of infection after gynecologic procedures. Obstet Gynecol 2018;131(6):e172–89.

Pediatric Cutaneous Oncology
Genodermatoses and Cancer Syndromes

Jackson G. Turbeville, MD[a], Jennifer L. Hand, MD[a,b,c],*

KEYWORDS

- Basal cell nevus syndrome • Photosensitivity disorders • Lynch syndrome
- BAP1-related tumor syndrome • Gorlin syndrome • Skin cancer • Genodermatoses

KEY POINTS

- Early onset skin cancers raise the possibility of an inherited cancer predisposition.
- Dermatologists play a primary role in the management of conditions with predisposition to skin cancer. With adequate management, many affected patients have a normal lifespan.
- This article reviews relevant genodermatoses with an increased risk of skin cancer in young patients and discusses approaches to management.
- Basal Cell Nevus syndrome, Rothmund–Thomson syndrome, Xeroderma Pigmentosum, Lynch syndrome, BAP1 tumor predisposition syndrome, and others are specifically addressed.

Since the complete sequencing of the human genome in 2003, the list of heritable conditions associated with skin cancer continues to expand. Recognition of syndromes by their clinical features gives dermatologists the ability to make a unifying diagnosis. In patients with skin cancer, certain features such as young age of onset, multi-focal primary lesions, and specific pathology signal that further workup for a genetic cause is warranted. Here, we review clinical features of genetic syndromes most likely encountered in a skin cancer-focused practice.

RECOGNIZING INHERITED CANCER SYNDROMES

Most mutations that cause cancer syndromes are present at conception or in the "germ-line." In dermatology patients, certain recognizable characteristics make the presence of a heritable syndrome more likely. For example, multifocal tumors are one such characteristic. Epidermoid cysts when associated with familial adenomatous polyposis (Gardner variant), caused by a germline mutation in the *FAP* gene, usually appear in multiple and possibly atypical locations.[1] In another example, *BAP1*-inactived melanocytic tumors (BIMTs) are atypical appearing dome-shaped, skin-colored to pink to reddish brown papules. The presence of multiple BIMTs in the same individual is considered a marker for the possible presence of a germ-line *BAP1* mutation.[2]

Similarly, cancers related to a genetic syndrome are likely to present with multiple primary tumors of the same or entirely different type. For example, pancreatic cancer and melanoma in the same individual are suspicious of melanoma-pancreatic cancer syndrome caused by a mutation in the *CDKN2A* gene. Another distinction of a genetic syndrome is an earlier age of cancer onset. For

a Department of Dermatology, Mayo Clinic – Rochester, 200 1st Street SW, Rochester, MN 55905, USA;
b Department of Clinical Genomics, Mayo Clinic – Rochester, 200 1st Street SW, Rochester, MN 55905, USA;
c Department of Pediatric and Adolescent Medicine, Mayo Clinic – Rochester, 200 1st Street SW, Rochester, MN 55905, USA
* Corresponding author. Department of Dermatology, Mayo Clinic – Rochester, 200 1st Street Southwest; Rochester, MN 55905.
E-mail address: hand.jennifer@mayo.edu
Twitter: @jlh8515 (J.L.H.)

Dermatol Clin 41 (2023) 175–185
https://doi.org/10.1016/j.det.2022.07.013

example, breast cancer in a patient younger than age 50 is more likely to be associated with a germ-line BRCA mutation.[3] In BAP1 germ-line mutation carriers, the average age of uveal melanoma diagnosis is younger at age 53 years compared with 62 years in the general population.[2]

For dermatologists who prefer visual learning and patterns, a pedigree is an especially useful tool for the assessment of family cancer history. When assessing a cancer-affected family, younger ages at cancer diagnosis or a second primary cancer in the same family member each increase the likelihood of a heritable mutation. Certain rare cancer types can also herald genetic predisposition. For example, mesothelioma increases the chance of a *BAP1* germline mutation being present.[4] When following patients with multiple nevi or melanoma, an annual update of their family history is recommended.[5]

Finally, environmental exposures directly influence cancer risk independently of genetics. Ionizing radiation and cigarette smoke are carcinogens that increase somatic mutations leading to cancer. For patients with skin cancer, taking a history that includes ultraviolet light exposure is essential. A patient with an outdoor occupation and history of tanning bed use may present with multiple primary skin cancers independent of a single gene inherited disorder and is not necessarily a good candidate for testing.

In patients with multiple skin cancers and an extensive history of UV light exposure and in whom a single gene cancer predisposition is unlikely, the inheritance pattern is considered "multifactorial." That is, a combination of shared familial factors both genetic or nongenetic increases the patient and family's risk for cancer. Skin cancer prevention recommendations for patients with an extensive skin cancer history due to either environmental exposure or a predisposing genetic mutation are mostly similar.

BASAL CELL NEVUS SYNDROME

Basal cell nevus syndrome (BCNS), also called Nevoid basal-cell carcinoma syndrome or Gorlin–Goltz syndrome is a multisystem disorder of autosomal dominant inheritance. The most common genetic cause is a heterozygous, pathogenic variant in either *PTCH1* (known as patched 1) or *SUFU* (suppressor of fused) genes.[6] Mutations in these genes disrupt the sonic hedgehog regulatory pathway. This critical pathway regulates mammalian embryogenesis. Somatic as well as inherited or germ-line disruption of the sonic hedgehog pathway contributes to tumor formation, especially basal cell skin cancers. The

estimated prevalence of BCNS is 1 in 40,000 to 1 in 60,000 people, affecting men and women equally.

Individuals with BCNS are predisposed to the early development of basaloid neoplasms and carcinomas (BCC), jaw keratocysts, and ectopic intracranial calcifications in tissues such as the falx cerebri. Characteristic skin findings that affect some, but not all patients include distinctive, asymmetric palmoplantar pits. These individuals are often affected by abnormalities of the ocular, skeletal and genitourinary systems. White patients typically develop more BCCs compared with darker skinned individuals.

BCCs appear at a much earlier age in BCNS compared with the general population, often affecting individuals younger than 20 years of age.[7] For treatment, Mohs micrographic surgery (MMS) has demonstrated efficacy by providing strong cure rates with minimal recurrence rates. However, MMS is problematic in BCNS because follicular-based benign basal cell nevi can obscure the true tumor border, and often a negative margin is virtually impossible to obtain (Fig 1). An impactful report appeared in 2014 documenting 40 years of history in a woman with BCNS who underwent simple excision of 730 basal cell carcinomas. Many excisions had positive margins which were not removed with a second procedure.[7] This article advocated that narrow margins are adequate without MMS. The patient was pictured in youth and juxtaposed against herself at a much older age with an excellent cosmetic outcome using this conservative approach.

For small basal cell nevi that are stable and behave in a benign manner, treatment is not needed. For those that become inflamed and grow, destructive treatment is warranted with the consideration of chemotherapeutic treatment

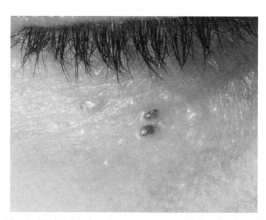

Fig. 1. Multiple, closely approximated follicular-based basal cell nevi in an individual with basal cell nevus syndrome.

such as topical 5-fluorouracil or imiquimod. Cure rates for single lesions are higher than field treatment of multiple lesions. Targeted genetic inhibitors offer another tactic for the treatment of metastatic and especially aggressive tumors. Vismodegib is an FDA-approved systemic treatment of multiple and recurrent BCCs. The use of vismodegib is not without complications and is limited by dose-dependent adverse effects. Side effects such as dysgeusia, alopecia, muscle cramps, weight loss, and others prompted half of patients included in a clinical trial to discontinue the medication. Also, tumors recurred when resistance to vismodegib developed over time.[8] Another systemic inhibitor of the sonic hedgehog pathway, sonidegib, showed a similar problematic side effect profile in patients with advanced BCC.[9]

PHOTOSENSITIVITY SYNDROMES
Rothmund–Thomson Syndrome

In 1957, the American dermatologist Taylor proposed the eponym Rothmund–Thompson Syndrome (RTS) to characterize a cohort of patients with features of poikiloderma, growth retardation, juvenile cataracts, and skeletal defects.[10] This novel syndrome combined the observations from 2 earlier publications—the first by the German ophthalmologist Rothmund in 1868 and the second by the English dermatologist Thompson in 1936.[11,12]

RTS is an autosomal recessive disorder caused by pathogenic mutations that affect the RecQ family of helicases. Due to their critical importance in DNA maintenance and stability, RecQ helicases are considered guardians of the genome. Specific mutations associated with RTS are *ANAPC1* (Type 1) or *RECQL4* (Type 2).[13,14] The former encodes a subunit of the anaphase-promoting complex while the latter encodes a DNA helicase. These mutations ultimately lead to defects in DNA repair and cell cycle progression.

Classically, dermatologic findings present within the first 3 to 6 months of life with marked photosensitivity of the cheeks, hands, feet, and buttocks. This acute phase creates erythema, edema, and occasionally bullae which then eventuate into a chronic poikiloderma.[15] Many individuals possess dental anomalies, alopecia of the scalp, and sparse eyebrows or eyelashes, especially of the lower lids. The condition affects boys twice as often as girls.[16] RTS Type 1 seems to predispose to the development of juvenile cataracts while RTS type 2 is more strongly associated with skeletal deformities and an increased risk of osteosarcoma.[14] Complicating the diagnosis,

significant phenotypic overlaps occur, and not all features are present in all patients.

Overall skin cancer risk is increased in RTS including both nonmelanoma and melanoma skin cancers with an estimated prevalence of about 5%.[17,18] Skin cancer tends to affect these individuals at an earlier age compared with the general population with a mean age of 34.4 years at onset. Careful follow-up skin examinations are required because around 30% of patients develop hyperkeratotic, verrucous papules about the hands, feet, elbows, and knees by adolescence which demonstrates an increased risk of transformation to squamous cell carcinoma in adulthood.[15] Routine cancer screening examinations should occur at least annually with the frequency increased depending on the clinical situation. Skin cancers may be hard to distinguish from surrounding poikilodermatous skin and hyperkeratosis. Confirmed skin cancers may be managed with standard techniques including topical agents (such as 5-flurouracil or imiquimod), electrodessication and curettage, excision, or MMS. With diligent management of these comorbidities, individuals with RTS often have a normal life span.

Xeroderma Pigmentosum

Xeroderma pigmentosum (XP), first described by Hebra and Kaposi in 1874, is a rare, autosomal recessive condition characterized by extreme photosensitivity and increased risk of UV-induced DNA damage and carcinogenesis.[19] James Cleaver elucidated the genetic basis of the condition in 1968 as a defect in DNA repair.[20] The incidence varies across different populations. Early estimates placed the incidence of XP in the United States at 1 in 250,000 births while rates as high as 1 in 20,000 births have been more recently reported in Japan.[21,22] The condition is usually diagnosed within the first 2 years of life secondary to the marked photosensitivity observed in these individuals that includes characteristic lentigines with a freckled appearance.[23] Many genes have been implicated in the pathogenesis of XP; these mutations are traditionally divided into 7 complementation groups (XP-A through G). Each of these encodes a protein associated with a particular step in nucleotide excision repair. With the advent of molecular genetic testing, complementation groups have become outdated. Mutations in *POLH*, which causes XPV, disrupt DNA polymerase eta involved in translesional synthesis.[24] Skin cancers typically have signature mutations of UV light damage. Nucleotide excision repair proteins function to identify and remove UV-induced pyrimidine–

pyramine dimers within damaged DNA; transle-sional synthesis normally allows specialized DNA polymerases to replicate UV-damaged DNA. As such, these ineffective processes each indepen-dently lead to accumulating UV-induced DNA de-fects in cutaneous cells.[25]

Skin cancer risk in affected individuals is increased by orders of magnitude. XP engenders an estimated 10,000-fold increased risk of nonme-lanoma skin cancers and 600 to 8000-fold increased risk of melanoma.[26,27] Skin cancer diag-nosis first occurs at a median age of 8 years.[26] Oral cancers, most commonly on the tip of the tongue due to UV exposure, also occur at an increased frequency with an estimated risk 3000 to 10,000 times higher than the general population.[28] Clini-cally, in about 60% of cases, XP manifests as se-vere photosensitivity often within the first few weeks of life after sun exposure.[21] Severe blis-tering sunburn reactions are seen and can wrongly be confused with neglect or infectious etiologies such as cellulitis or impetigo.[27] This extreme photosensitivity is seen in XP subtypes XPA, XPB, XPD, XPF, and XPG; while XPC, XPE, and XPV subtypes have a normal sunburn response but experience abnormal skin pigmentary changes.[29] In early childhood, signs of chronic UV-induced damage present with lentigines (which should be distinguished from more typical ephelides), skin atrophy, actinic keratoses, and stucco keratoses. The cornea is also vulnerable to pain associated with UV exposure. Many pa-tients suffer from photophobia.[27]

The prognosis of this condition rests on the abil-ity to minimize UV exposure and to quickly detect potential malignant skin changes in their earliest stages. The strictest modes of sun protection are used for these patients including physical barrier protection with UV-blocking clothing, UV-protective goggles, and the use of high SPF sun-screens. Individuals may need to be screened for vitamin D deficiency and require significant psy-chosocial support due to the severe lifestyle re-strictions that are required.[30] Actinic keratoses and small, localized BCC may be treated with cryotherapy, topical 5-fluorouracil or imiquimod. A series of 18 patients with XP and 45 primary facial BCC documented adequate response to cryotherapy and only one case of recurrence after a mean follow-up period of 30 months.[31] Surgical excision is preferred for larger lesions and SCC. Given the high tumor burden associated with this condition, narrow margins are preferred with frequent clinical follow-up and re-excision as necessary. MMS offers the ability to obtain irrefut-ably negative margins, but this procedure may be impractical in a patient who requires frequent surgical excisions.[32] With the burden of actinic damage at a young age, regular skin cancer screening examinations are essential in the early detection of possible malignant change.

Oculocutaneous Albinism

Oculocutaneous albinism (OCA), refers to a group of autosomal recessive disorders characterized by abnormalities in melanin biosynthesis, visual acu-ity, and a generalized reduction in the pigmenta-tion of the skin, hair, and eyes.[33] Since tyrosine metabolites are required in the embryonic period for proper formation of the optic chiasm and binocular vision, decreased visual acuity is a debil-itating feature of this diagnosis. OCA can be sub-divided into 8 forms (OCA1-8) each corresponding to distinct gene mutations. OCA1 and OCA2 are the most common forms account-ing for 30% and 50% of cases, respectively, although prevalence vary widely according to pop-ulation.[33–35] OCA1 is caused by mutations in the TYR gene that encode tyrosinase. Tyrosinase is the key rate-limiting step in melanin synthesis. OCA2 is caused by OCA2 mutations. The OCA2 gene encodes a transmembrane protein respon-sible for normal melanosome function.[36] These 2 subtypes are most associated with increased risk of skin cancer development. OCA3-4 account for nearly all remaining cases of oculocutaneous albi-nism worldwide as OCA5-8 has only been re-ported in single individuals or family cohorts.[37–40] The overall prevalence of OCA is thought to range between 1:17,000 and 1:20,000 in the Western world, and 1 in 70 individuals is thought to be a carrier of an OCA-mutated allele.[41]

Classically, OCA1 can be split into 2 subtypes based on either absent (OCA1a) or reduced (OCA1b) activity of the tyrosinase enzyme. OCA1a is clinically characterized by the total absence of pigmentation as affected individuals are unable to synthesize melanin due to the pres-ence of 2 null OCA1 alleles. These patients demonstrate milk-white skin, white hair, and blue irides regardless of familial skin phenotype.[42] Ocular symptoms include photophobia, nystagmus, strabismus, and decreased visual acuity resulting in legal blindness for most of these patients.[43] Markers of cutaneous UV-induced photodamage develop in young adulthood and include actinic damage and cutaneous malig-nancies. OCA1b demonstrates a less severe phenotype with variable pigmentation secondary to variability in tyrosinase activity. Infants with this phenotype may have white terminal hair at birth that then darkens with age due to staining from minerals in water and environmental exposure.[33] OCA2 most commonly affects Black individuals and has a variable phenotype characterized by different degrees of melanin expression.[44] The skin ranges in color from pink to cream; the hair is yellowish-brown; and the eyes are blue to yellowish-brown.[33] These individuals may develop pigmented nevi over time. SCC is the most common type of skin cancer to develop in these patients; however, BCC and melanoma occur at higher rates than those seen in the general population.[45] With the absence or reduced pigmentation, melanoma poses a particular diagnostic challenge. Heightened vigilance is required to detect changes in pink and red lesions. These amelanotic melanomas may be more advanced at the time of diagnosis (owing to their difficulty in recognition) and are reported to occur most frequently on the back and legs.[46]

Due to the risk of skin cancer, OCA-affected individuals must use life-long photoprotection including avoiding peak hours of UV exposure, use of protective clothing, frequent application of sunscreens containing at least sun protective factor 30, and avoidance of photosensitizing medications when possible.[47] With such strict sun protective measures, vitamin D levels should be screened. Skin cancer surveillance should start in adolescence at routine 6-to-12-month intervals. During these surveillance visits, dermoscopy may help delineate clinically suspicious lesions from benign melanocytic nevi. A recent study in 37 OCA children reported "structureless homogenous" or "globular" as the most common dermatoscopic patterns in benign nevi.[48] Comparatively, dermoscopic analysis of vessels can also help to identify high-risk lesions. Patterns that should prompt further investigation include linear, irregular vessels, and polymorphous-appearing vessels over a central disposition of dotted vessels.[49] With the management of these potential comorbidities, and accommodations for patients with decreased visual acuity OCA typically enjoy a normal life span.

LYNCH SYNDROME

An especially common and relevant cancer syndrome for dermatologists is Lynch syndrome (hereditary nonpolyposis colorectal cancer). Lynch syndrome is the most common form of hereditary colorectal carcinoma with an estimated prevalence of 1:279 from a 2017 study by Win and colleagues.[50] This syndrome accounts for approximately 3% of new cases of colorectal carcinoma and 2% to 3% of endometrial cancer.[51] Most pertinent to dermatologists are the cutaneous manifestations. Historically, Muir–Torre syndrome described a subset of patients with Lynch syndrome with characteristic skin manifestations including sebaceous neoplasms and keratoacanthoma. This subset of patients is now grouped into the larger domain of Lynch syndrome.

In patients with Lynch syndrome, symptoms of colorectal carcinoma such as gastrointestinal bleeding, abdominal pain, or a change in bowel habits are often the first sign of disease.[52] Among these individuals, about 9% have cutaneous characteristics consistent with the Muir–Torre variant of Lynch syndrome.[53] Cutaneous malignancies develop in affected individuals at an average age of 53 (range 23–89).[54] Inactivating mutations in genes which encode proteins implicated in mismatch repair underpin Lynch syndrome. The most well-known genes include *MLH1*, *MSH2*, *MSH6*, and *PMS2*.[55,56] Microsatellite regions of DNA are made up of highly repetitive sequences that commonly "mismatch" during cell division. The result of this defective mismatch repair leads to microsatellite instability and tumor formation. In cases associated with the characteristic skin lesions, most of the patients harbor mutations in *MSH2*.[55] Typical cutaneous lesions include sebaceous tumors such as sebaceous adenoma and sebaceous carcinoma.[57] The most specific cutaneous lesion from this condition is the sebaceous adenoma (**Fig. 2**).[58] In nonsyndromic patients, sebaceous neoplasms have a predilection for the face, and examination reveals yellowish to pink papules often with a central dell. In patients with Lynch syndrome, these characteristic skin lesions are frequently present on the trunk.[59] Molecular testing of these skin tumors is critical for early diagnosis as these sebaceous tumors will precede the development of visceral malignancy in more than 50% of affected patients.[57]

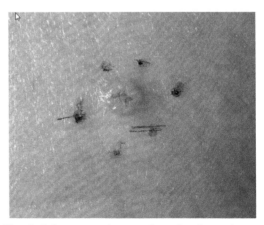

Fig. 2. Sebaceous adenoma in a Lynch syndrome-affected patient with characteristic pink to yellow color and telangiectasias.

Tumor testing is distinct from germ-line mutation testing of blood or saliva. The genetic derangement that characterizes cancer typically occurs well *after* conception. Typically, these somatic tumor mutations are not transmissible to future generations. In skin cancer, somatic genetic changes are often characteristic of ultraviolet (UV) light damage.[60] Somatic mutation testing usually takes place on actual tumor tissue, although, increasingly, next-generation technology can distinguish tumor DNA that makes its way into the blood or other body fluid. Mutations detected in this way are considered postzygotic and not heritable because they represent mutations specific to the tumor. For some specific somatic mutations, however, detection in tumor tissue raises the possibility but does not confirm inheritance from birth. Cutaneous sebaceous carcinomas are a relevant example for dermatologists. On a sebaceous carcinoma tumor specimen, immunohistochemical stains for mismatch repair mutations (eg, *MLH1*, *MSH2*, *MSH6*, or *PMS2*) reveal the presence or absence of somatic mutations associated with Lynch syndrome.[61] Universal immunohistochemical staining is not currently performed on all sebaceous tumors, though at least one study supports its usefulness.[61] A heterozygous pathogenic mismatch repair mutation (eg, *MLH1*, *MSH2*, *MSH6* or *PMS2*), when present in the germline, causes Lynch syndrome. That is, molecular diagnosis of Lynch syndrome requires confirmation in another tissue. Tumor staining establishes the presence or absence of a Lynch syndrome somatic mutation. Follow-up germline testing of blood or saliva is then required to confirm if a Lynch syndrome diagnosis is present. If so, extra-cancer surveillance according to established guidelines is recommended.

Simple excision may be undertaken for the management of benign sebaceous adenoma to prevent recurrence and possible malignant transformation. Management of sebaceous carcinoma is typically pursued via MMS to ensure complete tumor removal; however, if this procedure is not available, WLE with 1 cm margins down to the deep fascial plain is recommended.[62,63] Prolonged and frequent follow-up is recommended for these patients with a history of sebaceous carcinoma every 6 months for 3 years then annually thereafter.[63]

CANCER AND CONSTITUTIONAL MISMATCH REPAIR DEFICIENCY SYNDROME

A rare cancer syndrome, directly related to Lynch Syndrome, with special relevance to pediatric dermatologists is Cancer and Constitutional Mismatch Repair Deficiency Syndrome (CCMRD). The condition is inherited recessively and caused by biallelic mutations in mismatch repair genes, most commonly *PMS2* and *MHS6*.[64] The first reports, which were published in 1999, described the clinical characteristics of offspring from consanguineous marriages of Lynch Syndrome families.[65,66] A particularly virulent cancer syndrome, hematologic malignancies develop during early childhood in these offspring. These affected individuals were also noted to have cutaneous stigmata of neurofibromatosis. Since that original description, Wimmer and colleagues characterized the first cohort of 146 patients with this condition.[67] The most commonly reported tumors in this group of patients include CNS tumors (glioblastoma multiforme, high-grade glial tumors, medulloblastoma), hematologic malignancies, and/or polyposis. Nearly all affected patients were diagnosed in childhood before 18 years of age. High mortality, at more than 70%, is reported among those affected with this condition.[68] The cutaneous features of this condition include café-au-lait macules (CALM) and hypopigmented macules. The CALM tend to have jagged borders as opposed to the smooth borders typically associated with neurofibromatosis.[69] Diagnostic criteria for this condition have been proposed which include: (1) café-au-lait spots and/or hypopigmented skin lesions (2) history of parental consanguinity, or (3) positive family history of hereditary nonpolyposis colon cancers.[67] This condition highlights the importance of a broad differential and the need to obtain a thorough history when evaluating patients with multiple CALM.

BAP1 TUMOR PREDISPOSITION SYNDROME

BRCA1-associated protein (*BAP1*) tumor mutations are similarly relevant to dermatologists. BAP1-inactivated benign melanocytic nevi or "melanocytomas" have been reported as an identifying feature in some individuals who carry a germ-line null mutation in *BAP1*.[70] Increased cancer surveillance for uveal melanoma, mesothelioma, cutaneous melanoma, and renal cancer is recommended for individuals confirmed to carry germ line, pathogenic *BAP1* mutations. Apart from these well-known examples of tumor testing potentially revealing a germ-line mutation that requires follow-up confirmatory testing, few studies describe whether patients should be offered germ-line testing for other somatic mutations detected by tumor testing.

Clinically, BAP1-inactivated benign melanocytic nevi present as well-marginated, skin-colored to red/brown, pedunculated or dome-shaped papules typically distributed most commonly on the head and neck, followed by trunk and extremities.[71,72] Multiple lesions are characteristically present in individuals with germline mutations (ranging from 5 to 50 lesions in individual members of affected families).[73] Dermatoscopic findings associated with these lesions have been reported. Interestingly, structureless with eccentric dots/globules pattern and network with raised structureless areas pattern was significantly associated with germline mutations.[72] Ultimately, diagnosis relies on the histopathologic evaluation of biopsy specimen. Excisional biopsy is the preferred method to ensure accurate histopathologic diagnosis. No specific guidelines exist for the management of these lesions once histopathologically confirmed, often re-excision is pursued to guarantee complete removal. Once a diagnosis is established, genetic testing should be considered if a patient has a history of multiple such lesions, a strong family history of such lesions exists, or the lesion is diagnosed in a young patient.[74]

INTERNAL CANCER SYNDROMES (EG, BRCA, DICER 1)
Familial Melanoma

Some authors divide melanoma-related single gene cancer predisposition disorders into "melanoma dominant" and "melanoma subordinate." Melanoma dominant mutations describe those which predominantly increase melanoma risk and may increase the risk of other specific cancers, but not to the same degree as melanoma. CDKN2A is considered the most commonly inherited mutation in 30% to 40% of families that present with multiple melanomas in multiple members and meet diagnostic criteria.[75]

Since a mutation in CDKN2A primarily increases melanoma risk and increases pancreatic cancer risk, but to a lesser degree, it is considered "melanoma dominant."[4] Another "melanoma dominant" mutation is BAP1 which increases the risk of mesothelioma but to a lesser degree than melanoma. An example of a melanoma subordinate mutation is BRCA which increase melanoma risk but not to the same degree as breast and ovarian cancer[4,76]. Since patients with "melanoma dominant" and "melanoma subordinate" mutations may present in dermatology clinics with the same phenotype of multiple primary or early onset melanomas, this overlap impacts testing strategies for a genetic diagnosis.[4] When features of single gene cancer syndromes overlap, targeted multi-gene panels that interrogate many different well-known cancer genes at once are an efficient testing option.

RESOURCES

For patients with a suspected cancer predisposition, consultation with a genetics professional is recommended.[76] A typical visit includes a three-generation targeted family history and drawn pedigree. Pretest counseling requires discussion about potential equivocal or noninformative results, insurance discrimination based on a new diagnosis, and disclosure of nonpaternity and impact on the family. Potential benefits are also discussed, especially the potential for enhanced screening based on results to detect cancers at an early and curable stage. If the patient chooses to proceed, targeted testing is offered for relevant mutations according to the patients' personal and family history. A multi-gene panel is an efficient choice due to overlapping phenotypes of cancer syndromes, especially in an individual who develops more than one melanoma.[76]

SUMMARY

Childhood skin cancer is rare, and its diagnosis should spark the clinical suspicion of an underlying genetic cancer predisposition syndrome. In many of these conditions, the skin is often the first clue to a potential diagnosis. Dermatologists play a crucial role in the detection and treatment of skin cancers; thus, working knowledge of these genodermatoses and their extracutaneous clinical associations is necessary to recommend management and improve care. For example, several conditions discussed impact vision. Affected patients typically worry about skin surgery that could impact one or both eyes making them temporarily blind due to bandage placement. Establishing a correct diagnosis in these patients ultimately may involve referral to genetics professional services for testing, and the threshold for referral should be based on heightened clinical suspicions.

Advances in genomics have provided information underlying genetic pathways implicated in these conditions and afford insight into potential therapeutic targets. Genetic testing offers the ability to confirm clinical suspicion, and, with accurate diagnosis, the risks of future cancer development can be mitigated with appropriate strategies. While these exciting developments have increased understanding of these conditions, the results of genetic testing can be mired in myriad psychosocial concerns including the potential for discrimination. Early referral to geneticists who can guide appropriate investigations is recommended in these cases to review the benefits of testing and discuss potential ramifications. Additionally, those experienced in clinic genomics can develop comprehensive, personalized management plans for each patient.

CLINICS CARE POINTS

- Diagnosis of a BCC at a young age should prompt concern for BCCN syndrome. The presence of palmoplantar pits may serve as a clinical clue.
- Mohs micrographic surgery may not be the first choice for the treatment of BCC in patients with BCCN due to the inability to obtain negative margins.
- The presence of poikiloderma in childhood should heighten suspicion of a photosensitivity disorder such as RTS
- Skin cancer may arise in hyperkeratotic or poikilodermatous lesions of patients with RTS
- Blistering sunburns in infancy are a hallmark of XP
- Lentigines may be a presenting sign of XP and distinguish from other photosensitivity disorders
- In OCA, pink to red nevi deserve extra-diagnostic scrutiny to exclude amelanotic melanoma
- Skin cancer prevention with strict sun protection and regular screening examinations allow individuals with photosensitivity disorders to have a normal life span
- Sebaceous neoplasms occurring outside of the head and neck, especially sebaceous adenoma, raise the possibility of Lynch Syndrome
- CCMRD syndrome shares phenotypical overlap with neurofibromatosis
- Obtain relevant family history including cancer history in patients with multiple CALMs
- "Melanoma dominant" mutations are associated with an increased primary risk of melanoma, examples include *CDNK2A* and *BAP-1* mutations
- Diagnosis of melanoma in patients with family histories of melanoma and/or pancreatic cancer may suggest *CDKN2A* mutations
- An example of a "melanoma subordinate" cancer mutation is *BRCA* which typically presents with breast and ovarian cancers
- Genetic testing can help guide appropriate screening measures and preventative care for patients with increased tendencies

DISCLOSURE

J.L. Hand is a section editor for Genetic skin disorders at UpToDate, Inc. The authors have no other disclosures.

REFERENCES

1. Ladd R, Davis M, Dyer JA. Genodermatoses with malignant potential. Clin Dermatol 2020;38:432–54.
2. Zocchi L, Lontano A, Merli M, et al. Familial Melanoma and Susceptibility Genes: A Review of the Most Common Clinical and Dermoscopic Aspect, Associated Malignancies and Practical tips for Management. J Clin Med 2021;10(16):3760.
3. Rodriguez JL, Thomas CC, Massetti GM, et al. CDC Grand Rounds: Family History and Genomics as Tools for Cancer Prevention and Control. MMWR 2016;65(46):1291–4.
4. Leachman SA, Lucero OM, Sampson JE, et al. Identification, genetic testing and management of hereditary melanoma. Cancer Metastasis Rev 2017;36:77–90.
5. Soura E, Eliades P, Shannon K, et al. Hereditary Melanoma: Update on Syndromes and Management-Emerging melanoma cancer complexes and genetic counseling. JAAD 2016;74(3):411–20.
6. Hosoya A, Shalehin N, Takebe H, et al. Sonic Hedgehog Signaling and Tooth Development. Int J Mol Sci 2020;21:1587.
7. Griner D, Sutphin D, Sargent LA. Surgical Management of Gorlin Syndrome: A 4-Decade Experience Using Local Excision Technique. Ann Plast Surg 2015;74(4):467–70.
8. Athar M, Li C, Kim AL, et al. Sonic hedgehog signaling in Basal cell nevus syndrome. Cancer Res 2014;74:4967–75.
9. Lear JT, Migden MR, Lewis KD, et al. Long-Term Efficacy and Safety of Sonidegib in Patients with Locally Advanced and Metastatic Basal Cell Carcinoma: 30-Month Analysis of the Randomized Phase 2 BOLT Study. J Eur Acad Dermatol Venereol 2018;32(3):372–81.
10. Taylor WB. Rothmund's syndrome-Thomson syndrome. Arch Dermatol 1957;75:236–44.
11. Rothmund A. Uber Cataracte in Verbindung mit einer eigenthuemlichen Hautdegeneration. Albrecht von Graefes Arch Klin Exp Ophthal 1868;14:159–82.
12. Thomson MS. Poikiloderma congenitale. Br J Dermatol 1936;48:221–34.
13. Ajeawung NF, Nguyen TTM, Lu L, et al. Mutations in ANAPC1, Encoding a Scaffold Subunit of the Anaphase-Promoting Complex, Cause Rothmund-Thomson Syndrome Type 1. Am J Hum Genet 2019;105(3):625–30.
14. Wang LL, Gannavarapu A, Kozinetz CA, et al. Association between osteosarcoma and deleterious

mutations in the RECQL4 gene in Rothmund-Thomson syndrome. J Natl Cancer Inst 2003;95(9): 669–74.

15. Wang LL, Plon SE. Rothmund-Thomson Syndrome. In: Adam MP, Ardinger HH, Pagon RA, et al, editors. GeneReviews® [Internet]. Seattle (WA): University of Washington, Seattle; 1993-2022; 1999. Available at: https://www.ncbi.nlm.nih.gov/books/NBK1237/.

16. Wang LL, Levy ML, Lewis RA, et al. Clinical manifestations in a cohort of 41 Rothmund-Thomson syndrome patients. Am J Med Genet 2001;102(1): 11–7. PMID: 11471165.

17. Howell SM, Bray DW. Amelanotic melanoma in a patient with Rothmund-Thomson syndrome. Arch Dermatol 2008;144(3):416–7.

18. Borg MF, Olver IN, Hill MP. Rothmund-Thomson syndrome and tolerance of chemoradiotherapy. Australas Radiol 1998;42(3):216–8.

19. Hebra F, Kaposi M. Xeroderma, parchment skin. In On diseases of the skin including exanthemata. Volume III. New Syndenham Soc 1874;61:252–8.

20. Cleaver JE. Defective repair replication of DNA in xeroderma pigmentosum. 1968. DNA Repair (Amst) 2004;3(2):183–7. PMID: 15344228.

21. Robbins JH, Kraemer KH, Lutzner MA, et al. Xeroderma pigmentosum: an inherited disease with sun-sensitivity, multiple cutaneous neoplasms, and abnormal DNA repair. Ann Intern Med 1974;80: 221–48.

22. Hirai Y, Kodama Y, Moriwaki S, et al. Heterozygous individuals bearing a founder mutation in the XPA DNA repair gene comprise nearly 1% of the Japanese population. Mutat Res 2006;601:171–8.

23. Tang J, Chu G. Xeroderma pigmentosum complementation group E and UV-damaged DNA-binding protein. DNA repair 2002;1:601–16.

24. Yuasa M, Masutani C, Eki T, et al. Genomic structure, chromosomal localization and identification of mutations in the xeroderma pigmentosum variant (XPV) gene. Oncogene 2000;19(41):4721–8.

25. Masutani C, Kusumoto R, Yamada A, et al. The XPV (xeroderma pigmentosum variant) gene encodes human DNA polymerase eta. Nature 1999;399: 700–4.

26. Jaju PD, Ransohoff KJ, Tang JY, et al. Familial skin cancer syndromes:increased risk of nonmelanotic skin cancers and extracutaneous tumors. J Amacad Dermatol 2016;74:437–51. quiz 452– 434.

27. Lehmann AR, McGibbon D, Stefanini M. Xeroderma pigmentosum. Orphanetj Rare Dis 2011;6:70.

28. Shah J. Atlas of clinical Oncology: cancer of the head and neck. 1st ed. Hamilton, Ontario: Decker; 2001.

29. Sethi M, Lehmann AR, Fawcett H, et al. Patients with xeroderma pigmentosum complementation groups C, E and V do not have abnormal sunburn reactions. Br J Dermatol 2013;169(6):1279–87.

30. Kuwabara A, Tsugawa N, Tanaka K, et al. High prevalence of vitamin D deficiency in patients with xeroderma pigmetosum-A under strict sun protection. Eur J Clin Nutr 2015;69(6):693–6. PMID: 25669318.

31. Zghal M, Triki S, Elloumi-Jellouli A, et al. 'apport de la cryochirurgie dans la prise en charge du xeroderma pigmentosum [Contribution of the cryosurgery in the management of xeroderma pigmentosum]. Ann Dermatol Venereol 2010;137(10):605–9.

32. Lambert WC, Lambert MW. Development of effective skin cancer treatment and prevention in xeroderma pigmentosum. Photochem Photobiol 2015; 91(2):475–83. Epub 2015 Feb 6. PMID: 25382223.

33. Grønskov K, Ek J, Brondum-Nielsen K. Oculocutaneous albinism. Orphanet J Rare Dis 2007;2:43.

34. Urtatiz O, Sanabria D, Lattig MC. Oculocutaneous albinism (OCA) in Colombia: first molecular screening of the TYR and OCA2 genes in South America. J Dermatol Sci 2014;76(3):260–2.

35. Marçon CR, Maia M. Albinism: epidemiology, genetics, cutaneous characterization, psychosocial factors. An Bras Dermatol 2019;94(5):503–20.

36. Montoliu L, Grønskov K, Wei AH, et al. Increasing the complexity: new genes and new types of albinism. Pigment Cell Melanoma Res 2014;27(1): 11–8. Epub 2013 Oct 17. PMID: 24066960.

37. Kausar T, Bhatti MA, Ali M, et al. OCA5, a novel locus for non-syndromic oculocutaneous albinism, maps to chromosome 4q24. Clin Genet 2013;84:91.

38. Wei AH, Zang DJ, Zhang Z, et al. Exome sequencing identifies SLC24A5 as a candidate gene for nonsyndromic oculocutaneous albinism. J Invest Dermatol 2013;133:1834.

39. Grønskov K, Dooley CM, Østergaard E, et al. Mutations in c10orf11, a melanocyte-differentiation gene, cause autosomal-recessive albinism. Am J Hum Genet 2013;92:415.

40. Pennamen P, Tingaud-Sequeira A, Gazova I, et al. Dopachrome tautomerase variants in patients with oculocutaneous albinism. Genet Med 2021;23:479.

41. Witkop CJ. Albinism: hematologic-storage disease, susceptibility to skin cancer, and optic neuronal defects shared in all types of oculocutaneous and ocular albinism. Ala J Med Sci 1979;16(4):327–30. PMID: 546241.

42. King RA, Pietsch J, Fryer JR, et al. Tyrosinase gene mutations in oculocutaneous albinism 1 (OCA1): definition of the phenotype. Hum Genet 2003; 113(6):502–13.

43. Winsor CN, Holleschau AM, Connett JE, et al. A cross-sectional examination of visual acuity by specific type of albinism. J AAPOS 2016;20(5): 419–24.

44. Oetting WS, King RA. Molecular basis of albinism: mutations and polymorphisms of pigmentation genes associated with albinism. Hum Mutat 1999; 13(2):99–115.

45. Kiprono SK, Chaula BM, Beltraminelli H. Histological review of skin cancers in African Albinos: a 10-year retrospective review. BMC Cancer 2014;14:157. PMID: 24597988; PMCID: PMC3975641.

46. Ruiz-Sanchez D, Garabito Solovera EL, Valtueña J, et al. Amelanotic melanoma in a patient with oculocutaneous albinism. Dermatol Online J 2020;26(5): 13030. qt2gv5w93x. PMID: 32621707.

47. Moreno-Artero E, Morice-Picard F, Bremond-Gignac D, et al. Management of albinism: French guidelines for diagnosis and care. J Eur Acad Dermatol Venereol 2021;35(7):1449–59. Epub 2021 May 27. PMID: 34042219.

48. Ramos AN, Fraga-Braghiroli N, Ramos JGR, et al. Dermoscopy of naevi in patients with oculocutaneous albinism. Clin Exp Dermatol 2019;44(5): e196–9. Epub 2019 Jan 17. PMID: 30656729.

49. De Luca DA, Bollea Garlatti LA, Galimberti GN, et al. Amelanotic melanoma in albinism: the power of dermatoscopy. J Eur Acad Dermatol Venereol 2016; 30(8):1422–3. Epub 2015 Aug 20. PMID: 26290313.

50. Win AK, Jenkins MA, Dowty JG, et al. Prevalence and penetrance of major genes and polygenes for colorectal cancer. Cancer Epidemiol Biomarkers Prev 2017;26(3):404–12.

51. Moreira L, Balaguer F, Lindor N, et al, EPICOLON Consortium. Identification of Lynch syndrome among patients with colorectal cancer. JAMA 2012;308(15):1555–65.

52. Møller P, Seppälä T, Bernstein I, et al, Mallorca Group. Cancer incidence and survival in Lynch syndrome patients receiving colonoscopic and gynaecological surveillance: first report from the prospective Lynch syndrome database. Gut 2017; 66(3):464–72. Epub 2015 Dec 9. PMID: 26657901; PMCID: PMC5534760.

53. Le S, Ansari U, Mumtaz A, et al. Lynch Syndrome and Muir-Torre Syndrome: An update and review on the genetics, epidemiology, and management of two related disorders. Dermatol Online J 2017; 23(11):13030. qt8sg5w98j. PMID: 29447627.

54. Ponti G, Pellacani G, Seidenari S, et al. Cancer-associated genodermatoses: skin neoplasms as clues to hereditary tumor syndromes. Crit Rev Oncol Hematol 2013;85(3):239–56. Epub 2012 Jul 21. PMID: 22823951.

55. Mahalingam M. MSH6, Past and Present and Muir-Torre Syndrome-Connecting the Dots. Am J Dermatopathol 2017;39(4):239–49. PMID: 28323777.

56. Ponti G, Ponz de Leon M. Muir-Torre syndrome. Lancet Oncol 2005;6(12):980–7.

57. Ponti G, Losi L, Di Gregorio C, et al. Identification of Muir-Torre syndrome among patients with sebaceous tumors and keratoacanthomas: role of clinical features, microsatellite instability, and immunohistochemistry. Cancer 2005;103(5):1018–25. PMID: 15662714.

58. Abbas O, Mahalingam M. Cutaneous sebaceous neoplasms as markers of Muir-Torre syndrome: a diagnostic algorithm. J Cutan Pathol 2009;36(6):613–9.

59. Singh RS, Grayson W, Redston M, et al. Site and tumor type predicts DNA mismatch repair status in cutaneous sebaceous neoplasia. Am J Surg Pathol 2008;32(6):936–42. PMID: 18551751.

60. Liu-Smith F, Jia J, Zheng Y. UV-Induced Molecular Signaling Differences in Melanoma and Non-melanoma Skin Cancer. Adv Exp Med Biol 2017; 996:27–40.

61. Schon K, Rytina E, Drummond J. Evaluation of universal immunohistochemical screening of sebaceous neoplasms in a service setting. Clin Exp Derm 2018;43(4):410–5.

62. Hou JL, Killian JM, Baum CL, et al. Characteristics of sebaceous carcinoma and early outcomes of treatment using Mohs micrographic surgery versus wide local excision: an update of the Mayo Clinic experience over the past 2 decades. Dermatol Surg 2014; 40(3):241–6. Epub 2014 Jan 25. PMID: 24460730.

63. Owen JL, Kibbi N, Worley B, et al. Sebaceous carcinoma: evidence-based clinical practice guidelines. Lancet Oncol 2019;20(12):e699–714.

64. Aronson M, Colas C, Shuen A, et al. Diagnostic criteria for constitutional mismatch repair deficiency (CMMRD): recommendations from the international consensus working group. J Med Genet 2022; 59(4):318–27.

65. Ricciardone MD, Ozcelik T, Cevher B, et al. Human MLH1 deficiency predisposes to hematological malignancy and neurofibromatosis type 1. Cancer Res 1999;59:290–3.

66. Wang Q, Lasset C, Desseigne F, et al. Neurofibromatosis and early onset of cancers in hMLH1-deficient children. Cancer Res 1999;59:294–7.

67. Wimmer K, Kratz CP, Vasen HFA, et al. Diagnostic criteria for constitutional mismatch repair deficiency syndrome: suggestions of the European consortium 'Care for CMMRD' (C4CMMRD). J Med Genet 2014; 51:355–65.

68. Lavoine N, Colas C, Muleris M, et al. Constitutional mismatch repair deficiency syndrome: clinical description in a French cohort. J Med Genet 2015; 52(11):770–8. Epub 2015 Aug 28. PMID: 26318770.

69. Özyörük D, Cabı EÜ, Taçyıldız N, et al. Cancer and constitutional Mismatch Repair Deficiency syndrome due to homozygous MSH 6 mutation in children with Café au Lait Spots and review of literature. Turk J Pediatr 2021;63(5):893–902. PMID: 34738371.

70. Walpole S, Pritchard AL, Cebulla CM, et al. Comprehensive Study of the Clinical Phenotype of Germline BAP1 Variant-Carrying Families Worldwide. JNCI 2018;110(12):1328–41.

71. Zhang AJ, Rush PS, Tsao H, et al. BRCA1-associated protein (BAP1)-inactivated melanocytic tumors. J Cutan Pathol 2019;46:965–72.

72. Yélamos O, Navarrete-Dechent C, Marchetti MA, et al. Clinical and dermoscopic features of cutaneous BAP1-inactivated melanocytic tumors: Results of a multicenter case-control study by the International Dermoscopy Society. J Am Acad Dermatol 2019;80(6): 1585–93.

73. Cabaret O, Perron E, Bressac-de Paillerets B, et al. Occurrence of BAP1 germline mutations in cutaneous melanocytic tumors with loss of BAP1-expression: a pilot study. Genes Chromosomes Cancer 2017;56(9):691–4.

74. Rai K, Pilarski R, Cebulla CM, et al. Comprehensive review of BAP1 tumor predisposition syndrome with report of two new cases. Clin Genet 2016;89(3):285–94. Epub 2015 Jul 14. PMID: 26096145; PMCID: PMC4688243.

75. Casula M, Paliogiannis P, Ayala F, et al. Germline and somatic mutations in patients with multiple primary melanomas: a next generation sequencing study. BMC Cancer 2019;19:772.

76. Abdo JF, Sharma A, Sharma R. Role of Heredity in Melanoma Susceptibility: A Primer for the Practicing Surgeon. Surg Clin N Am 2020;100(13–28).

A Practical Review of the Presentation, Diagnosis, and Management of Cutaneous B-Cell Lymphomas

Nikhil Goyal, BS[a], Daniel O'Leary, MD[b], Joi B. Carter, MD[c],
Nneka Comfere, MD[d,e], Olayemi Sokumbi, MD[f,g],
Amrita O'Leary Goyal, MD[h],*

KEYWORDS

- Cutaneous lymphoma • Primary cutaneous B- cell lymphoma • Cutaneous B- cell lymphoma
- Primary cutaneous marginal zone lymphoma • Primary cutaneous follicle center lymphoma
- Primary cutaneous diffuse large B- cell lymphoma • Intravascular large B- cell lymphoma
- EBV+ mucocutaneous ulcer

KEY POINTS

- Primary cutaneous B-cell lymphomas are rare but important diagnostic entities in dermatology that require accurate histopathologic diagnosis and a thorough workup to rule out systemic involvement.
- The cutaneous B-cell lymphomas (CBCLs) include primary cutaneous marginal zone B-cell lymphoma, primary cutaneous follicle center B-cell lymphoma, primary cutaneous diffuse large B-cell lymphoma, and intravascular large B-cell lymphoma. Epstein–Barr virus-positive mucocutaneous ulcer is a new provisional entity in this category.
- Each of the CBCLs has a distinct clinical presentation, pathobiology, and management strategy.
- There have been numerous recent advances in the molecular biology underlying the development and progression of CBCL which may have prognostic significance.
- Management of a patient with CBCL requires coordination between dermatology, pathology, hematology/oncology, and radiation oncology.

INTRODUCTION

Cutaneous B-cell lymphomas (CBCLs) are a rare but important diagnostic entity in dermatology.[1] CBCLs may be divided into primary cutaneous (those arising primarily in the skin) vs. secondary cutaneous lymphomas (systemic lyphomas with skin involvement). The World Health Organization (WHO)/EORTC classification of cutaneous lymphomas includes four diagnostic entities: primary cutaneous marginal zone lymphoma (PCZML), primary cutaneous follicle center lymphoma (PCFCL), primary cutaneous diffuse large B-cell lymphoma, leg-type (PCDLBCL, LT), and intravascular large B-cell lymphoma (IVLBCL) (Table 1).[2] Of note, the first three of these are primary

[a] Perelman School of Medicine, University of Pennsylvania, Philadelphia, PA, USA; [b] Division of Hematology, Oncology, and Transplantation, University of Minnesota, 420 Delaware Street SE, MMC480, Minneapolis, MN 55455, USA; [c] Department of Dermatology, Dartmouth Geisel School of Medicine, Hanover, NH, USA; [d] Department of Dermatology, Mayo Clinic, 18 Old Etna Rd, Lebanon, NH 03766, USA; [e] Department of Laboratory Medicine & Pathology, Mayo Clinic, Rochester, MN, USA; [f] Department of Dermatology, Mayo Clinic, Jacksonville, FL, USA; [g] Departmen of Laboratory Medicine & Pathology, Mayo Clinic, Jacksonville, FL, USA; [h] Department of Dermatology, University of Minnesota, 6545 France Avenue, Ste 564, Edina, MN 55435, USA
* Corresponding author.
E-mail address: goyal046@umn.edu

Dermatol Clin 41 (2023) 187–208
https://doi.org/10.1016/j.det.2022.07.014

Table 1
Clinical characteristics of cutaneous B-cell lymphomas

	PCMZL	PCFCL	PCDLBCL	IVLBCL
Indolent or aggressive	Indolent	Indolent	Aggressive	Aggressive
Percentage of cases of CBCL[1,54]	25%–30%	30%–60%	20%–40%	<1%
Percentage of cases of all cutaneous lymphomas[1]	7.1%	8.5%	11.4%	<1%
Median age (years)	30s–60s	50s–60s	70s	60s
Male:female ratio	3:2	3:2	1:2	1:1
Lesion morphology	Solitary or multiple erythematous to violaceous domed papules, plaques, nodules, or tumors	Solitary or grouped erythematous-to-violaceous domed papules, plaques, nodules, or tumors	Solitary or multiple red or blue-red tumors	Western–cutaneous and central nervous system (CNS) manifestations Eastern–hemophagocytic syndrome
Location[7]	Upper limb (31%) Trunk (27%) Face (27%) Scalp/neck (8%) Lower limb (7%)	Scalp/neck (37%) Face (33%) Trunk (19%) Upper limb (8%) Lower limb (3%)	Lower limb (29%) Scalp/neck (22%) Face (22%) Trunk (16%) Upper limb (11%)	Systemic See text for discussion of the utility of random skin biopsies in diagnosis.
Associated symptoms	None	None	Typically none	B symptoms, neurologic abnormalities, hemophagocytic syndrome
Common therapeutic options	Solitary: Low-dose RT (preferred), excision, intralesional corticosteroids, wait-and-see Multifocal: Low-dose RT, intralesional corticosteroids, rituximab	Solitary: Low-dose RT (preferred), intralesional corticosteroids Multifocal: Low-dose RT, rituximab	Systemic chemotherapy + radiation[36]	Combination chemotherapy, allogeneic hematopoietic stem cell transplant if patient is a candidate

Likelihood of cutaneous relapse[25]	50%	30% Often adjacent to previous areas of involvement.	65%	Systemic at diagnosis
Likelihood of visceral dissemination	5% Visceral dissemination may be more common in non-class-switched (IgM-restricted) cases[10,11]	5%–10%[25]	35%[25]	Systemic at diagnosis
5-y disease-specific survival	99%[25]	95%[25]	30%–50% w/o R-CHOP 70%–80% w/R-CHOP[32]	50%[60]
5-y overall survival	94%[25]	87%[25]	20% w/o R-CHOP 60% w/R-CHOP[32]	45%[60]

cutaneous; IVLBCL is a systemic lymphoma that often presents in the skin.[3] Epstein–Barr virus-positive (EBV+) mucocutaneous ulcer (EBVMCU) was first described as a lymphoproliferative disorder in 2010[4] and was added to the classification of cutaneous lymphomas as a provisional entity in 2018.[2]

This review is divided into two sections. Part 1 will be an overview of CBCLs, which will address the clinical presentation and management of each lymphoma, recent advances in the pathobiology of the CBCLs, and evidence regarding the treatment of each of the CBCLs. Part 2 is a detailed guide to the steps in diagnosis and workup of a newly diagnosed CBCL according to the International Society for Cutaneous Lymphoma/European Organization for Research and Treatment of Cancer (ISCL/EORTC)[5] and National Comprehensive Cancer Network (NCCN) guidelines.[6]

PART 1: OVERVIEW OF THE CUTANEOUS B-CELL LYMPHOMAS
Primary Cutaneous Marginal Zone Lymphoma

Clinical presentation
Primary cutaneous marginal zone B-cell lymphoma (PCMZL) is an indolent, primary cutaneous B-cell lymphoma (PCBCL) which most commonly presents as solitary or multiple erythematous to violaceous domed papules, plaques, nodules, or tumors on the upper limbs (31%), trunk (27%), and face (27%) (**Figs. 1 and 2**).[7] This extranodal non-Hodgkin lymphoma (NHL) falls in the class of extranodal B-cell lymphomas of mucosa-associated lymphoid tissue, or MALT lymphomas.

Approximately 30% to 50% of patients present with a solitary lesion (T1 disease), and 50% to 70% with multifocal disease; of the patients with multifocal disease, approximately 60% had regional skin involvement (T2 disease) and 40% had generalized skin lesions (T3 disease).[8,9]

PCMZL responds extremely well to conservative therapies like involved-field low-dose radiation therapy and excision. Overall, approximately 90% of patients will experience a complete remission after initial treatment with conservative therapy, including 93% of patients with solitary or localized disease and 71% of patients with multifocal or generalized disease.[8] Cutaneous relapse after treatment is very common, occurring in 40% to 50% of patients. Relapse is more likely in multifocal disease.[8,9] Approximately 4% to 5% of patients may develop extracutaneous dissemination. Systemic dissemination may be more common in patients with IgM-restricted disease.[10,11]

In our experience, patients respond very well to re-treatment of relapsed areas, particularly with localized disease. The median *disease-free* survival for patients with PCMZL is 47 months. Five-year overall survival is approximately 93%, with a disease-specific survival of nearly 99%.[9]

Histopathology
The histopathology and immunohistochemical (IHC) characteristics of PCMZL is described in detail in **Table 2** and by Drs. Sarah E. Gibson and Steven H. Swerdlow in the *American Journal of Surgical Pathology* (2021).[12]

Treatment for primary cutaneous marginal zone lymphoma, including radiation therapy for indolent cutaneous B-cell lymphoma
Treatment for PCMZL may differ depending on the extent of cutaneous involvement and the development of extracutaneous spread.

Treatment for solitary or localized lesions of PCMZL includes low-dose radiation therapy, excision, intralesional corticosteroid injection, and watchful waiting. Corticosteroid injections have a complete remission rate of only 44% and may require multiple rounds of injections; topical corticosteroids are typically ineffective.[13] Although excision can be definitive, PCMZL has a high propensity for local recurrence,[14–16] making field therapy with radiation preferable, as it can treat the area immediately surrounding the tumor and has less morbidity than excision.

Radiation therapy options for indolent PCBCL include standard-dose radiation therapy and very low-dose radiation therapy. A series of PCMZL patients treated with standard-dose radiation (range 20–46 Gy, administered over 12–20 fractions) showed a 99% complete remission rate and 95% 5-year survival. Approximately 60% of patients experienced a localized relapse. For PCFCL, these rates were 99%, 29%, and 97%, respectively (**Fig. 3**).[17] A subsequent study by Goyal and colleagues compared very low-dose radiation (VLD-RT, 2–4 Gy in two treatments) to standard dose therapy (SD-RT, 24–40 Gy in 12–20 treatments). This showed similar efficacy (94.1% vs 97.3% initial complete response, $P = 0.49$), with 1-year relapse rates of 6.7% and 5.6%, respectively. The rate of side effects (localized erythema and pruritus) was significantly lower for VLD-RT patients than SD-RT (15.7% vs 78.4%, $P < 0.0001$). This data highlights that VLD-RT is very effective, less burdensome for the patient, and associated with fewer side effects than SD-RT, making it a very attractive treatment option for indolent primary CBCL (PCMZL and PCFCL).[18] Radiation offers an excellent option for areas of the

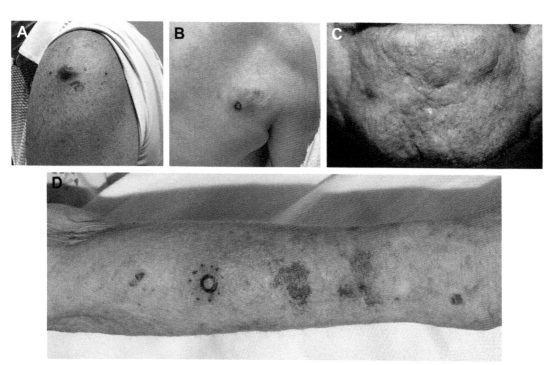

Fig. 1. Clinical images of primary cutaneous marginal zone lymphoma (PCMZL). (*A*) PCMZL, presenting as an indurated, red nodule on the shoulder of a 42 year-old man. (*B*) PCMZL, presenting as coalescent pink-red indurated nodules on the posterior shoulder of a 79 man.(*C*) PCMZL, presenting as an infiltrated plaque on the chin of an older man. (*D*) PCMZL, presenting as indurated nodules on the arm of an older person in a background of senile purpura. (*Courtesy of* [A] Wayne Day, MD, Nashville, TN; [B] Mark P. Eid, MD, FAAD, Fredericksburg, VA.)

body where an excision scar would be cosmetically suboptimal (eg, face) or where healing may be challenging (eg, lower leg).

Multifocal disease may be treated with radiation or with systemic agents, including rituximab. Treatment of systemic involvement of PCMZL would be carried out by hematology/oncology and require systemic therapy. An estimated 4%–5% of patients with PCMZL may develop systemic dissemination at some point in their disease course.

One special circumstance which may necessitate additional consideration: the rare occurrence of PCMZL in children. This population has excellent survival, so the cumulative risk of imaging studies and age-related toxicities of treatment, particularly radiation, must be carefully considered.[19]

Recent advances

- *Prognostic significance of IgM-restriction vs. class-switching.* Recent advances in immunohistochemistry and genetic analysis have revealed that there may be two types of PCMZL: (1) IgM-restricted cases that have not undergone class-switching and (2) class-switched cases expressing IgG, IgA, and/or IgD. There is evidence that IgM-restricted

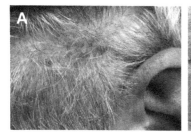
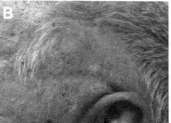
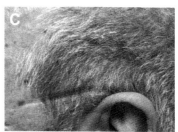

Fig. 2. Radiation therapy is effective for treatment of cutaneous lesions of primary cutaneous B-cell lymphomas. (*A*) PCFCL presenting as a nodule on the hair-bearing scalp of a 63-year-old man, pre-treatment. (*B*) 1 month after radiation treatment with 4 Gy x 2 sessions, resulting in complete remission. (*C*) The patient experienced excellent regrowth of hair in the treated area 6 months after treatment, more than expected.

Table 2
Histopathologic characteristics of cutaneous B-cell lymphomas

	PCMZL	PCFCL	PCDLBCL	IVLBCL
Distribution of lymphoid infiltrate	Dense, nodular, dermal, and subcutaneous infiltrate	3 patterns: 1. Follicular 2. Diffuse 3. Follicular and diffuse	Diffuse infiltrates or confluent sheets of large cells	Intravascular
Presence or absence of follicles	Colonized follicles overrun with neoplastic marginal zone cells Normal reactive lymphoid follicles typically present	Expanded neoplastic follicles and/or diffuse sheets of cells Reactive follicles typically absent	Follicle formation absent	Absent
Presence of admixed T-cells	Abundant around follicles	Often abundant	Sparse, mainly perivascular	Absent
Cytology	Centrocyte-like marginal zone B cells Variable plasma and lymphoplasmacytoid cells Rare immunoblasts	Medium-to-large centrocytes and centroblasts	Large cells resembling immunoblasts or centroblasts	Large atypical lymphocytes in vascular lumina
Remnants of follicular dendritic cell networks (best seen with CD21 immunohistochemical staining)	Intact networks typically present	Sometimes present	Absent	Absent (neoplastic cells are intravascular)
Immunohistochemical features of neoplastic cells[61]	CD20+ BCL2+ BCL6- CD10- MUM1-	CD20+ BCL2- BCL6+ CD10+ MUM1- IgM- IgD- FOXP1-	CD20+ BCL2+ BCL6-/+ CD10- MUM1+ IgM+ IgD+/- FOXP1+ CD5- FOXP1 expression may be associated with worse survival in patients with extranodal DLBCL.[40]	CD20+ BCL2+ BCL6-/+ CD10- MUM1+ CD5+ (22%–38%)

Light-chain restriction	Present in plasma cells in 70% of cases	Absent in plasma cells	May be present in neoplastic cells, absent in plasma cells	May be present in neoplastic cells, absent in plasma cells
Immunoglobulin rearrangement	IgM-restricted in 20%, class-switched in 80% (most often IgG; may be IgA, IgD, or biclonal)	Clonal rearrangement present		
Typical histopathologic description in a report	Sheets of neoplastic marginal zone B-cells and aggregates of lymphoplasamcytoid cells Mature plasma cells with light chain restriction Numerous surrounding non-neoplastic reactive T-cells.	Ill-defined expanded follicles composed of neoplastic centrocytes and centroblasts with disrupted follicular dendritic cell meshworks and absent mantle zones	Monomorphous sheets of large neoplastic B-cells	Intravascular neoplastic B-cells

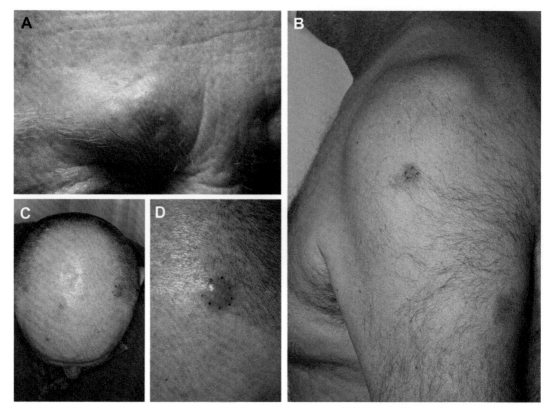

Fig. 3. Clinical images of primary cutaneous follicle center lymphoma (PCFCL). (*A*) PCFCL presenting as infiltrated plaques on arm. (*B*) PCFCL presenting as an erythematous nodule above the medial eyebrow. (*C*) PCFCL presenting as multiple violaceous nodules on the scalp. (*D*) Close-up photo of the lesions from C.

cases may show a worse prognosis with a higher likelihood of extracutaneous spread. Some have proposed that class-switched PCMZL be considered a lymphoproliferative disorder (potentially related to chronic antigenic stimulation), with the classification of lymphoma limited to IgM-restricted cases.[10,20]

• *Presentation of PCMZL as amyloidoma.* There have been reports of PCMZL presenting as amyloid light chain (AL) amyloidoma in the skin, characterized by dermal/subcutaneous deposits of amyloid, associated with sparse to moderately dense perivascular infiltrates of lymphocytes and monotypic plasma cells.[21]

Primary Cutaneous Follicle Center B-Cell Lymphoma

Clinical presentation

PCFCL is an indolent B-cell NHL that presents as solitary or grouped erythematous-to-violaceous domed papules, plaques, nodules, or tumors, most commonly on the scalp/neck (37%) and face (33%) (**Fig. 4**).[7] The median age of patients is 50 to 60 years, and there is a slight male predominance (M:F 3:2). Approximately 60% of cases will present with localized disease (T1), 20% to 30% with regional disease (T2), and 10% to 20% with multifocal disease (T3).[22–24]

PCFCL has an excellent prognosis, with a 5-year overall survival of 87% and a 5-year disease-specific survival of 95%. Approximately 5% to 10% of patients may experience systemic involvement.[25] As with PCMZL, recurrence after treatment is common, particularly local recurrences immediately outside of prior treatment fields.

Histopathology

The histopathology and IHC characteristics of PCFCL is described in detail in **Table 2** and in the *Archives of Pathology and Laboratory Medicine* by Skala and colleagues.[22]

Treatment

Treatment of localized lesions of PCFCL may include excision or radiation therapy. Very low dose radiation therapy (2–4 Gy in 2 sessions) has been shown to be very effective for PCFCL.[18] An additional consideration for PCFCL is that it commonly occurs on the scalp, where hair loss

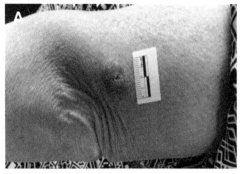

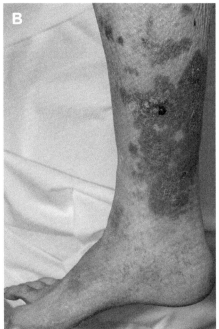
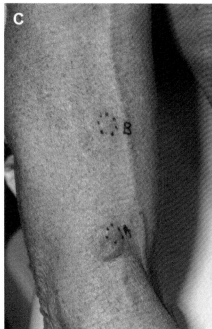

Fig. 4. Clinical images of primary cutaneous diffuse large B-cell lymphoma (PCDLBCL). (A) PCDLBCL presenting as a focally ulcerated erythematous nodule on the posterior upper arm of a 65 year-old woman. (B) PCDLBCL presenting as hemorrhagic plaques and nodules on the lower leg of an older patient; the differential diagnosis in this case included stasis dermatitis or acroangiodermatitis, until a nodule grew in one of the erythematous plaques. (C) PCDLBCL presenting as multiple erythematous nodules on the arm. (Courtesy of [A] Whitney D. Tope, MPhil, MD, FAAD. [B] K Hollandsworth, PA-C, Nashville, TN.)

may be of significant concern for patients treated with radiation, in our experience, the hair loss associated with VLD-RT is minimal and reversible.

Multifocal disease may be treated with radiation or with systemic agents, including rituximab. Treatment of disseminated involvement of PCFCL by hematology/oncology would require systemic therapy, as per protocols for systemic follicular lymphomas.[6]

Recent advances

- *Molecular criteria for identifying patients at higher risk of systemic spread of PCFCL.*

Recent work examining the genomic landscape of PCFCL has revealed molecular markers that may help identify patients with PCFCL who are more likely to experience cutaneous dissemination, or patients who may have systemic involvement below a detectable threshold at the time of diagnosis.[26] This algorithm is not yet in general clinical use.

- *Molecular features distinguishing PCFCL, diffuse type, and PCDLBCL-LT.* Various molecular studies have revealed factors that may help resolve this differential. Although 65% to 80% of cases of PCDLBCL show expression of MYC on IHC, this is typically absent in PCFCL[27]; use of MYC IHC staining is currently gaining clinical use. Gene expression profiling should show a germinal center B-cell (GCB)-type profile in PCFCL and an activated B-cell (ABC)-type profile in PCDLBCL.[28] Mutations in MYD88 (part of the NFkB signaling pathway) are seen in 60% of cases of PCDLBCL but absent in PCFCL.[29–31] Gene expression profiling and mutational analysis are not in widespread diagnostic use at this time.

Primary Cutaneous Diffuse Large B-Cell Lymphoma, Leg-Type

Clinical presentation of primary cutaneous diffuse large B-cell lymphoma, leg-type

PCDLBCL is a rare, aggressive extranodal B-cell NHL that classically presents as solitary or multiple red or blue-red tumors (**Fig. 5**). Although lesions most commonly occur on the legs (29%), the majority of lesions occur in other areas, including the scalp/neck (22%), face (22%), trunk (16%), and upper limb (11%).[7]

PCDLBCL is aggressive: 35% will experience systemic dissemination. Disease-specific survival ranges from 30% to 50% in the absence of systemic chemotherapy with R-CHOP, and 70% to 80% with R-CHOP. Overall survival is approximately 60% with R-CHOP but drops to approximately 20% without R-CHOP.[32] Of note, there is evidence that DLBCL, LT occurring on the leg does have a worse prognosis than DLBCL, LT occurring at other body sites. Additional poor prognostic factors include elevated lactate dehydrogenase (LDH),[33] disseminated cutaneous spread,[34] and extracutaneous progression.[33]

Histopathology

The histopathology and IHC characteristics of PCDLBCL are described in detail in **Table 2** and by Xie and colleagues in their review in *Seminars in Hematology*.[35]

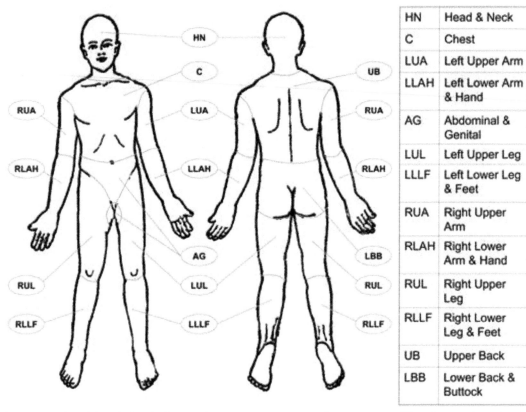

HN	Head & Neck
C	Chest
LUA	Left Upper Arm
LLAH	Left Lower Arm & Hand
AG	Abdominal & Genital
LUL	Left Upper Leg
LLLF	Left Lower Leg & Feet
RUA	Right Upper Arm
RLAH	Right Lower Arm & Hand
RUL	Right Upper Leg
RLLF	Right Lower Leg & Feet
UB	Upper Back
LBB	Lower Back & Buttock

Fig. 5. Map identifying distinct body areas for use in TNM staging of cutaneous B-cell lymphomas, from the ISCL/EORTC staging guidelines. (*From* Kim YH, Willemze R, Pimpinelli N, Whittaker S, Olsen EA, Ranki A, Dummer R, Hoppe RT; ISCL and the EORTC. TNM classification system for primary cutaneous lymphomas other than mycosis fungoides and Sezary syndrome: a proposal of the International Society for Cutaneous Lymphomas (ISCL) and the Cutaneous Lymphoma Task Force of the European Organization of Research and Treatment of Cancer (EORTC). Blood. 2007 Jul 15;110(2):479-84.)

Treatment of primary cutaneous diffuse large B-cell lymphoma, leg-type

Patients with PCDLBCL require both localized therapy for the lesion (typically radiation) and systemic chemotherapy.[6]

Systemic chemotherapy with rituximab is a key component of treatment. Patients who received rituximab with multiagent chemotherapy had 3-year and 5-year survival rates of 80% and 74%, as compared with 48% and 38% for patients who received less intensive therapy.[32]

Involved field radiation therapy has been shown to significantly improve outcomes for patients with PCDLBCL. R-CHOP (rituximab, cyclophosphamide, doxorubicin, vincristine, and prednisone) *with* involved-field radiation therapy (IFRT) was associated with a longer median progression-free survival compared with R-CHOP without IFRT as front-line therapy for PCDLBCL, LT, 41.8 months versus 13.7 months, respectively. Median overall survivals were 74.8 months and. 38.2 months, respectively.[36]

Recent advances in primary cutaneous diffuse large B-cell lymphoma, leg-type

In the last decade, a tremendous amount of information about the underlying molecular mechanisms driving PCDLBCL has been gleaned from genetic studies. Many of these advances have significant implications for prognosis and treatment.

- *CDKN2A and MYD88 alterations are associated with worse prognosis in PCDLBCL-LT.* Approximately two-thirds of patients show loss of CDKN2A either by gene deletion or promoter methylation, as well as the presence of MYD88 L265P mutations. These alterations have both been associated with inferior prognosis.[30,37]
- *NFkB pathway activating mutations, B-cell signaling, and immune evasion mechanisms in PCDLBCL-LT.* Recent work done by Zhou and colleagues showed that 77% of cases of PCDLBCL-LT had NFkB-activating MYD88 mutations oroncogenic mutations activating the NFkB pathway (NFKBIE or REL). Mutations in other canonical cancer pathways (BRAF, MED12, PIK3R1, and STAT3) were also identified,[38] as were mutations in different components of the B-cell receptor signaling pathway, including CARD11 (10%), CD79 B (20%), and TNFAIP3/A20 (40%).[29,39] The second most commonly mutated pathways were implicated in immune evasion via mutations to downregulate antigen processing (B2M, CIITA, HLA) or T-cell costimulation (CD58).[38] This may suggest

utility of therapeutic approaches such as BRAF or PI3K inhibitors.
- *Therapeutic implications of genetic similarity of PCDLBCL-LT to testicular and CNS DLBCL.* Work by Zhou and colleagues[38] showed that PCDLBCL shows significant genetic similarities to primary testicular and primary CNS DLBCLs. As with those lymphomas, 40% of DLBCL-LT had PDL1/PDL2 translocations, resulting in overexpression of PD-L1 or PD-L2 in 50% of cases. This data suggests that checkpoint inhibitors and other therapies currently being developed for other genetically similar lymphomas may be useful in the treatment of PCDLBCL-LT.
- *FOXP1 expression.* FOXP1 expression may be associated with worse survival in patients with extranodal DLBCL, a group that includes PCDLBCL.[40]

Intravascular Large B-Cell Lymphoma

Clinical presentation

IVLBCL is a rare, clinically aggressive B-cell NHL characterized by the proliferation of large neoplastic B-cells within the lumen of blood vessels of all sizes.

There are three primary variants of IVLBCL: (1) classical, (2) hemophagocytic, and (3) cutaneous. The classical variant, more common in western countries, presents with nonspecific symptoms such as fever of unknown origin, central nervous system abnormalities, and skin involvement. The hemophagocytic variant, more common in Asian countries, often presents with hepatosplenic involvement and cytopenias. The cutaneous variants, most common in western countries, appear to be skin limited and may have a better prognosis.[3] The prognosis of IVLBCL is generally poor, and though it has improved with the advent of rituximab, the disease course is typically marked by relapse, particularly in patients with CNS manifestations.[41]

Historically, the majority of patients were identified on autopsy[42]; however, with greater awareness of the disease and improved diagnostic methods, approximately 80% of cases are now identified antemortem.[43] Neoplastic cells are generally not seen on peripheral blood smears (absent in 95% of cases).[44] Peripheral blood flow cytometry may be necessary to identify the neoplastic population of cells, and diagnosis requires bone marrow biopsy.

Classical variant: The median age of patients with classic IVLBCL is 70 years (range 34–90 years) and may present with fever of unknown origin (45%), pain, organ-specific symptoms,

B-symptoms (>50%, only manifestation in 25%), or multiorgan failure and often show rapid deterioration in performance status.[3] Cutaneous lesions may be present in 40% of patients, and range from painful indurated lesions, poorly circumscribed violaceous plaques, "peau d'orange" change, nodular discolorations, tumors, ulcerated nodules, and areas of desquamation and erythema; often in the inframammary region, breast, extremities, and lower abdomen.[42] Neurologic symptoms are present in 35% of cases and may include sensory and motor deficits, neuropathies, transient visual loss, vertigo, and altered mental status. Neuroimaging often reveals ischemic foci and signs of vasculitis.[42]

Cutaneous variant. The cutaneous variant of IVLBCL accounts for 25% of cases and presents with skin lesions in the absence of systemic findings.[45] These patients typically have normal white cell and platelet count with a median age of 59 years, and the disease course is typically less aggressive. Only 30% of patients have systemic symptoms, and 3-year overall survival is 56% (as compared with 22% for patients with systemic involvement).[45]

Hemophagocytic syndrome-associated variant. This syndrome is characterized by bone marrow involvement, fever, hepatosplenomegaly, and thrombocytopenia. Peripheral blood smears and bone marrow smears typically show the presence of nonneoplastic hemophagocytic histiocytes.[46] This variant is extremely aggressive and has a median survival of 2 to 8 months.[3]

Laboratory assessment

The diagnosis of IVLBCL requires bone marrow biopsy and peripheral blood flow cytometry. Random skin biopsy may be helpful in suspected cases (patients with unexplained neurologic abnormalities, fever of unknown origin, concern for vasculitis on CNS imaging). Complete blood count (CBC) typically reveals anemia (63%), thrombocytopenia (29%), and leukopenia (24%). Thrombocytopenia is typically associated with bone marrow infiltration and hepatosplenic involvement. 15% of patients may have abnormalities of liver, renal, or thyroid function, likely reflecting organ involvement.[3]

Histopathology

IVLBCL is characterized by the presence of large, neoplastic B cells in vessels of various diameters, as summarized in **Table 2** and by Ponzoni and colleagues.[3]

Treatment

Treatment of IVLBCL depends on rituximab-based combination chemotherapy, as directed by a hematologist/oncologist.

Recent Advances

- *Random incisional skin biopsies with adipose tissue may be helpful in suspected cases of IVLBCL.* The diagnosis of IVLBCL is challenging. For many years it was thought that biopsies of cherry angiomas may be more likely to reveal a diagnosis of IVLBCL.[47,48] However, recent work has shown that neoplastic intravascular cells are most likely to be detected in the capillaries of subcutaneous adipose tissue.[49,50] Work done in Japan by Matsue and colleagues[49] found that incisional biopsies of *normal skin* (including adipose tissue), taken in fatty areas such as the thigh, abdomen, and upper arm of patients with suspected IVLBCL have a sensitivity of 77.8%, specificity of 98.7%, positive predictive value of 96.6%, and negative predictive value of 90.6% for the diagnosis of IVLBCL. Reports also highlight the importance of performing multiple skin biopsies.[51]

Epstein–Barr virus-positive mucocutaneous ulcer (provisional)

EBVMCU was first described as an EBV + lymphoproliferative disorder in 2010[4,52] and was subsequently added to the classification of cutaneous lymphomas as a provisional entity in 2018.[2] Details of this entity are presented in **Table 3**.

PART 2: GUIDE TO DIAGNOSIS AND WORKUP OF CUTANEOUS B-CELL LYMPHOMA
Establishing the Diagnosis of Cutaneous B-Cell Lymphoma

Although a diagnosis of CBCL may be clinically suspected based on morphology, location, and history, the final diagnosis of CBCL is dependent on histopathology. Of note, although classically certain lymphomas have been characterized as predominantly occurring in particular locations (eg, PCMZL on the trunk and extremities, PCFCL on the scalp, PCDLBCL on the leg), there is significant overlap in spatial distribution of the lymphomas, and this is not a reliable diagnostic characteristic.[7]

Biopsy technique

Obtaining an adequate biopsy specimen is crucial to diagnosis. The specimen must be large and deep enough to show the architecture of the infiltrate and to allow for ancillary studies, hence, a minimum of a 4 mm punch biopsy is recommended (6 mm or larger preferred), with preference for incisional or excisional biopsies.[6] A shave biopsy is generally insufficient to allow for adequate

Table 3
Features of EBV + mucocutaneous ulcer (EBVMCU)

Classification	Indolent EBV + B-cell Lymphoproliferative Disorder
Demographics	Median age 66.4 y Slight female predominance
Clinical presentation	Isolated, sharply well-circumscribed ulcerations with symptoms directly attributable to the ulcer:[74,75] • Oropharyngeal mucosa (52%) • Skin (29%) • Gastrointestinal tract (19%) Absence of:[74,76] • EBV viremia • Systemic symptoms • Lymphadenopathy • Organomegaly • Bone marrow involvement
Predisposing factors	Iatrogenic immunosuppression (56%)[76] Advanced age-associated immunosenescence (40%) Primary immunosuppression (4%)
Proposed pathogenesis	Iatrogenic and/or senescence-related immune suppression results in reduced levels of cytotoxic T-cell activity against EBV-induced B-cell proliferations, permitting the development of localized EBV-driven lymphoid proliferations *without* systemic viremia[77–79]
Histopathology[4,52,74,80]	Ulceration Atypical lymphoid infiltrate composed of EBV-positive, variably sized, atypical B-cells that may resemble Hodgkin and Reed-Sternberg (HRS)-like cells Mixed inflammatory infiltrate with lymphocytes, histiocytes, plasma cells, eosinophils Commonly, a rim of reactive T-cells around EBV-positive B-cell areas
Differential diagnosis	Diffuse large B-cell lymphoma (DLBCL) Classic Hodgkin lymphoma (cHL) Post-transplant lymphoproliferative disorder (PTLD) Plasmablastic lymphoma Anaplastic large cell lymphoma (ALCL)
Workup	Histopathology: IHC or ISH for EBV-related antigens Systemic imaging: CT neck/chest/abdomen/pelvis with contrast or integrated full-body PET scan Serology: Rule out EBV viremia (need viral load, not just IgM, IgG) Bone marrow biopsy: May be considered
Management	May have complete resolution with reduction in iatrogenic immune suppression
Prognosis	Excellent, generally benign and responds to conservative management

architectural assessment. Tissue samples must be handled very carefully to avoid crushing artifacts.

Histopathology and immunohistochemistry

Tissue should be placed in formalin immediately and sent for evaluation by a dermatopathologist or hematopathologist with experience in diagnosing cutaneous lymphomas. If hematoxylin and eosin (H&E) stained sections raise suspicion for a hematolymphoid proliferation, additional IHC stains may be ordered.[6] For proliferations with numerous plasma cells, plasmacytic differentiation, or otherwise suspicious for MZL, ISH, or IHC for kappa and lambda light chains may be helpful (see **Table 2**).

Ancillary molecular diagnostic studies

A variety of ancillary studies may be performed by the pathologist to facilitate diagnosis (**Table 4**).

Table 4
Molecular features of CBCLs

	PCMZL	PCFCL	PCDLBCL	IVLBCL
Gene expression profile	Expression of both some early (PAX-5, PU-1) and mature (Oct2, BOB.1) B-cell transcription factors seen in small neoplastic cells; notable absence of mature transcription factor of BCL-6 in neoplastic cells[62]	GBC-type[28]	ABC-type[28]	ABC-type (83%) GCB-type (17%)[63]
Mutations	FAS/CD95 (63%)[64] Mutations in FAS/CD95 could potentially help distinguish PCMZL from pseudolymphoma MYD88 mutation present in a subset of IgM-restricted PCMZL cases[64]	MYD88 mutation absent[31] MYD88 may be helpful in differentiating PCFCL and PCDLBCL	NFkB pathway activating mutations:[29–31] -MYD88 (60%) -CD79 B (20%) -CARD11 (10%) -TNFAIP3/A20 (40%) Mutations in the NFkB pathway may be oncogenic in PCDLBCL and sDLBCL[65]	MYD88 (44%) CD79b (26%)[3]
Deletions		IgH (68%)[66,67] CDKN2A CDKN2B	CDKN2A Inactivation of CDKN2A by either deletion or methylation of its promoter may be a negative prognostic factor for PCDLBCL[66,67]	
Amplifications		REL (63%)[68]	BCL2[2]	
MYC expression		Negative	Positive (65%–80%) Presence of MYC expression may support a diagnosis of PCDLBCL over PCFCL[27]	Cases of MYC expression reported[69]
Translocations	IGH-MLT t(14;18) (q32;q21) and IGH-FOXP1 it(3;14) (p14.1;q32) translocations have been reported in a proportion of PCMZL[70]		IGH (50%) BCL6 (30%) MYC (35%)	Minimal data available. Reports of t(14; 18) and t(11; 22) (q23; q11)[71,72] Possible recurrent alterations of chromosome 6[3]

| Genetic changes in primary cutaneous vs systemic disease | Most MALT lymphomas are IgM restricted: ~80% of PCMZL are class-switched (IgG, IgA, IgD) and 20% are IgM restricted. [10,11] Often present in sMZL but typically absent in PCMZL [64]
• Translocations of MALT1, BCL2, or BCL10
• Aberrant somatic hypermutation of Ig genes
• Mutations in protooncogenes PIM1 or cMYC
• Activating mutations in MYD88
These genetic alterations may be of pathobiologic significance but not currently in use clinically. | t(14;18) absent in PCFCL but typically present in sFL *Clinically helpful in differentiating PCFCL and sFL.* [2] BCL2 rearrangement (8% of skin-restricted PCFCL, 92% of systemically disseminated PCFCL, 89% of sFL) *May be clinically important, as presence of BCL2 rearrangement in combination with CREBBP, KTMT2D, EZH2, or EP300 mutations may suggest increased likelihood of systemic dissemination or presence of sFL that is below detection threshold* [26] | Gains of 1p, 7p, 12q24.21–12q24.31, and 22q and chromosome X; loss of chromosome 4, 6q, and 18q22.3–23 are more common in extranodal than nodal DLBCLs Amplification of 18q and BCL2 overexpression are more common in nodal than extranodal DLBCL. [73] *These changes may be of pathobiologic significance but not currently in use clinically.* |

This table summarizes many of the recent advancements in exploration into the genomic landscape of the CBCLs; it is not intended to be comprehensive, but rather to include genetic changes that may have pathobiological, diagnostic, or prognostic significance.

PCMZL with IgM restriction (non-class-switched) may represent disease more similar to other MALTs, with higher incidence of extracutaneous dissemination. Given the indolent nature of class-switched cases, a distinction between IgM-restricted cases as PCMZL and class-switched cases as an indolent lymphoproliferative disorder is under consideration. Routine assessment of Ig expression may be considered for cases of PCMZL. [14]

Table 5
Components of the histopathologic diagnosis of CBCL

Essential components of diagnosis of CBCL	Comments
Adequate biopsy (punch, incisional, excisional)	Performed by dermatology *Because tissue architecture is critical to pathologic diagnosis, care must be taken not to crush the specimen. Samples of at least 4 mm diameter are preferred. If multiple morphologies are present, sampling of each type is recommended.*
Adequate immunophenotyping panel to establish diagnosis: CD3, CD20, CD10, BCL2, BCL6, IRF4/MUM1, CD21	Ordered by pathology as part of histopathologic assessment
Review by a dermatopathologist/ hematopathologist with expertise in cutaneous B-cell lymphomas	May be requested by dermatology or pathology
Useful in selected circumstances	
Expanded ICH panels: *Suspected PCMZL:* kappa/lambda (ISH or IHC); CD23; IgM, IgG, IgA, and IgD (to assess for class-switching) *Suspected PC-DLBCL vs PCFCL:* Ki-67; EBER (ISH); IgM; IgD; FOXP1; MYC *Rule-out CLL:* CD5, CD43, CD23 *Rule-out mantle cell lymphoma:* CyclinD1	Ordered by pathology as needed as part of histopathologic assessment
Cytogenetics (FISH and karyotype) • Systemic FL: t(14;18) translocation • PCDLBCL: BCL6 (30%), MYC (35%), IGH (50%) translocations	Typically ordered by pathology as needed as part of histopathologic assessment
Mutational analysis DLBCL: MYD88 (60%), CD79 B (20%), CARD11 (10%), TNFAIP3/A20 (40%)	Typically ordered by pathology as needed as part of histopathologic assessment
Tissue flow cytometry	Ordered by dermatology; requires fresh tissue in saline *May be helpful for establishing clonality in select cases*
Tissue IgH gene rearrangement	May be ordered by dermatology or pathology *May be helpful for establishing clonality in select cases*

Establishing the diagnosis of CBCL requires a variety of cutaneous and systemic tests to identify the subtype of lymphoma. Generally, clinical correlation is required to distinguish between primary cutaneous and secondary cutaneous disease, although some genetic factors (eg, t(14;18) translocation in systemic FL) may favor the systemic disease. Close communication between the clinician and pathologist is key to accurate diagnosis of CBCLs.[5,6]

Examples of expanded IHC panels are included in **Table 5**.

Tissue flow cytometry

Tissue flow cytometry may be helpful in assessing for clonality in challenging cases, to help differentiate from cutaneous lymphoid hyperplasia or other reactive infiltrates. This technique requires fresh tissue submitted in saline and may thus require an additional biopsy. Before submitting tissue, it is best to ensure that the clinical laboratory is able to run this test.[53]

Workup of CBCLs: evaluation for systemic disease

Once a tissue diagnosis of B-cell lymphoma has been established, the workup of CBCL requires assessment for evidence of systemic malignancy and of any factors that may impact therapy (**Table 6**). The diagnosis of "primary cutaneous" lymphomas requires the absence of systemic involvement at the time of diagnosis.[54]

In general, there are no histopathologic or IHC features that would allow a pathologist to definitively distinguish a primary cutaneous lymphoma and secondary cutaneous involvement

Table 6
Components of workup for cutaneous B-cell lymphoma

Essential Components of the Workup for CBCL	Comments
History and physical examination: Including complete skin examination	Performed by dermatology at initial and *all* follow-up visits
Laboratory studies: *All patients:* CBC with differential, comprehensive serum chemistry, serum lactate dehydrogenase (LDH) *PCMZL:* SPEP and quantitative immunoglobulins *Candidates for systemic therapy:* HIV, Hepatitis B and C; serum HCG for persons able to become pregnant	Ordered by dermatology; studies for candidates for systemic therapies may be ordered by hematology/oncology
Imaging studies: CT of chest, abdomen, and pelvis with contrast, or with whole-body PET (18F-FDG) AND CT or ultrasound of neck if clinically indicated *Versus* Whole-body integrated PET/CT *DLCBL:* Testicular ultrasound may be considered to evaluate for primary testicular DLBCL with secondary cutaneous involvement, as the testicles may be difficult to evaluate on CT or PET imaging	Ordered by dermatology or hematology/oncology, depending on provider preference *Lymph nodes that are >1.0 cm in short axis and/or have significantly increased PET activity should be sampled for histopathologic examination (an excisional biopsy is preferable whenever possible).*
Bone marrow biopsy and aspirate: Required for CBCL with intermediate to aggressive clinical behavior (per WHO-EORTC classification, eg, DLCBL, IVLBCL): *And* Considered for CBCL with indolent clinical behavior (per WHO-EORTC classification, eg, PCMZL, PCFCL); not required unless indicated by other staging assessments	Requires hematology/oncology consultation
Peripheral blood flow cytometry: Recommended if CBC shows lymphocytosis or systemic lymphoma suspected	Ordered by dermatology or hematology/oncology, depending on provider preference

Once a tissue diagnosis of B-cell lymphoma has been established, the workup of CBCL requires assessment for evidence of systemic malignancy and assessment of any factors that may impact therapy. A diagnosis of *primary cutaneous* B-cell lymphoma requires exclusion of systemic malignancy based on clinical assessment. Close team-work between dermatology and hematology/oncology may be needed in the workup of CBCLs.[5,6]

of a systemic malignancy. Rather, a diagnosis of PCBCLs requires exclusion of systemic malignancy based on clinical assessment and clinical correlation.[5,6]

Of note, some B-cell lymphomas do not have primary cutaneous variants and are always secondary cutaneous, including mantle cell lymphoma,[55] Hodgkin lymphoma,[56] and Burkitt lymphoma.[57]

History and physical examination

The workup of CBCL includes a detailed history and physical examination at the time of diagnosis, at a minimum of annually after diagnosis, and with any change in disease presentation. The history should include the chronology of the skin disease,

a complete review of systems including B-symptoms (weight loss, fatigue, night sweats), medical and oncologic history, and medications.[5] Any past biopsy results or records should be reviewed and forwarded to the pathologist. A full-body skin examination, including genital and complete lymph node assessment, is needed.

Laboratory evaluation

All patients with a new diagnosis of CBCL should undergo a CBC with differential, peripheral blood smear, comprehensive metabolic panel (CMP), and serum LDH.[5,6] Lymphocytosis should trigger the performance of peripheral blood flow cytometry to identify any atypical cells.[5]

Hematology/oncology referral

In general, patients diagnosed with a CBCL should be given an initial referral to hematology/oncology. Patients with indolent variants of the primary cutaneous disease may or may not need subsequent follow-up with an oncologist, but an initial visit is generally recommended.

Imaging studies

In general, the ISCL/EORTC recommends either a CT of the chest/abdomen/pelvis *and* CT/ultrasound of the neck *or* a whole body integrated PET/computed tomography (CT) scan at the time of diagnosis to assess for lymphadenopathy or visceral involvement. These scans may be ordered by dermatology or hematology/oncology, depending on the provider's comfort with addressing any imaging findings.

Lymph node biopsy

If lymphadenopathy is identified on imaging or physical examination, lymph-node biopsy should be performed. Sampling via *excisional biopsy* to assess for nodal involvement of lymphoma is recommended by the ISCL/EORTC for lymph nodes that are >1.0 cm in the short axis and/or have significantly increased PET activity. Fine needle aspiration is not sufficient to allow evaluation of lymph node architecture and should not be performed.

Peripheral blood flow cytometry

Peripheral blood flow cytometry may be helpful in patients with peripheral blood lymphocytosis. This test is required for the diagnosis of patients with suspected IVLBCL. This may be ordered by dermatology or oncology, depending on the practitioner's degree of comfort in interpreting the report.

Bone marrow biopsy

Bone marrow biopsy may be considered in some patients, particularly those with DLBCL, unexplained cytopenias, bone marrow enhancement on CT, suspected IVLBCL, or other evidence of widespread or systemic lymphoma. Bone marrow biopsy is typically not done for PCMZL or PCFCL, with the exception of unexplained cytopenias, unclear diagnosis, atypical clinical presentation, or unexplained B symptoms.[58,59] Evaluation for the need for bone marrow biopsy is determined via referral to hematology/oncology.

Staging of Primary Cutaneous B-Cell Lymphomas

Once a diagnosis of *primary cutaneous* CBCL is established (ie, systemic disease excluded), staging is performed according to the ISCL/EORTC

Table 7
Staging of cutaneous B-cell lymphomas (CBCL)

T	T1	Solitary skin involvement
		T1a Solitary lesion <5 cm diameter
		T1b Solitary >5 cm diameter
	T2	Regional skin involvement: multiple lesions limited to 1 body region or 2 contiguous body regions
		T2a All-disease-encompassed in a <15 cm diameter circular area
		T2b All-disease-encompassed in a >15 and < 30 cm diameter circular area
		T2c All-disease encompassed in a >30 cm circular area
	T3	Generalized skin involvement
		T3a Multiple lesions involving 2 non-contiguous body areas
		T3b Multiple lesions involving ≥3 body regions
N	N0	No clinical or pathologic lymph node involvement
	N1	Involvement of 1 peripheral lymph node region that drains an area of current or prior skin involvement
	N2	Involvement of 2 or more peripheral lymph node regions or involvement or any lymph node region that does not drain an area of current or prior skin involvement
	N3	Involvement of central lymph nodes
M	M0	No evidence of extracutaneous non-lymph node disease
	M1	Extracutaneous non-lymph node disease present

International Society for Cutaneous Lymphoma/European Organization for Research and Treatment of Cancer (ISCL/EORTC) Tumor-Node-Metastasis (TNM) classification for cutaneous B-cell lymphoma (CBCL).
Adapted from Kim YH, Willemze R, Pimpinelli N, Whittaker S, Olsen EA, Ranki A, Dummer R, Hoppe RT; ISCL and the EORTC. TNM classification system for primary cutaneous lymphomas other than mycosis fungoides and Sezary syndrome: a proposal of the International Society for Cutaneous Lymphomas (ISCL) and the Cutaneous Lymphoma Task Force of the European Organization of Research and Treatment of Cancer (EORTC). Blood. 2007 Jul 15;110(2):479-84.

guidelines, in the tumor-node-metastasis (TNM) format (**Table 7**).[5,6] Staging of PCBCLs is recorded in the tumor-node-metastasis (TNM) format. T stage is determined by the extent of cutaneous involvement of the lymphoma, assessed via the circumference of a circular area drawn around the involved tissue and the number and distribution of areas of involvement (see **Fig. 5**).[5] N is defined by the extent of lymph node involvement, which includes the number of lymph node basins involved and their location relative to the skin primary. M is determined by the presence or absence of visceral non-lymph node involvement, as assessed by imaging and typically confirmed by biopsy.

SUMMARY

The diagnosis and management of a patient with CBCL is a multidisciplinary challenge, requiring cooperation between dermatology, pathology, hematology/oncology, and radiation oncology. Both establishing a tissue diagnosis and ruling out systemic involvement are critical and necessary steps in the diagnosis and management of a primary cutaneous lymphoma. Management options differ significantly by the type of lymphoma.

CLINICS CARE POINTS

- There are four cutaneous lymphomas recognized by the WHO/EORTC, each with unique clinical and histopathologic features and separate treatment algorithms.
- The diagnosis of lymphomas in the skin is based on histopathologic analysis of biopsy tissue, best read by a dermatopathologist with experience in the cutaneous lymphomas. Punch biopsies of at least 6 mm are preferred. The tissue may be fragile and care must be taken not to crush it.
- Distinguishing primary cutaneous lymphoma and secondary cutaneous involvement by a systemic lymphoma is critical to selecting appropriate treatment, and requires a detailed history and physical, lab work, and potentially imaging.
- Referral to hematology/oncology is often helpful, and in some cases (pcDLBCL, IVLBCL) absolutely necessary.
- There have been many recent advances in our understanding of the molecular underpinnings of these lymphomas, but the majority of them are not in clinical use yet. Careful attention should be paid to advances in the field.

DISCLOSURE

This study was funded in part by National Cancer Institute of the National Institutes of Health (T32 HL007062) at the University of Minnesota. The content is solely the responsibility of the authors and does not necessarily represent the official views of the National Institutes of Health.

REFERENCES

1. Bradford PT, Devesa SS, Anderson WF, et al. Cutaneous lymphoma incidence patterns in the United States: a population-based study of 3884 cases. Blood 2009;113(21):5064–73.
2. Willemze R, Cerroni L, Kempf W, et al. The 2018 update of the WHO-EORTC classification for primary cutaneous lymphomas. Blood 2019;133(16):1703–14.
3. Ponzoni M, Campo E, Nakamura S. Intravascular large B-cell lymphoma: a chameleon with multiple faces and many masks. Blood 2018;132(15):1561–7.
4. Dojcinov SD, Venkataraman G, Raffeld M, et al. EBV Positive Mucocutaneous Ulcer—A Study of 26 Cases Associated With Various Sources of Immunosuppression. Am J Surg Pathol 2010;34(3):405–17.
5. Kim YH, Willemze R, Pimpinelli N, et al. TNM classification system for primary cutaneous lymphomas other than mycosis fungoides and Sézary syndrome: a proposal of the International Society for Cutaneous Lymphomas (ISCL) and the Cutaneous Lymphoma Task Force of the European Organization of Research and Treatment of Cancer (EORTC). Blood 2007;110(2):479–84.
6. Network NCC. Primary cutaneous lymphomas. Version 1. Available at: https://www.nccn.org/professionals/physician_gls/pdf/primary_cutaneous.pdf. Accessed Jan 26, 2022.
7. O'Leary D, Goyal N, Rubin N, et al. Characterization of Primary and Secondary Cutaneous B-Cell Lymphomas: a Population-Based Study of 4758 patients. Clin Lymphoma Myeloma Leuk; 2021.
8. Hoefnagel JJ. Primary Cutaneous Marginal Zone B-Cell Lymphoma. Arch Dermatol 2005;141(9):1139.
9. Servitje O, Muniesa C, Benavente Y, et al. Primary cutaneous marginal zone B-cell lymphoma: Response to treatment and disease-free survival in a series of 137 patients. J Am Acad Dermatol 2013;69(3):357–65.
10. Edinger JT, Kant JA, Swerdlow SH. Cutaneous Marginal Zone Lymphomas Have Distinctive Features and Include 2 Subsets. Am J Surg Pathol 2010;34(12):1830–41.
11. Carlsen ED, Swerdlow SH, Cook JR, et al. Class-switched Primary Cutaneous Marginal Zone Lymphomas Are Frequently IgG4-positive and Have Features Distinct From IgM-positive Cases. Am J Surg Pathol 2019;43(10):1403–12.
12. Gibson SE, Swerdlow SH. How I Diagnose Primary Cutaneous Marginal Zone Lymphoma. Am J Clin Pathol 2020;154(4):428–49.

13. Perry A, Vincent BJ, Parker SRS. Intralesional corticosteroid therapy for primary cutaneous B-cell lymphoma. Br J Dermatol 2010;163(1):223–5.

14. Olsen S, Burdick JF, Keown PA, et al. Primary acute renal failure ("acute tubular necrosis") in the transplanted kidney: morphology and pathogenesis. Medicine (Baltimore) 1989;68(3):173–87.

15. Hamilton SN, Wai ES, Tan K, et al. Treatment and Outcomes in Patients With Primary Cutaneous B-Cell Lymphoma: The BC Cancer Agency Experience. Int J Radiat Oncol 2013;87(4):719–25.

16. Kheterpal M, Mehta-Shah N, Virmani P, et al. Managing Patients with Cutaneous B-Cell and T-Cell Lymphomas Other Than Mycosis Fungoides. Curr Hematol Malig Rep 2016;11(3):224–33.

17. Senff NJ. Results of Radiotherapy in 153 Primary Cutaneous B-Cell Lymphomas Classified According to the WHO-EORTC Classification. Arch Dermatol 2007;143(12):1520.

18. Goyal A, Carter JB, Pashtan I, et al. Very low-dose versus standard dose radiation therapy for indolent primary cutaneous B-cell lymphomas: A retrospective study. J Am Acad Dermatol 2018; 78(2):408–10.

19. Amitay-Laish I, Tavallaee M, Kim J, et al. Paediatric primary cutaneous marginal zone B-cell lymphoma: does it differ from its adult counterpart? Br J Dermatol 2017;176(4):1010–20.

20. van Maldegem F, van Dijk R, Wormhoudt TAM, et al. The majority of cutaneous marginal zone B-cell lymphomas expresses class-switched immunoglobulins and develops in a T-helper type 2 inflammatory environment. Blood 2008;112(8):3355–61.

21. Walsh NM, Lano IM, Green P, et al. Amyloidoma of the Skin/Subcutis. Am J Surg Pathol 2017;41(8): 1069–76.

22. Skala SL, Hristov B, Hristov AC. Primary Cutaneous Follicle Center Lymphoma. Arch Pathol Lab Med 2018;142(11):1313–21.

23. Bekkenk MW, Vermeer MH, Geerts M-L, et al. Treatment of Multifocal Primary Cutaneous B-Cell Lymphoma: A Clinical Follow-Up Study of 29 Patients. J Clin Oncol 1999;17(8):2471.

24. Suárez AL, Pulitzer M, Horwitz S, et al. Primary cutaneous B-cell lymphomas. J Am Acad Dermatol 2013;69(3):329.e1–13.

25. Willemze R. Primary cutaneous B-cell lymphomas. Belgian J Hematol 2017;8(6):213–21.

26. Zhou XA, Yang J, Ringbloom KG, et al. Genomic landscape of cutaneous follicular lymphomas reveals 2 subgroups with clinically predictive molecular features. Blood Adv 2021;5(3):649–61.

27. Schrader AMR, Jansen PM, Vermeer MH, et al. High Incidence and Clinical Significance of MYC Rearrangements in Primary Cutaneous Diffuse Large B-Cell Lymphoma, Leg Type. Am J Surg Pathol 2018; 42(11):1488–94.

28. Hoefnagel JJ, Dijkman R, Basso K, et al. Distinct types of primary cutaneous large B-cell lymphoma identified by gene expression profiling. Blood 2005;105(9):3671–8.

29. Koens L, Zoutman WH, Ngarmlertsirichai P, et al. Nuclear Factor-κB Pathway–Activating Gene Aberrancies in Primary Cutaneous Large B-Cell Lymphoma, Leg Type. J Invest Dermatol 2014;134(1): 290–2.

30. Pham-Ledard A, Beylot-Barry M, Barbe C, et al. High Frequency and Clinical Prognostic Value of MYD88 L265P Mutation in Primary Cutaneous Diffuse Large B-Cell Lymphoma, Leg-Type. JAMA Dermatol 2014;150(11):1173.

31. Pham-Ledard A, Cappellen D, Martinez F, et al. MYD88 Somatic Mutation Is a Genetic Feature of Primary Cutaneous Diffuse Large B-Cell Lymphoma, Leg Type. J Invest Dermatol 2012;132(8):2118–20.

32. Grange F, Joly P, Barbe C, et al. Improvement of Survival in Patients With Primary Cutaneous Diffuse Large B-Cell Lymphoma, Leg Type, in France. JAMA Dermatol 2014;150(5):535.

33. Joly P, Vasseur E, Esteve E, et al. Primary cutaneous medium and large cell lymphomas other than mycosis fungoides. An immunohistological and follow-up study on 54 cases. Br J Dermatol 2006; 132(4):506–12.

34. Brice P, Cazals D, Mounier N, et al. Primary cutaneous large-cell lymphoma: analysis of 49 patients included in the LNH87 prospective trial of polychemotherapy for high-grade lymphomas. Leukemia 1998;12(2):213–9.

35. Xie Y, Pittaluga S, Jaffe ES. The Histological Classification of Diffuse Large B-cell Lymphomas. Semin Hematol 2015;52(2):57–66.

36. Kraft RM, Ansell SM, Villasboas JC, et al. Outcomes in primary cutaneous diffuse large B-cell lymphoma, leg type. J Clin Oncol 2021;39(15_suppl):e19547.

37. Senff NJ, Zoutman WH, Vermeer MH, et al. Fine-Mapping Chromosomal Loss at 9p21: Correlation with Prognosis in Primary Cutaneous Diffuse Large B-Cell Lymphoma, Leg Type. J Invest Dermatol 2009;129(5):1149–55.

38. Zhou XA, Louissaint A, Wenzel A, et al. Genomic Analyses Identify Recurrent Alterations in Immune Evasion Genes in Diffuse Large B-Cell Lymphoma, Leg Type. J Invest Dermatol 2018;138(11):2365–76.

39. Pham-Ledard A, Prochazkova-Carlotti M, Andrique L, et al. Multiple genetic alterations in primary cutaneous large B-cell lymphoma, leg type support a common lymphomagenesis with activated B-cell-like diffuse large B-cell lymphoma. Mod Pathol 2014;27(3):402–11.

40. Yu B, Zhou X, Li B, et al. FOXP1 expression and its clinicopathologic significance in nodal and extranodal diffuse large B-cell lymphoma. Ann Hematol 2011;90(6):701–8.

41. Liu Z, Zhang Y, Zhu Y, et al. <p>Prognosis of Intravascular Large B Cell Lymphoma (IVLBCL): Analysis of 182 Patients from Global Case Series</p>. Cancer Manag Res. 2020;Volume 12:10531–10540.

42. Ponzoni M, Ferreri AJM. Intravascular lymphoma: a neoplasm of 'homeless' lymphocytes? Hematol Oncol 2006;24(3):105–12.

43. Brunet V, Marouan S, Routy J-P, et al. Retrospective study of intravascular large B-cell lymphoma cases diagnosed in Quebec. Medicine (Baltimore) 2017; 96(5):e5985.

44. Ponzoni M, Ferreri AJM, Campo E, et al. Definition, Diagnosis, and Management of Intravascular Large B-Cell Lymphoma: Proposals and Perspectives From an International Consensus Meeting. J Clin Oncol 2007;25(21):3168–73.

45. Ferreri AJM, Campo E, Seymour JF, et al. Intravascular lymphoma: clinical presentation, natural history, management and prognostic factors in a series of 38 cases, with special emphasis on the 'cutaneous variant' [1]. Br J Haematol 2004;127(2): 173–83.

46. Murase T, Nakamura S, Kawauchi K, et al. An Asian variant of intravascular large B-cell lymphoma: clinical, pathological and cytogenetic approaches to diffuse large B-cell lymphoma associated with haemophagocytic syndrome. Br J Haematol 2000; 111(3):826–34.

47. Satoh S, Yamazaki M, Yahikozawa H, et al. Intravascular large B cell lymphoma diagnosed by senile angioma biopsy. Intern Med 2003;42(1):117–20.

48. Adachi Y, Kosami K, Mizuta N, et al. Benefits of skin biopsy of senile hemangioma in intravascular large B-cell lymphoma: A case report and review of the literature. Oncol Lett. 2014;7(6):2003–2006.

49. Matsue K, Abe Y, Kitadate A, et al. Sensitivity and specificity of incisional random skin biopsy for diagnosis of intravascular large B-cell lymphoma. Blood 2019;133(11):1257–9.

50. Asada N, Odawara J, Kimura S, et al. Use of Random Skin Biopsy for Diagnosis of Intravascular Large B-Cell Lymphoma. Mayo Clin Proc 2007; 82(12):1525–7.

51. Kiyohara T, Kumakiri M, Kobayashi H, et al. A case of intravascular large B-cell lymphoma mimicking erythema nodosum: the importance of multiple skin biopsies. J Cutan Pathol. 2000;27(8):413–418.

52. Ikeda T, Gion Y, Yoshino T, et al. A review of EBV-positive mucocutaneous ulcers focusing on clinical and pathological aspects. J Clin Exp Hematop 2019;59(2):64–71.

53. Lima M. Cutaneous primary B-cell lymphomas: from diagnosis to treatment. An Bras Dermatol 2015; 90(5):687–706.

54. Willemze R. WHO-EORTC classification for cutaneous lymphomas. Blood 2005;105(10):3768–85.

55. Goyal A, O'Leary D, Foreman RK, et al. Assessing the diagnosis of "primary cutaneous mantle cell lymphoma": A systematic review and population-based analysis. J Am Acad Dermatol 2021.

56. Dhull AK, Soni A, Kaushal V. Hodgkin's lymphoma with cutaneous involvement. Case Rep 2012;(nov28 1):2012. bcr2012007599.

57. Thakkar D, Lipi L, Misra R, et al. Skin involvement in Burkitt's lymphoma. Hematol Oncol Stem Cell Ther 2018;11(4):251–2.

58. Vachhani P, Neppalli VT, Cancino CJ, et al. Radiological imaging and bone marrow biopsy in staging of cutaneous B-cell lymphoma. Br J Haematol 2019; 184(4):674–6.

59. Quereux G, Frot AS, Brocard A, et al. Routine bone marrow biopsy in the initial evaluation of primary cutaneous B-cell lymphoma does not appear justified. Eur J Dermatol 2009;19(3):216–20.

60. Goyal A, Goyal K, Bohjanen K. Mortality in intravascular large B-cell lymphoma: A SEER analysis. J Am Acad Dermatol 2018;79(6):1163–5.

61. Carter JB. Atlas of Cutaneous Lymphomas. Atlas of Cutaneous Lymphomas. 2015.

62. Hoefnagel JJ, Mulder MMS, Dreef E, et al. Expression of B-cell transcription factors in primary cutaneous B-cell lymphoma. Mod Pathol 2006;19(9): 1270–6.

63. Murase T, Yamaguchi M, Suzuki R, et al. Intravascular large B-cell lymphoma (IVLBCL): a clinicopathologic study of 96 cases with special reference to the immunophenotypic heterogeneity of CD5. Blood 2007;109(2):478–85.

64. Maurus K, Appenzeller S, Roth S, et al. Panel Sequencing Shows Recurrent Genetic FAS Alterations in Primary Cutaneous Marginal Zone Lymphoma. J Invest Dermatol 2018;138(7):1573–81.

65. Visco C, Tanasi I, Quaglia FM, et al. Oncogenic Mutations of MYD88 and CD79B in Diffuse Large B-Cell Lymphoma and Implications for Clinical Practice. Cancers (Basel) 2020;12(10):2913.

66. Dijkman R, Tensen CP, Jordanova ES, et al. Array-Based Comparative Genomic Hybridization Analysis Reveals Recurrent Chromosomal Alterations and Prognostic Parameters in Primary Cutaneous Large B-Cell Lymphoma. J Clin Oncol 2006;24(2):296–305.

67. Dijkman R, Tensen CP, Buettner M, et al. Primary cutaneous follicle center lymphoma and primary cutaneous large B-cell lymphoma, leg type, are both targeted by aberrant somatic hypermutation but demonstrate differential expression of AID. Blood 2006;107(12):4926–9.

68. Chimenti S, Fink-Puches R, Peris K, et al. Cutaneous involvement in lymphoblastic lymphoma. J Cutan Pathol 1999;26(8):379–85.

69. Ogasawara T, Ebata N, Hamasaki J, et al. [BCL2, BCL6, and MYC-positive intravascular large B-cell

lymphoma presenting with bilateral adrenal gland lesions]. Rinsho Ketsueki 2019;60(6):570–6.

70. Streubel B, Vinatzer U, Lamprecht A, et al. T(3; 14)(p14.1;q32) involving IGH and FOXP1 is a novel recurrent chromosomal aberration in MALT lymphoma. Leukemia 2005;19(4):652–8.

71. Mandal AKJ, Savvidou L, Slater RM, et al. Angiotropic lymphoma: Associated chromosomal abnormalities. Eur J Intern Med 2007;18(5):432–4.

72. Shigematsu Y, Matsuura M, Nishimura N, et al. Intravascular Large B-cell Lymphoma of the Bilateral Ovaries and Uterus in an Asymptomatic Patient with a t(11;22)(q23;q11) Constitutional Translocation. Intern Med 2016;55(21):3169–74.

73. Al-Humood SA, Al-Qallaf AS, AlShemmari SH, et al. Genotypic and Phenotypic Differences between Nodal and Extranodal Diffuse Large B-Cell Lymphomas. J Histochem Cytochem 2011;59(10): 918–31.

74. Dojcinov S, Fend F, Quintanilla-Martinez L. EBV-Positive Lymphoproliferations of B- T- and NK-Cell Derivation in Non-Immunocompromised Hosts. Pathogens 2018;7(1):28.

75. Ikeda T, Gion Y, Sakamoto M, et al. Clinicopathological analysis of 34 Japanese patients with EBV-positive mucocutaneous ulcer. Mod Pathol 2020;33(12): 2437–48.

76. Roberts TK, Chen X, Liao JJ. Diagnostic and therapeutic challenges of EBV-positive mucocutaneous ulcer: a case report and systematic review of the literature. Exp Hematol Oncol. 2015;5(1):13.

77. Natkunam Y, Goodlad JR, Chadburn A, et al. EBV-Positive B-Cell Proliferations of Varied Malignant Potential. Am J Clin Pathol 2017;147(2):129–52.

78. Gali V, Bleeker JS, Lynch D. Epstein-Barr Virus Positive Mucocutaneous Ulcer: A Case Report. S D Med. 2018;71(6):252–255.

79. Satou A, Nakamura S. EBV-positive B-cell lymphomas and lymphoproliferative disorders: Review from the perspective of immune escape and immunodeficiency. Cancer Med 2021;10(19):6777–85.

80. Isnard P, Bruneau J, Sberro-Soussan R, et al. Dissociation of humoral and cellular immune responses in kidney transplant recipients with EBV mucocutaneous ulcer. Transpl Infect Dis 2021;23(3).

A Practical Guide to the Diagnosis, Evaluation, and Treatment of Cutaneous T-Cell Lymphoma

Serena Shimshak, BA[a], Olayemi Sokumbi, MD[b,c], Nasro Isaq, MD[d],
Amrita O'Leary Goyal, MD[e], Nneka Comfere, MD[d,f],*

KEYWORDS

- Mycosis fungoides • Sezary syndrome • Lymphomatoid papulosis • Large cell lymphoma
- Adult T- cell leukemia/lymphoma • Gamma delta lymphoma • Peripheral T- cell lymphoma

KEY POINTS

- Diagnostic classification of cutaneous T-cell lymphomas requires the careful correlation of the clinical features, disease course, histopathologic, immunophenotypic, and molecular genetic attributes.
- Management and prognosis of cutaneous T-cell lymphomas are dependent on accurate diagnostic classification and staging.
- Management of cutaneous T-cell lymphoma relies on a multidisciplinary care model that includes dermatology, hemato-oncology, palliative medicine, and radiation oncology expertise.

INTRODUCTION

Cutaneous T-cell lymphomas (CTCLs) encompass a group of clinically heterogenous non-Hodgkin lymphomas characterized by the infiltration of the skin by neoplastic T-lymphocytes. CTCL constitutes 75% of all cutaneous lymphomas and mycosis fungoides (MF) represents more than half of all CTCL. In this article, our primary objective is to present the pertinent clinicopathologic features and treatment approaches for the main subtypes of CTCL.

Diagnostic Evaluation

Evaluation of a patient suspected of having CTCL requires the correlation of clinical and histopathologic data. A complete skin and lymph node (LN) examination, including the estimation of body surface area (BSA) are important for an accurate assignment of the T stage (**Tables 1** and **2**).[1] A common method for the estimation of BSA involves using the patient's palm including digits which approximates 1% BSA.

Skin Biopsy

Skin biopsies are required for diagnosis and may include punch (at least 6 mm), incisional, and/or excisional biopsies of the most representative lesion(s). If multiple lesion morphologies are present, sampling each type of lesion is advised.[1,2] Treatment with topical steroids, ultraviolet light, or

[a] Mayo Clinic Alix School of Medicine, 4500 San Pablo Road, Jacksonville, FL 32224, USA; [b] Department of Dermatology, Mayo Clinic, 4500 San Pablo Road, Jacksonville, FL 32224, USA; [c] Department of Laboratory Medicine and Pathology, Mayo Clinic, 4500 San Pablo Road, Jacksonville, FL 32224, USA; [d] Department of Dermatology, Mayo Clinic, 200 First Street Southwest, Rochester, MN 55905, USA; [e] Department of Dermatology, University of Minnesota, 516 Delaware Street Southeast, Minneapolis, MN 55455, USA; [f] Department of Laboratory Medicine and Pathology, Mayo Clinic, 200 First Street Southwest, Rochester, MN 55905, USA
* Corresponding author. Mayo Clinic, 200 First Street Southwest, Rochester, MN 55905.
E-mail address: Comfere.nneka@mayo.edu

Dermatol Clin 41 (2023) 209–229
https://doi.org/10.1016/j.det.2022.07.019

Table 1
TNMB classification of cutaneous T-cell lymphoma

TNMB Classification	Description of TNMB
Skin (T)	
T1	Limited patches/plaques involving ≤10% of total skin surface
T2	Generalized patches/plaques involving ≥10% of total skin surface
T3	Tumors (one or more tumors with diameter ≥1 cm)
T4	Erythroderma (confluent erythema involving ≥80% BSA)
Lymph node (N)	
N0	No clinically abnormal lymph nodes; negative pathology
N1	Clinically abnormal lymph nodes; negative pathology for CTCL
N2	Clinically abnormal lymph nodes; negative pathology for CTCL
N3	Clinically abnormal lymph nodes; pathology positive for CTCL
NX	Clinically abnormal peripheral or central lymph nodes, no histologic confirmation
Visceral (M)	
M0	No visceral involvement
M1	Visceral involvement (must have pathologic confirmation)
Blood (B)	
B0	No circulating atypical (Sézary) cells or (<5% of lymphocytes)
B1	Low blood tumor burden (≥5% of lymphocytes are Sézary cells but not B2)
B2	High blood tumor burden (≥1000/mcl Sézary cells + positive clone)

From Olsen EA. Evaluation, Diagnosis, and Staging of Cutaneous Lymphoma. Dermatol Clin. 2015 Oct;33(4):643-54.

Table 2
Clinical staging of CTCL

Stages	T	N	M	B
Stage IA	1	0	0	0–1
Stage IB	2	0	0	0–1
Stage IIA	1–2	1	0	0–1
Stage IIB	3	0–1	0	0–1
Stage III	4	0–1	0	0–1
Stage IVA1	1–4	2–3	0	2
Stage IVA2	1–4	3	0	0–2
Stage IVB	1–4	N-any	1	0–2

obtaining skin biopsies to maximize the diagnostic yield.[1] It is not uncommon that biopsies of erythroderma or early patch stages of CTCL may yield nonspecific findings in up to 30% of cases and may require serial biopsies to establish a definitive diagnosis.

Immunophenotype and Molecular Genetics

Immunophenotypic characterization of the atypical T-cell infiltrates in skin biopsies includes assessment for T-cell markers: CD2, CD3, CD4, CD5, CD7, CD8, CD20, CD30, T-cell receptor (TCR) beta F1, and TCR gamma or delta.[1–3] Molecular analysis to detect clonal TCR gene rearrangements in the skin is an important component of the workup. The presence of a T-cell clone alone is insufficient for a diagnosis of lymphoma, as inflammatory dermatoses may also demonstrate clonal TCR rearrangement (eg, PLEVA, pigmented purpuric dermatosis).[1] Thus, careful correlation of the clinical, histopathologic, immunophenotypic, and molecular genetic features is necessary to establish a diagnosis of CTCL.

Laboratory Evaluation

An appropriate laboratory workup may include complete blood count (CBC) with differential, peripheral smear, lactate dehydrogenase (LDH), complete metabolic panel (CMP), and peripheral blood TCR gene rearrangement assay.[1,3] Sezary cell counts performed on peripheral blood smears are generally no longer performed as they are highly user dependent. Flow cytometry is considered the standard for the assessment of circulating disease involvement for patients with stages T2-T4 and those with suspected extracutaneous involvement.[3] Flow cytometry may be performed for patients with T1 disease depending on the clinical index of suspicion for peripheral blood involvement.

systemic immunosuppressants may diminish or eliminate neoplastic T-cells in lesional skin, hampering diagnosis. Therefore, if there is clinical suspicion for CTCL, recommendations are to discontinue all treatment for 2 to 4 weeks before

Imaging

Computed tomography (CT) of the chest, abdomen, and pelvis (and potentially the neck) is performed at the time of diagnosis for patients with stage II or higher disease. Repeat imaging may be indicated if patients demonstrate a clinical change (new tumors or new peripheral blood involvement). CT may be considered in patients with early-stage CTCL based on clinical assessment.[2] Any clinically suspicious LNs as well as large LNs of diameter greater than 1.5 cm should be biopsied via excisional or incisional methods. Core needle biopsy and fine needle aspiration are not sufficient as they do not allow for the assessment of LN architecture.[1] Cervical LNs are preferred followed by axillary then inguinal nodes. LN excision specimens should be analyzed by histopathology, flow cytometry, and molecular genetic analysis for T-cell receptor gene rearrangement. Performing a bone marrow (BM) biopsy is not a standard element of the work-up for MF and should be limited to patients with unexplained hematologic abnormalities.[1,2] Staging patients with MF and Sézary syndrome (SS) is important as it dictates management and has prognostic significance.

MYCOSIS FUNGOIDES
Introduction

MF is the most common CTCL accounting for 60% of CTCLs and 50% of all primary cutaneous lymphomas.[3] It is characterized by pink to erythematous patches and plaques that can be localized or generalized as well as tumors and erythroderma.[1] (Fig. 1) There are several subtypes of MF discussed later in discussion. The natural history of MF is characterized by an indolent course with waxing and waning lesions.[1,3]

MF typically presents between the ages of 55 and 60 years and demonstrates a male to female ratio of 2:1.[1–3] Incidence rates in the US and Europe are approximately 6.4 cases per million per year, representing 4% of all cases of non-Hodgkin lymphomas.[4] Rates of diagnosis have been increasing likely due to improvements in the surveillance and detection of skin lesions with the highest incidence rates occurring in males and African Americans.[3,4] The overall 5-year survival rate for MF is 88%, but survival varies by subtype, stage, and the presence of large cell transformation.[2–4]

MF is characterized by a clonal expansion of resident CD4+ T-helper or memory T-cells (CD45RO+) that normally reside in the skin. Numerous studies examining the genetic and environmental underpinnings of MF have identified a heterogenous group of associations. Hence, our understanding of the factors that initiate MF and promote disease progression remains limited.

Clinical and Histopathologic Features

MF classically progresses through patch, plaque, and tumor stages, however, may present de novo as any lesion type.[1] Early stages of MF are complicated by significant overlapping clinical and histopathologic features with inflammatory dermatoses such as eczema, psoriasis, parapsoriasis, and drug hypersensitivity reactions resulting in diagnostic delays. The median time from disease presentation to the diagnosis of MF can range from 2 to 10 years.[1]

MF is characterized by persistent and progressive patches and plaques that develop in a "bathing suit" distribution with variable sizes, shapes, and colors (see Fig. 1A, C, D, F). Although tumors are often accompanied by a background of patches and plaques, rarely they can be observed in the absence of other lesions. Tumors are often accompanied by ulceration and may be solitary, localized, or generalized.[1] In classic presentations of MF, lesions are frequently large, may be pruritic, and multifocal. However, there is a broad range of clinical variants with distinguishing features based on differences in lesion distribution, pigmentation, and epitheliotropism.

MF variants included in the WHO-EORTC classification are folliculotropic MF, pagetoid reticulosis, and granulomatous slack skin.[3] (see Fig. 1H, I) Table 3 summarizes MF variants and their clinical mimics that clinicians should consider in their differential diagnoses.[5] The most common variant is folliculotropic MF (FMF) which accounts for 13% of MF.[3] It often presents as follicular papules or plaques on the head and neck region with associated alopecia. The prognosis of FMF is worse as compared with classic MF with a 5-year overall survival of 70% to 80%.[3] Granulomatous slack skin is an extremely rare variant and is characterized by erythematous plaques that become bulky and pendulous in the intertriginous areas.[3] Other clinical variants of MF to be aware of include erythrodermic, palmoplantar, poikilodermatous, unifocal/solitary, hypo- and hyperpigmented, bullous, and papular.[2,3] (see Fig. 1B, J) MF may undergo large-cell transformation (MF-LCT) and follow an aggressive clinical course.[1] (see Fig. 1G) MF-LCT is a histopathologic diagnosis and can occur in 10% to 25% of patients with MF.[6] It has variable outcomes with many patients experiencing rapid clinical deterioration. It is important for clinicians to be aware of MF-LCT as it impacts prognosis as well as management. Additionally, visceral or extracutaneous involvement of LNs, lung, spleen,

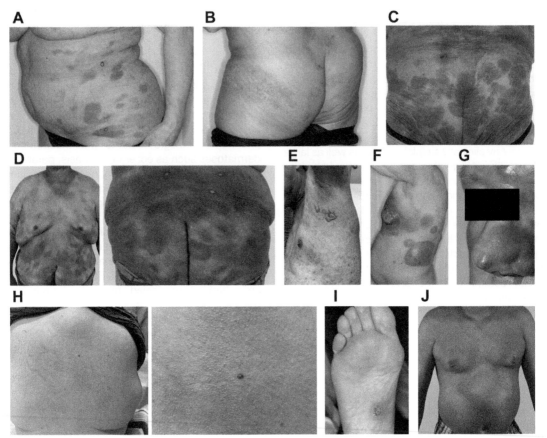

Fig. 1. (*A*) Mycosis fungoides. Patches and plaques on torso. (*B*) Mycosis Fungoides. Poikilodermatous patches on buttocks (*C*) Mycosis fungoides. Patches and plaques on buttocks. (*D*) Mycosis fungoides. Plaques with hyperpigmentation on i) torso and ii) buttocks (*E*) Mycosis fungoides. Diffuse small patches and cluster of tumor nodules on torso (*F*) Mycosis fungoides. Patches, plaques, and ulcerated tumor on torso. (*G*) Mycosis fungoides with large cell transformation. Facial plaques and tumor on nose. (*H*) Mycosis fungoides – folliculotropic variant. Erythematous patches with follicular prominence on back. (*I*). Mycosis fungoides - Pagetoid reticulosis variant. Solitary erythematous hyperkeratotic plaque on plantar foot. (*J*). Mycosis fungoides – Erythrodermic variant. Diffuse violaceous erythema with scale on torso.

and liver can rarely occur usually late in the disease course.[2]

Opportunistic infections are common due to immune dysfunction and skin barrier breakage leading to the introduction of microorganisms.[1] Sepsis and/or pneumonia are major causes of mortality in advanced stage MF.[1,2]

Histopathologic diagnosis of early-stage MF can be challenging. Practicing clinicians should be aware of the barriers associated with rendering a pathologic diagnosis of MF and the conditions that histopathologically mimic MF. Early MF is characterized by a patchy, variably dense lichenoid atypical lymphoid infiltrate with epidermotropism. Lymphocyte tagging along the dermoepidermal junction, epidermotropism, and the formation of intraepidermal aggregates of neoplastic lymphoid cells (Pautrier's microabscess) are typically present. An expanded papillary dermis with fibrosis and coarse bundles of collagen is often identified. Plaques of MF are characterized by a dense band-like infiltrate involving the upper dermis and tumors are characterized by dense nodular or diffuse infiltrate involving the entire dermis and usually the subcutaneous fat. Tumors of MF may lose epidermotropism typically found in patch and plaque MF. The neoplastic cells are characteristically CD3+CD4+CD8-and demonstrate variable loss of pan-T-cell antigens CD2, CD5, and CD7. A minority of MF cases exhibit a T-cytotoxic lineage CD3+CD4-CD8+ with no clinical differences. In these cases, correlation with clinical presentation is critical to rule out an aggressive cytotoxic lymphoma. In general, cytotoxic markers such as TIA-1 and granzyme B are negative in MF. Determination of T-cell clonality further supports a

Table 3
Clinical variants of MF and their mimics. The clinical mimics should be considered in the differential diagnosis of MF subtypes

Clinical Variants of MF	Clinical Mimics
Folliculotropic	Alopecia mucinosa, alopecias (alopecia areata, trichotillomania, lichen planopilaris, folliculitis decalvans), adult-onset acne, acne conglobata, rosacea (papulopustular or granulomatosis), Favre-Rouchot syndrome, chloracne, keratosis pilaris, lichen spinulosus, lymphomatoid papulosis, drug eruption
Pagetoid Reticulosis	Psoriasis, Paget's disease, cutaneous tuberculosis, lupus, eczema, blastomycosis, leishmania, tinea, verruca vulgaris, squamous cell carcinoma, leukemia cutis, pseudolymphoma, cutaneous B-cell lymphoma
Granulomatous slack Skin	Psoriasis, Paget Disease, Granuloma annulare, other benign granulomatous dermatitis, Rosai-Dorfman disease, acquired cutis laxa, sarcoidosis
Hypopigmented	Vitiligo, pityriasis alba, tinea versicolor, pityriasis lichenoides chronica, progressive macular hypomelanosis, post-inflammatory hypopigmentation, syphilis, onchocerciasis, leprosy
Poikilodermatous	Dermatomyositis, steroid-induced atrophy, radiation dermatitis
Granulomatous	Sarcoidosis, Granuloma annulare
Erythrodermic MF	Sezary syndrome, pityriasis rubra pilaris, scabies, graft-versus-host-disease, psoriatic erythroderma, atopic dermatitis, chronic contact dermatitis, hypereosinophilic syndrome

diagnosis of MF. The detection of identical clones from two different sites is quite specific for MF.[7]

SÉZARY SYNDROME
Introduction

Sezary Syndrome (SS) is the rare leukemic variant of CTCL that frequently affects men in their 50s and comprises 1% to 5% of all CTCLs.[1,3]

Clinical and Histopathological Features

Clinically, it presents with erythroderma (confluent erythema of ≥80% of BSA), generalized lymphadenopathy, and a clonal neoplastic T-cell proliferation with cerebriform nuclei in the peripheral blood.[1-3] (**Fig. 2**) Patients have associated intractable pruritus, alopecia, onychodystrophy, palmoplantar hyperkeratosis, ectropion, and blepharoconjunctivitis.[3] Immune system dysfunction increases the risk for opportunistic infections as well as secondary malignancies.[3] SS diagnostic criteria proposed by International Society for Cutaneous Lymphoma (ISCL) requires the integration of clinical, histopathologic, immunophenotyping, and molecular studies.[1,8] Patients with clinical signs of SS require the same diagnostic workup discussed for CTCL. Sezary cell counts by flow cytometry is required for the diagnosis of SS. It is important to note that Sezary cell counts should

be expressed in absolute terms.[3] In addition, Sezary cells can be detected in normal donors and under benign conditions; hence it is not specific to only CTCL. Per ISCL diagnostic criteria for SS

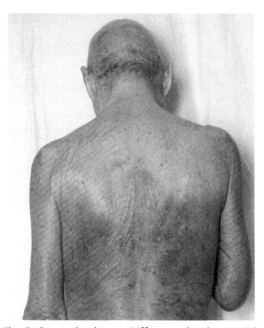

Fig. 2. Sezary Syndrome. Diffuse erythroderma with erosions and associated alopecia.

include, absolute Sezary cell count >/ = 1000/ul, CD4/CD8 ratio >/ = 10, aberrant pan T-cell antigen expression (CD2, CD3, CD4, CD5, CD7, and CD26), and demonstration of T-cell clonality.[8] Loss of CD7 and CD26 is sensitive and highly specific for SS.[8] At minimum, the WHO-EORTC recommends the demonstration of T-cell clonality in combination with the ISCL criteria for diagnosis of SS. While SS is not the leukemic variant MF,[3] on rare occasions SS may be preceded by a previous history of classic MF. The ISCL recommends designating such cases as "SS preceded by MF."[8]

Treatment of Mycosis Fungoides and Sézary Syndrome

Treatment of MF is stage-dependent and requires multidisciplinary collaboration between dermatology, hematology oncology, radiation oncology, and palliative medicine. **Table 4** shows the available treatments for various stages of MF and SS. Continued topical therapy remains critical to maintaining the quality of life even for patients with advanced disease who are receiving systemic therapy. Topical anti-itch or menthol-based creams may be used to manage pruritus. Topical antiseptic washes and antibiotics serve as prophylaxis against skin infections. Oncologists are often unfamiliar with the management of the cutaneous aspects of MF, and it is important that dermatologists remain involved in the treatment of patients with advanced-stage disease and communicate openly with other providers.

Early-Stage Mycosis Fungoides

Topical therapies
Topical corticosteroids (CS), are the most commonly used first-line treatments for early MF. They have anti-inflammatory and anti-proliferative activity through the induction of apoptosis of

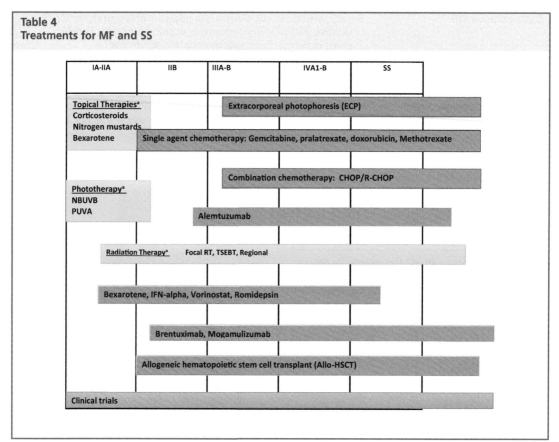

Table 4
Treatments for MF and SS

	IA-IIA	IIB	IIIA-B	IVA1-B	SS
Topical Therapies[a] Corticosteroids Nitrogen mustards Bexarotene			Extracorporeal photophoresis (ECP)		
		Single agent chemotherapy: Gemcitabine, pralatrexate, doxorubicin, Methotrexate			
			Combination chemotherapy: CHOP/R-CHOP		
Phototherapy[a] NBUVB PUVA		Alemtuzumab			
Radiation Therapy[a]	Focal RT, TSEBT, Regional				
Bexarotene, IFN-alpha, Vorinostat, Romidepsin					
Brentuximab, Mogamulizumab					
Allogeneic hematopoietic stem cell transplant (Allo-HSCT)					
Clinical trials					

Green, SDT. orange, Consider combining different treatment options if patients are not clinically responding or disease progresses.
Abbreviations: CHOP, cyclophosphamide; Doxorubicin, Vincristine; Prednisone, IFN-alpha; Interferon alpha, NBUVB; Narrowband-ultraviolet B, PUVA; Psoralen-ultraviolet A, R-CHOP; rituximab, Cyclophosphamide; Doxorubicin, Vincristine; Prednisone, RT; radiotherapy, TSEBT; total skin electron beam therapy.
[a] Skin-directed topical therapy should be offered to all MF/SS patients regardless of stage.

malignant T-cells.[8] Overall response rates are higher in early-stage MF (80%–90%).[8] Frequently reported side effects include cutaneous atrophy, telangiectasias, purpura, hypopigmentation, and striae which occur with prolonged use. If progressive clinical response is not observed with monotherapy within 3 months, then alternative skin-directed treatment (SDT) options are warranted either alone or in combination with other SDTs.[9]

Topical nitrogen mustard (mechlorethamine 0.02% gel or ointment) is an alkylating agent, which may act by halting mitotic activity in dividing cells. When applied once daily over a 12-month period it resulted in a sustained response of 85.5%. Irritant or allergic contact dermatitis is the most common side effect which typically requires the coadministration of topical CS. Treatment with topical nitrogen mustard should be continued as maintenance therapy for at least 6 months after clearance of skin lesions.[8,10] Mechlorethamine is useful when there is failure of response to topical Class I CS, patient preference to avoid the use of CS or for plaque lesions of MF.[9] Topical carmustine, also nitrogen mustard, is an alternative option and has similar efficacy as mechlorethamine but may be associated with systemic absorption and subsequent myelosuppression; thus, carmustine is not generally recommended for use on large BSAs.[8] Topical retinoids exert their effects by binding to intracellular receptors (retinoic acid receptors (RARs) or retinoid X receptors (RXRs)) and induce apoptosis of malignant T-cells.[8,10] Bexarotene 1% gel is the only topical retinoid that is FDA approved for the treatment of MF. It is well-tolerated and may be used in early-stage disease that is not responsive to the above therapies.[8] Bexarotene is cost prohibitive, and thus, a commonly used alternative topical retinoid is tazarotene. Tazarotene binds to RARs and monotherapy with the 0.1% cream formulation is associated with complete response in 60% of patients with early-stage disease with a mean time to response of 4 months.[9] The most important adverse reactions observed with topical retinoids include irritant contact dermatitis, burning or stinging at the application site, and pruritus.[8,10] These adverse effects can be mitigated by gradually increasing the frequency of application.[9]

Phototherapy

Phototherapy is a safe and effective treatment modality that can be used alone in early-stage disease or in combination with topical or systemic (oral) agents in advanced stage disease.[8,10] Treatment options include narrowband UVB (NBUVB, 311 nm) and psoralen plus ultraviolet A (PUVA). The therapeutic effects of phototherapy in MF are attributed to direct apoptosis of lymphocytes

by altering the proinflammatory microenvironment.[9] Treatment dose, schedule, and maintenance vary among institutions. The efficacy of phototherapy for MF is well established. The side effect profile between PUVA and NBUVB is comparable. However, psoralen was associated with nausea, headache, and worse phototoxic effects.[10] Additionally, cumulative doses of PUVA are associated with increased risk of skin cancer while similar rates of carcinogenicity have not been observed in NBUVB. Therefore, NBUVB is the safest and first choice in early MF.[11] PUVA is a great treatment modality for skin of color patients. Highest response is seen with the combination of PUVA and interferon-alpha but maintenance therapy is not generally recommended given the potential carcinogenic effect.[11]

Radiation Therapy

The neoplastic T-lymphocytes in MF are highly radiosensitive. RT may be used for curative or palliative purposes dependent on disease stage and degree of response to previous therapies. Localized (single or few lesions) MF may be treated with focal radiation therapy while generalized disease is best managed with total skin electron beam radiotherapy (TSEBT).[8] A single-center retrospective review of 572 patients with any stage of MF who received treatment with radiation therapy (focal or regional RT or TSEBT) demonstrated high response rates (99%).[12] Low dose TSEBT regimens (6–12 Gy) are commonly used due to their lower toxicity profile; particularly when combined with radiosensitizing adjuvant therapies, their similar efficacy in comparison to higher dose schedules and provision for multiple treatment courses over a patient's lifetime.[8] TSEBT is associated with a reduction in disease burden and improvement in quality of life.[13] Adverse effects associated with RT include erythema, desquamation, atrophy, and xerosis.

Advanced-Stage Mycosis Fungoides /Sezary Syndrome

Treatment of advanced stage disease is typically led by hematology-oncology including BM transplantation specialists. The discussion will focus on the most common systemic therapies that are co-managed by dermatologists, including bexarotene and extracorporeal photopheresis. Other systemic therapies including alemtuzumab, mogamulizumab, brentuximab, multiagent chemotherapy, and hematopoietic stem cell transplant are well described in these reviews.[8,10,14]

Patients with advanced-stage MF (Stage IIB or higher)/SS have poor prognosis, and it is recommended that immune preserving treatments such as oral retinoids or immunostimulatory therapies such as interferon are initiated first.[3] Failing adequate response, then targeted therapies may be utilized. Finally, patients at every stage of disease who are eligible for ongoing clinical trials should be enrolled in these studies, especially those with advanced or refractory disease.

Bexarotene

Bexarotene is approved for refractory CTCL and the recommended starting daily dose is 150 mg/m^2 for the first month that may be titrated upwards to a dose of 300 mg/m^2 based on tolerability. Bexarotene is commonly co-administered with other skin-directed therapies or systemic agents. Response rates of 55% were noted at a dose of 300 mg/m^2 with a median time to response of 6 months. Treatment response should be observed within 2 to 3 months.[8,10] Hypertriglyceridemia occurs in 82% of patients, and central hypothyroidism in 29% patients, typically within weeks of treatment initiation.[8] Thus, lipid panel, T3, and free T4 should be monitored regularly during therapy. Treatment with triglyceride lowering agents (typically fenofibrate; gemfibrozil is contraindicated in patients with MF on bexarotene) may be necessary, as may thyroid hormone supplementation.

Extracorporeal Photopheresis

In Extracorporeal photopheresis (ECP), lymphocytes are extracted from the patient via leukapheresis and treated with the photosensitizing agent 8-methoxypsoralen (8-MOP), then exposed to UVA light in a cassette, and reinfused into the patient. Psoralen cross-links DNA through covalent bonding after UVA exposure leading to apoptosis in lymphocytes via multiple mechanisms including the disruption of mitochondrial membrane potential, activation of extrinsic pathways, and activation of the bcl-2 family.[8,10,14] In addition, ECP leads to monocyte activation via gene expression, dendritic cell differentiation leading to enhanced antigen presentation and host cell immune response.[8,14] The standard regimen is one treatment on 2 consecutive days, every 2 to 4 weeks for 6-month followed by a maintenance schedule. Each treatment sessions last about 2 to 3 hours. ECP is managed by transfusion medicine specialists with close follow-up of response to therapy performed by hematology-oncology and dermatology. Overall responses are approximately 60% with complete response noted in 20% in case reports and series.[10] Higher response rates are seen when ECP is used with topical and systemic therapies (bexarotene or IFN).[8]

Prognosis of Mycosis Fungoides and Sézary Syndrome

Prognosis of MF is strongly dependent on the stage at presentation. Approximately 80% of patients with early-stage MF will have a chronic and indolent clinical course without extracutaneous involvement. Stage IA disease has a 10-year risk of disease progression of 12% compared with 83% in stage IVA1.[15] The estimated 5-year survival for advanced-stage disease is approximately 40%. Independent prognostic factors for advanced-stage MF and SS include age >60 years, large-cell transformation, and increased lactate dehydrogenase levels.[15] In a study comparing survival outcomes of 4459 patients from the US National Cancer Database with MF across racial groups, African Americans were noted to have a worse prognosis after controlling for disease characteristics, socioeconomic factors, and types of therapy.[16]

There is no cure for SS, and it has a grim prognosis even with aggressive treatment. The 5-year survival is 10% to 33% with median survival of 3 years.[1,3,15] Many of the available therapeutic options offer transient responses, and the disease rapidly relapses often with progression and eventually death.[2] Majority of the patients die from opportunistic infections due to immune dysfunction induced by the neoplastic cells.

Pruritus in Cutaneous T-Cell Lymphomas

Severe and persistent pruritus are common in SS and MF which poorly impacts the patient's quality of life. The management of pruritus is challenging and often unsatisfactory. Treatment to alleviate itch in CTCL relies on addressing the cause of itch in the skin. Hence, the most effective treatment to manage pruritus is achieving remission of the cutaneous lymphoma. Besides addressing the underlying malignancy to mitigate pruritus, it is crucial to include treatments that target itch. **Table 5** highlights the mechanism of action, dosages, and side effects of these recommended therapies.[17]

CD30+ Lymphoproliferative Disorders

CD30+ LPDs are the second most common (25% of CTCLs) group of CTCL after MF and comprise lymphomatoid papulosis (LyP) and primary cutaneous anaplastic large cell lymphoma (pcALCL). They exist on a spectrum and share overlapping clinical and histopathologic features.[18] Therefore, the clinical morphology of the lesions, clinical behavior, and course over time is critically

Table 5
Highlights the medications used to mitigate pruritus in CTCL

Medication	Mechanism of Action	Dosages	Adverse Reactions
Aprepitant	Antagonist of the neurokinin-1 receptor of substance P	80 mg daily Or 125 mg on day 1, then 80mg on days 2 and 3; repeat every 2 weeks	Fatigue, diarrhea, dyspepsia, abdominal pain, constipation, leukopenia, dehydration, and hypotension.
Naloxone	Antagonist of the mu-opioid receptor	0.2 mg subcutaneously every 3–4 h PRN	Agitation, anxiety, nausea, and vomiting.
Naltrexone	Antagonist of the mu-opioid receptor	50–100 mg PO daily for 1 mo	Agitation, anxiety, nausea, and vomiting.
Mirtazapine[a]	Antidepressant that blocks multiple receptors including a2-adrenergic autoreceptors/ hetereceptors, serotonergic 5-hydroxtriptamine (both 5-HT2 & 5-HT3) receptors, and H1 receptors	7.5–15 mg PO nightly	Somnolence, weight gain, and hypercholesterolemia.
Gabapentin	Blocks calcium influx by binding to $\alpha2\delta1$ subunit of a voltage gated calcium channel on the neurons cell membrane, thus preventing neurotransmitter release	Start 300 mg nightly and uptitrate as needed but not exceeding 2400 mg daily • 900–2400 mg daily may be needed to control itch in CTCL patients	Dizziness, somnolence, fatigue, and sedation.

[a] Mirtazapine is contraindicated in patients on monoamine oxidase inhibitors to avoid serotonin syndrome.
Adapted from Ahern K, Gilmore ES, Poligone B. Pruritus in cutaneous T-cell lymphoma: a review. J Am Acad Dermatol. 2012 Oct;67(4):760-8.

important in distinguishing between these entities. Careful clinicopathological correlation is essential to distinguish these entities from each other and from other nonneoplastic inflammatory and infectious dermatoses.

LYMPHOMATOID PAPULOSIS (LyP)
Introduction

LyP was initially described by Macaulay in 1980 and has since been classified by the WHO-EORTC under the category of cutaneous T-cell and NK-cell lymphomas.[19] It is estimated that LyP has an incidence of 1.2 to 1.9/1,000,000 people.[20] Adult males are predominantly affected with a peak in the 5th decade; however, it also occurs in children (median age 9 yrs).[20–22]

Clinical and Histopathologic Features

Clinically, patients with LyP present with recurrent crops of asymptomatic or pruritic papules ranging in size from 0.5 to 1 cm and in color from pink to violaceous.[20,21] These papulonodules may be singular or multiple and affect the trunk and/or limbs.[20,21] (**Fig. 3**) While they do tend to spontaneously regress in the weeks to months following the eruption, they can result in postinflammatory hyperpigmented macules or atrophic varioliform scars.[20] Despite the distinctive self-healing course of LyP, these patients must be routinely followed as approximately 10% may go on to develop a second lymphoproliferative disorder including CD30+ ALCL, Hodgkin lymphoma, or MF.[20] Older age and the presence of a T-cell clone in LyP lesions are noted risk factors for associated lymphomas.[23] An increased risk of non-hematologic malignancies have also been described including cutaneous squamous cell carcinoma, melanoma, gastrointestinal, lung, and bladder carcinomas.[24]

The WHO recognizes histopathologic subtypes of LyP (A-E) each of which has distinct histopathologic findings (**Table 6**).[3,20,21] Histopathologic

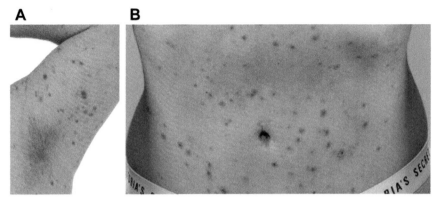

Fig. 3. Lymphomatoid papulosis. Papulonecrotic lesions and regressing erythematous macules on (A). arm and (B). abdomen.

subtype does not influence survival or clinical presentation; however, there may be overlapping histopathologic features that mimic other aggressive CTCLs.[21] Therefore, accurate recognition of the different subtypes of LyP is important to avoid misdiagnosis and inappropriate treatment. The histopathologic features are dependent on the stage/age of lesion that is sampled. Multiple subtypes may be seen in separate but concurrent lesions and in the same LyP lesion. The lymphoid infiltrate in LyP expresses CD3, CD4 (subtypes A, B, and C) or CD8 (subtypes D, E and with DUSP22-IRF4 rearrangement), CD25, CD30, CD45RO, with variable loss of expression of pan T-cell antigens such as CD2, CD5, and CD7.[20,21] Cytotoxic molecules such as TIA-1 and granzyme B are frequently expressed.[20,21]

Treatment

Therapeutic intervention in LyP has not been shown to significantly impact the course of disease or prevent the development of secondary neoplasms.[20,21] Observation is a reasonable first-line approach for mild disease. For more extensive disease, symptomatic treatment options include topical or intralesional steroids, phototherapy, or methotrexate.[20,21,25]

Table 6
Histopathologic subtypes of lymphomatoid papulosis

LyP Subtype	Primary Histopathologic Features	Differential Diagnosis
A	Wedge-shaped infiltrate composed of anaplastic CD30+ T-cells and inflammatory cells	C-ALCL, Tumor stage MF, Classic Hodgkin lymphoma
B	Epidermotropic infiltrate composed of atypical cells with cerebriform nuclei	Plaque stage MF
C	Nodular infiltrate composed of atypical CD30+ cells; inflammatory cell background	C-ALCL, Transformed MF (CD30+)
D	Epidermotropism, pagetoid distribution of CD8+/CD30+ atypical lymphocytes	CD8+ aggressive epidermotropic T-cell lymphoma
E	Angioinvasive infiltrates of atypical lymphocytes with hemorrhagic necrosis and ulceration	Extranodal NK/T-cell lymphoma
DUSP22-IRF4 rearrangement	Small epidermal CD30+ cerebriform lymphocytes, large dermal CD30+ transformed cells	Transformed MF

Abbreviations: C-ALCL, cutaneous anaplastic large cell lymphoma; LyP, lymphomatoid papulosis; MF mycosis, fungoides.
  Data from Willemze R, Cerroni L, Kempf W, et al. The 2018 update of the WHO-EORTC classification for primary cutaneous lymphomas. Blood. 2019;133(16); Moy A, Sun J, Ma S, Seminario-Vidal L. Lymphomatoid Papulosis and Other Lymphoma-Like Diseases. Dermatol Clin. 2019;37(4); and Martinez-Cabriales SA, Walsh S, Sade S, Shear NH. Lymphomatoid papulosis: an update and review. J Eur Acad Dermatol Venereol. 2020;34(1).

Prognosis

The primary role of monitoring is surveillance for secondary LPDs. The prognosis for LyP is excellent with a 10-year disease-specific survival of close to 100%.[20]

PRIMARY CUTANEOUS ANAPLASTIC LARGE CELL LYMPHOMA
Introduction

Primary cutaneous anaplastic large cell lymphoma (pcALCL), accounts for approximately 8% to 10% of all cases of ALCL.[26] The median age of onset is 60 years and the male:female ratio is 2 to 3:1.

Clinical and Histopathologic Features

Unlike the waxing and waning, grouped ulceronecrotic papules of LyP, pcALCL typically presents with solitary or grouped rapidly progressive, ulcerative nodules, tumors, or plaques (**Fig. 4**). Although partial regression of lesions of pcALCL may occur in 20% to 40% of cases, the lesions typically do not resolve completely and almost always recur.[27,28] These lesions tend to occur on the upper half of the body and can rarely be multifocal.[27,28] Extracutaneous dissemination typically to the LNs, occurs in 10% to 15% of cases.[3] Multiple lesions at presentation, early skin relapse and nodal progression are risk factors noted to portend a worse prognosis in this patient population.[29]

pcALCL and LyP, type C may be indistinguishable on pathology: both are characterized by a diffuse infiltrate of large, pleomorphic CD30+ T cells in the dermis.[27,28,30] The atypical lymphoid cells have an anaplastic cytomorphology, with round or oval irregular or horse-shoe shaped nuclei, prominent eosinophilic nucleoli, and abundant cytoplasm.[27] The neoplastic cells also express CD4 and cytotoxic markers including TIA-1, granzyme B, and perforin; variable loss of mature T-cell markers CD2, CD5 or CD3 may be seen. An admixture of background inflammatory cells which may be prominent and neutrophil-rich in the pyogenic variant of ALCL is also present. pcALCL may occasionally demonstrate epidermotropism or involvement of the adnexae.[27] CD30 is expressed in all lesions, typically in >75% of the tumor cells. It is critically important to distinguish pcALCL from systemic ALCL with secondary cutaneous involvement. Most pcALCL cases do not carry translocations involving the ALK gene, and thus, are negative for ALK; however, systemic ALCL characteristically expresses ALK. Thus, the presence of ALK expression is highly suggestive of secondary cutaneous involvement by systemic ALCL. Immunohistochemistry alone is not sufficient though to rule out systemic ALCL, and a thorough staging evaluation is necessary for all patients with cutaneous involvement of ALCL. Molecular rearrangements involving the DUSP22-IRF4 locus are noted in 25% of pcALCL and a small subset of LyP but do not have any prognostic significance in contrast to systemic ALCL. DUSP22-IRF4 and TP63 translocations have been noted to portend a favorable and poor prognosis, respectively, in ALK-negative ALCL.[31,32]

Treatment

Solitary or grouped tumors of pcALCL may be managed with surgical excision and/or radiotherapy.[27,28] Multiagent chemotherapy, single agents, or targeted therapies including methotrexate, pralatrexate, systemic retinoids, brentuximab vedotin (anti-CD30 monoclonal antibody–drug conjugate) are indicated for multifocal or relapsing disease.[27]

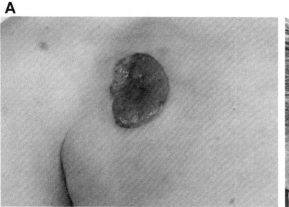
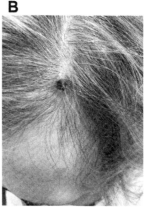

Fig. 4. Primary cutaneous anaplastic large cell lymphoma. (*A*). Large ulcerated tumor on upper chest and (*B*). Ulcerated nodule on frontal scalp.

Prognosis

The prognosis for pcALCL is excellent, with 5-year survival is 90%-97.5% for T1 disease. Extracutaneous spread of disease, extensive limb involvement, and advanced age are associated with worse long-term prognosis.[27,33] It is pertinent to note that isolated spread to locally draining LNs is not associated with worse outcomes as compared to skin involvement alone.[27,28,33]

SUBCUTANEOUS PANNICULITIS-LIKE T-CELL LYMPHOMA
Introduction

Subcutaneous panniculitis-like T-cell lymphoma (SPTCL) is a rare, indolent cytotoxic CD8+ T-cell lymphoma that primarily involves the subcutis. A subcutaneous lymphoma mimicking panniculitis and associated with hemophagocytic syndrome with an aggressive disease course was initially described by Gonzalez and colleagues in 1991.[34] However, subsequent evidence supported the division of SPTCL which was initially considered a provisional diagnosis by the REAL classification and European Organization for Research and Treatment of Cancer (EORTC) classification for cutaneous lymphoma into cases with an alpha-beta phenotype and an indolent course and those with a gamma delta phenotype and a poor prognosis.[18,34] SPTCL with an α/β T-cell phenotype was subsequently distinguished from that with a $\gamma\delta$ TCR (PCGDTCL) in the WHO-EORTC classification system in 2005 given their markedly different clinical presentations and survival.[35] SPTCL accounts for less than 1% of all CTCLs, and the median age at diagnosis ranges from 36 to 46.5 years with a female predominance.[36,37]

Clinical and Histopathologic Features

Patients present with nodular skin lesions or deep plaques which may be generalized with leg, arm, and/or trunk involvement.[36,37] Lesions are rarely ulcerative; however, residual lipoatrophy after lesion resolution is common.[36,37] (Fig. 5) B-symptoms, autoimmune disease (20% of cases), and hemophagocytic lymphohistiocytosis (HLH) in 18% of cases, are variably present.[36,37] SPTCL may resemble lupus erythematosus panniculitis (LEP) both clinically and histopathologically; therefore, distinguishing the 2 can be challenging.[37] On histopathology, SPTCL is characterized by a subcuticular infiltrate consisting of pleomorphic T-cells with adipotropism and rimming of fat cells resembling a lobular panniculitis.[36,37] Variable fat necrosis and karyorrhexis are typically present.[36]

Admixed histiocytes and small reactive T-lymphocytes are also typically present. Neoplastic T-cells are CD3+, CD4-, CD8+, CD56-, and βF1+. Cytotoxic proteins (granzyme B, TIA-1, and perforin) are strongly expressed.[36,37] Epstein Barr virus (EBV) negativity can help in distinguishing SPTCL from extranodal NK/T-cell lymphoma, nasal type.[36]

Treatment

There are no standard treatment guidelines for SPTCL. Treatment options for SPTCL include radiation, systemic CS, cyclosporine, and methotrexate. Systemic CS alone or in combination with either cyclosporine or low-dose methotrexate were commonly used as first-line therapies in SPTCL with a complete response rate of 85%. In cases with associated HLH or with refractory disease, doxorubicin-based multiagent chemotherapy, and hematopoietic stem cell transplantation have been used.[36,37]

Prognosis

Overall, the prognosis for SPTCL is very favorable, with a 5-year overall survival of 82%.[36] The presence of HLH is associated with worse survival, despite attempts at aggressive treatment.[36,37]

PRIMARY CUTANEOUS GAMMA-DELTA T-CELL LYMPHOMA
Introduction

Primary cutaneous gamma-delta T-cell lymphoma (PCGDTCL) was initially recognized as a provisional entity by the WHO-EORTC classification scheme in 2005 and subsequently reclassified as its own entity in 2008 when the distinction from other cutaneous lymphomas, namely subcutaneous panniculitis-like TCL (SPTCL) was made.[18,38] This rare lymphoma accounts for less than 1% of all PCTLs.[39–42] PCGDTCL is an aggressive lymphoma that occurs most commonly in adults (median age 60 years), with no significant gender predilection.[41]

Clinical and Histopathologic Features

Patients typically present with disseminated, rapidly progressive papules, plaques, and nodules that demonstrate ulceration and necrosis, predominantly affecting the extremities (Fig. 6). Associated symptoms that are commonly seen include fever, weight loss and in patients with panniculitis, hemophagocytic syndrome may be the presenting symptom. Although PCGDTCL is classically thought of as subcutaneous panniculitis- like TCL, the presentation is highly variable and may

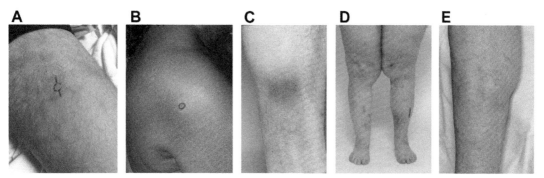

Fig. 5. Subcutaneous panniculitis-like T-cell lymphoma. (*A*). Multiple erythematous dermal and subcutaneous nodules on thigh. (*B*). Skin-colored subcutaneous nodule on upper arm. (*C*). Erythematous subcutaneous nodule on lower leg. (*D*). Erythematous subcutaneous nodule on lower leg with associated induration and (*E*). Residual lipoatrophy.

demonstrate prominent epidermal or dermal involvement with varying degrees of necrosis and angioinvasion/angiodestruction.[41,43] Neoplastic cells are medium to large in size with coarsely clumped chromatin. Areas of apoptosis or necrosis are frequent.[41] Two histopathologic patterns may be seen including an exclusively epidermotropic or a deep dermal/subcutaneous pattern.[44]

Immunophenotypically, the neoplastic T-cells are defined by the expression of a gamma/delta TCR. The T-cells are positive for CD2, CD3, and TCRδ but almost always lack both CD4 and CD8. CD30 and CD56 are variably expressed.[43] Staining for βF1 (marker of alpha/beta T cells) is absent.[39] Cytotoxic markers such as granzyme B and perforin are usually expressed, and activating mutations of STAT3 or STAT5B may be identified.[41,45]

It is important to note that although TCRγ expression is required for a diagnosis of PCGD-TCL, it is not a specific finding, given that TCRγ may be expressed in other primary CTCL.[41]

Treatment and Prognosis

There is no standard of care for the treatment of PCGDTCL, and treatments range from radiation of localized disease to doxorubicin-based multi-agent chemotherapy with allogenic or autologous stem-cell transplant for advanced disease.[25,41] The predominantly epidermotropic variant of PCGDTCL portends a better prognosis as compared with dermal/subcutaneous presentations.[46] Despite aggressive interventions, the prognosis is poor, with a tendency to metastasize to the lung, brain, testis, or oral cavity.[40] The

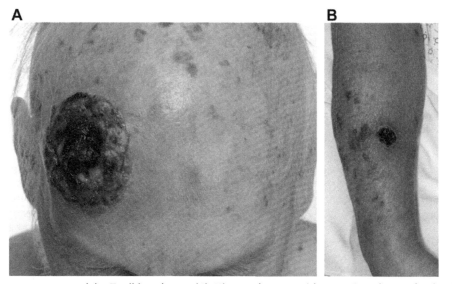

Fig. 6. Cutaneous gamma delta T-cell lymphoma. (*A*). Ulcerated tumor with necrotic eschar on forehead. (*B*) Ulcerated nodule with black eschar on forearm.

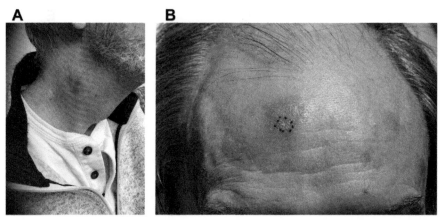

Fig. 7. Cutaneous Extranodal NK-T-cell Lymphoma. (*A*). Infiltrated erythematous patches and plaques on forehead (*B*). Erythematous plaque on neck.

median survival ranges from 15 to 31 months with an estimated 5-year overall survival of 11%-19.9%.[25,41,42]

EXTRANODAL NK/T-CELL LYMPHOMA, NASAL-TYPE
Introduction

Extranodal NK/T-Cell Lymphoma Nasal-Type (ENKTCL) is a lymphoma characterized by its derivation from NK cells and association with EBV.[47] While this lymphoma is relatively rare in North America, comprising 1% of non-Hodgkin lymphomas, it is more common in areas of higher prevalence of EBV infection, such as South America and East Asia, where ENKTCL accounts for up to 10% of non-Hodgkin lymphomas.[47–49] ENKTCL often carries the descriptive classification as "nasal type" when it presents as classic ulcerative plaques or tumors in the nasal cavity or upper aerodigestive tract ("lethal midline granuloma" with palatal or septal perforation).[25,48] Skin or subcutaneous involvement is typically a secondary presentation of advanced disease, along with gastrointestinal, BM, and peripheral blood involvement.[48] (**Fig. 7**) When there is evidence of NK/TCL at nonnasal sites, PET-CT should be performed to evaluate for the presence of an occult primary nasal NK/TCL. If nasal involvement is noted, then the appropriate designation for such cases should be nasal, disseminated type NK/TCL.[50]

Clinical and Histopathological Features

Cutaneous and mucosal lesions of ENKTCL exhibit marked angiocentricity, angiodestruction, and necrosis.[48,51] The epidermis, dermis, and subcutis may be variably involved.[51] The neoplastic cells express CD2, cytoplasmic CD3, CD56, and cytotoxic markers (perforin, granzyme B, TIA 1).[48,49,51] Invariable demonstration of Epstein Barr Virus (EBV) infection of neoplastic cells as assessed by in situ hybridization for EBV early RNA (EBER) is noted in most cases.[52]

Treatment

Treatment of ENKTCL is largely dependent on the stage of disease.[48] Traditional anthracycline-based chemotherapy is not effective in ENKTCL due to the expression of multidrug-resistant p-glycoprotein on NK cells, therefore, should not be used. L-asparaginase-based chemotherapy, however, has emerged as an effective treatment of both early stage (I/II) and advanced stage (III/IV) and relapsed or refractory disease. Additional therapies include radiotherapy in combination with chemotherapy which can be given concurrently or sequentially.[47,48] For relapsed or refractory disease, immunotherapies including pembrolizumab have shown promising results.[53] Allogeneic stem-cell transplant has demonstrated superior outcomes in patients with L-asparaginase refractory disease.[54]

Prognosis

Despite aggressive therapy, the prognosis for ENKTCL is poor. The 5-year OS is estimated to be between 38% and 50% with a median survival of 27 months for skin-limited disease and 4 months for advanced, extracutaneous disease.[25,48] The presence of cutaneous involvement at initial diagnosis of ENKTCL has been associated with a poorer prognosis as compared to oral/nasal presentations (5-year overall survival of 17% and 61%, respectively), likely reflecting more advanced-stage disease.[55]

Table 7
Summary of provisional CTCLs

CTCL	Demographics (M:F, Age)	Clinical Presentation	Clinical Course	Treatment	Prognosis	5-y Survival
CD8+ AECTCL	M > F, Elderly	Sudden onset, rapidly progressive widely distributed ulcerative and hemorrhagic plaques, papulo-nodules, or tumors	Aggressive, Metastatic spread to extracutaneous sites	Multiagent chemotherapy (CHOP, hyper-CVAD), HSCT	Poor, high rate of recurrence	18%–32%
pcSMPLPD	M = F, 50s	Slow-growing, erythematous or violaceous solitary papule, plaque, nodule, or tumor confined to the face, neck, or upper trunk	Indolent	Surgical excision, intralesional steroids, or local radiotherapy	Excellent	100%
pcATCL	M > F, 50s	Solitary or multiple slowly progressive nodules affecting acral sites (ie, ears). **(Fig. 8)**	Indolent	Radiation and surgical excision	Excellent	100%

Abbreviations: CD8+ AECTCL CD8+, aggressive epidermotropic cutaneous T-cell lymphoma; pcATCL, primary cutaneous acral CD8+ T-cell lymphoma; pcSMPTCL, primary cutaneous small-medium pleomorphic T-cell lymphoproliferative disorder.

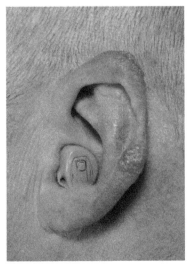

Fig. 8. Primary cutaneous acral CD8+ T-cell lymphoma. Erythematous papules on helix of ear.

PERIPHERAL T-CELL LYMPHOMA – NOT OTHERWISE SPECIFIED

Introduction

Peripheral T-cell lymphoma – not otherwise specified (PTCL-NOS) refers to the group of CTCLs that fail to fulfill the criteria for cutaneous lymphoma entities defined in the updated WHO 2018 and updated WHO-EORTC classifications. This heterogenous group of CTCLs is rare, and their numbers have progressively diminished with increasing understanding of CTCLs beyond MF.[56] Current descriptions of their clinicopathologic features are well-documented in retrospective studies conducted by Kempf and colleagues and Tolkachjov and colleagues, in addition to various case reports and review articles.[25,56–60]

Clinical and Histopathologic Features

As it is essentially a diagnosis of exclusion, PTCL-NOS manifests heterogeneously. In a multicenter

Table 8
Features of adult T-cell leukemia/lymphoma

Classification	Aggressive Mature Peripheral T-cell Lymphoma
Etiology	Chronic infection with HTLV-1 retrovirus
Demographics	Endemic regions: Southwest Japan, Central and South America, central Africa, the Middle East, Far East, and central Australia Age: 6th or 7th decade of life
Clinical Features	~50% of patients with ATLL develop cutaneous disease Multiple or generalized, pruritic nodulotumoral > papules and plaques > purpuric and erythrodermic lesions resembling MF/SS
Predisposing Factors	Patients who acquired HTLV-1 in childhood, likely through breastfeeding
Histopathologic Features	"Flower cells" or circulating lymphocytes with lobated nuclei on peripheral blood smear Superficial or diffuse angiocentric/angioinvasive dermal infiltrates of medium-to-large neoplastic T-cells with pleomorphic or polylobated nuclei, and epidermotropism
Differential Diagnosis	Mycosis Fungoides Sezary Syndrome
Diagnostic Clues	(+) HTLV-1 serology in a patient with the feature of MF/SS in HTLV-1 endemic region CTCL not classifiable as another cutaneous or peripheral T-cell lymphoma Clonal TCR gene rearrangement and HTLV-1 proviral genome integration
Management	Skin-localized disease: topical corticosteroids, phototherapy, or local radiotherapy Extensive cutaneous disease: multiagent chemotherapy and allogeneic HSCT Systemic treatments: oral retinoids, antiviral agents (zidovudine or IFN-alpha) Emerging targeted therapies: anti-CCR4 monoclonal antibody
Prognosis	Dependent on clinical subtype and degree and nature of cutaneous involvement: • Smoldering and chronic types: 4-y OS 36%-52% • Lymphomatous and acute types: 4-y OS 11%-16% • Nodulotumoral and erythrodermic disease: 5-y survival 0% • Multipapular, plaque, or patch disease: 5-y survival 40%

Abbreviations: ATLL, adult T-cell leukemia/lymphoma; CCR4, chemokine receptor 4; HTLV-1, human T-cell lymphotropic virus-1; MF, mycosis fungoides; OS, overall survival; SCT, hematopoietic stem cell transplantation; SS, Sezary syndrome; TCR, T-cell receptor.
Data from[18,25,61–70]

Table 9
Recent diagnostic and therapeutic advances in CTCL

CTCL	Diagnostic and Therapeutic Advances
Mycosis Fungoides	Diagnostic Whole genome sequencing for oncogenic pathway mutations • DNA damage repair – ATM, TP53 • Cell Cycle – CDKN2A, RB1 • Apoptosis – FAS, TNFRSF10 A • MAPK pathway – KRAS, BRAF, MAPK1 • Chromatin modifying genes – ARID1A, DNMT3A, KMT2C • TCR-NFkB signaling Somatic single nucleotide variations (SSNVs): TP53, RHOA, CD28, DNM3TA Therapeutic Anti-CTLA4 therapy (ipilimumab) for novel CD28-CTLA4 gene fusion Anti-PDL1 therapy for the deletion of PDCD1 on chromosome 2p JAK1/2 inhibitor (ruxolitinib) and JAK1/3 inhibitor (tofacitinib) for activating JAK/STAT pathway mutations
Sezary Syndrome	Chromosomal alternations leading to increased cell proliferation and leukemic behavior: • MYC oncogene and IL-2 receptor signaling pathway dysregulation • Activation of cytokine pathways • Inhibition of P53 Point mutations, single-gene alterations, copy number alterations involving TCR signaling, NF-kB and JAK/STAT pathways, apoptosis control, chromatin remodeling, and DNA damage response
Subcutaneous Panniculitis-Like T-cell lymphoma	Increased prevalence of HAVCR2 mutations especially among younger patients and those of Asian ancestry
Primary Cutaneous Gamma-Delta T-cell Lymphoma	Epidermotropic histopathologic variant is of Vdelta1 cellular origin Dermal-subcutaneous histopathologic variant is of Vdelta2 cellular origin

*Abbreviations:*CDKN2A, cyclin-dependent kinase inhibitor 2A; CTLA4, cytotoxic T-lymphocyte associated protein 4; DNMT3A, DNA methyltransferase 3A; HAVCR2, Hepatitis A virus cellular receptor 2; IL-2, interleukin 2; JAK, Janus kinase; KMT2C, lysine N-methyltransferase 2C; MAPK, mitogen-activated protein kinase; NK-kB, nuclear factor kappa B; PDCD1, programmed cell death 1; PDL1, programmed death-ligand 1; RB1, retinoblastoma protein; RHOA, Ras homolog family member A; STAT, signal transducer and activator of transcription; TNFRSF10 A, tumor necrosis factor receptor SF10 A; TP53, tumor protein p53.
Data from Refs.[42,71–80]

study of 30 patients with PTCL-NOS, Kempf and colleagues found that 70% of patients presented with disseminated papules and nodular lesions while 23% presents with a solitary nodule or tumoral plaque; rarely patients exhibit localized papules or nodules.[57] Lesions tended to involve the extremities and trunk.[57] Tolkachjov and colleagues carried out a similar retrospective review of 30 PTCL-NOS cases and identified similar findings with a predominance of multifocal lesions with plaques, papules, trunk and extremity involvement as the most common presentations.[56] Both studies reported male predominance.[56,57]

The diagnosis of PTCL-NOS is challenging as it must be distinguished from other CTCL subtypes. As such, extensive and detailed clinical examination, and review of the histopathologic and immunophenotypic profile is necessary. Histology tends

to display nodular or diffuse dermal and/or subcutaneous infiltrates composed predominantly of medium to large lymphocytes and infrequent or absent epidermotropism.[56,57,59,60] The immunophenotypic profile is diverse and may be dependent on the presentation as either solitary or disseminated disease.[57] The neoplastic T-cells are commonly immunoreactive for CD2, CD3, CD4, βF1 expression and demonstrate TCR gene rearrangements.[56,57] Kempf and colleagues described frequent double negative (CD4-/CD8-) T-cell phenotypes in solitary/localized disease and CD4+/CD8-immunophenotype in disseminated disease.[57]

Treatment and Prognosis

While treatment approaches are varied and not universally agreed on, anthracycline-based chemotherapy and potentially early autologous-SCT for appropriate candidates should be considered.[25,56,57,59] The prognosis of PTCL-NOS is varied based on current literature; however, more recent reviews have indicated it is poor with 5-year overall survival ranging from 16% to 61%.[25,56,57,59]

CLINICS CARE POINTS

- The cutaneous T-cell lymphomas are a heterogeneous group of non-Hodgkin T-cell lymphomas with distinct clinical presentations, pathophysiologies, prognoses, and treatments. Histopathologic diagnosis is central to guiding management and counseling for these malignancies.

- Mycosis fungoides is the most common of the CTCLs and is generally indolent. Skindirected therapies, particularly topical corticosteroids and phototherapy, are central to treatment of the majority of patients.

- Systemic agents may be necessary for a subset of patients with extensive, advanced, or aggressive disease. Early referral for evaluation for allogeneic hematopoietic stem cell transplant may be important for patients with aggressive or advanced-stage disease.

DISCLOSURE

The authors have nothing to disclose.

REFERENCES

1. Olsen EA. Evaluation, Diagnosis, and Staging of Cutaneous Lymphoma. Dermatol Clin 2015;33(4): 643–54. https://doi.org/10.1016/j.det.2015.06.001.
2. National Comprehensive Cancer Network. NCCN Guidelines, Primary Cutaneous Lymphomas. Available at: https://www.nccn.org/guidelines/guidelines-detail?category=1&id=1491. Accessed February 2, 2022.
3. Willemze R, Cerroni L, Kempf W, et al. The 2018 update of the WHO-EORTC classification for primary cutaneous lymphomas. Blood 2019;133(16). https://doi.org/10.1182/blood-2018-11-881268.
4. National Cancer Institute. SEER Database on Mycosis Fungoides. Available at: https://seer.cancer.gov/seertools/hemelymph/51f6cf57e3e27c3994bd5345/. Accessed February 2, 2022.
5. Martínez-Escala ME, González BR, Guitart J. Mycosis Fungoides Variants. Surg Pathol Clin 2014;7(2):169–89. https://doi.org/10.1016/j.path.2014.02.003.
6. Pulitzer M, Myskowski PL, Horwitz SM, et al. Mycosis fungoides with large cell transformation: clinicopathological features and prognostic factors. Pathology 2014;46(7). https://doi.org/10.1097/PAT.0000000000000166.
7. Thurber SE, Zhang B, Kim YH, et al. T-cell clonality analysis in biopsy specimens from two different skin sites shows high specificity in the diagnosis of patients with suggested mycosis fungoides. J Am Acad Dermatol 2007;57(5):782–90. https://doi.org/10.1016/j.jaad.2007.06.004.
8. Hristov AC, Tejasvi T, Wilcox RA. Mycosis fungoides and Sézary syndrome: 2019 update on diagnosis, risk-stratification, and management. Am J Hematol 2019;94(9):1027–41. https://doi.org/10.1002/ajh.25577.
9. Brumfiel CM, Patel MH, Puri P, et al. How to Sequence Therapies in Mycosis Fungoides. Curr Treat Options Oncol 2021;22(11):101. https://doi.org/10.1007/s11864-021-00899-0.
10. Kamijo H, Miyagaki T. Mycosis Fungoides and Sézary Syndrome: Updates and Review of Current Therapy. Curr Treat Options Oncol 2021;22(2):10. https://doi.org/10.1007/s11864-020-00809-w.
11. Olsen EA, Hodak E, Anderson T, et al. Guidelines for phototherapy of mycosis fungoides and Sézary syndrome: A consensus statement of the United States Cutaneous Lymphoma Consortium. J Am Acad Dermatol 2016;74(1):27–58. https://doi.org/10.1016/j.jaad.2015.09.033.
12. King BJ, Lester SC, Tolkachjov SN, et al. Skin-directed radiation therapy for cutaneous lymphoma: The Mayo Clinic experience. J Am Acad Dermatol 2020;82(3):634–41. https://doi.org/10.1016/j.jaad.2019.07.040.
13. Song A, Gochoco A, Zhan T, et al. A prospective cohort study of condensed low-dose total skin electron beam therapy for mycosis fungoides: Reduction of disease burden and improvement in quality of life. J Am Acad Dermatol 2020; 83(1):78–85. https://doi.org/10.1016/j.jaad.2020.01.046.
14. Photiou L, van der Weyden C, McCormack C, et al. Systemic Treatment Options for Advanced-Stage Mycosis Fungoides and Sézary Syndrome. Curr Oncol Rep 2018;20(4):32. https://doi.org/10.1007/s11912-018-0678-x.
15. Talpur R, Alberti-Violetti S, Schilti M, et al. Prognostic Factors, Staging and Treatments in Advanced Stage Mycosis Fungoides and Sézary Syndrome. Blood 2014;124(21):1673. https://doi.org/10.1182/blood.V124.21.1673.1673.
16. Su C, Nguyen KA, Bai HX, et al. Racial disparity in mycosis fungoides: An analysis of 4495 cases from the US National Cancer Database. J Am

Acad Dermatol 2017;77(3):497–502.e2. https://doi.
org/10.1016/j.jaad.2017.04.1137.

17. Ahern K, Gilmore ES, Poligone B. Pruritus in cutaneous T-cell lymphoma: A review. J Am Acad Dermatol 2012;67(4):760–8. https://doi.org/10.1016/j.
jaad.2011.12.021.

18. Willemze R. WHO-EORTC classification for cutaneous lymphomas. Blood 2005;105(10). https://doi.
org/10.1182/blood-2004-09-3502.

19. Macaulay WL. Lymphomatoid papulosis. A
continuing self-healing eruption, clinically benign–
histologically malignant. Arch Dermatol 1968;97(1).
https://doi.org/10.1001/archderm.97.1.23.

20. Martinez-Cabriales SA, Walsh S, Sade S, et al. Lymphomatoid papulosis: an update and review. J Eur
Acad Dermatol Venereol 2020;34(1). https://doi.
org/10.1111/jdv.15931.

21. Moy A, Sun J, Ma S, et al. Lymphomatoid Papulosis
and Other Lymphoma-Like Diseases. Dermatol Clin
2019;37(4). https://doi.org/10.1016/j.det.2019.05.
005.

22. Wieser I, Wohlmuth C, Nunez CA, et al. Lymphomatoid Papulosis in Children and Adolescents: A Systematic Review. Am J Clin Dermatol 2016;17(4):
319–27. https://doi.org/10.1007/s40257-016-0192-6.

23. Cordel N, Tressières B, D'Incan M, et al. Frequency and
Risk Factors for Associated Lymphomas in Patients
With Lymphomatoid Papulosis. Oncologist 2016;
21(1):76–83. https://doi.org/10.1634/theoncologist.
2015-0242.

24. Melchers RC, Willemze R, Bekkenk MW, et al. Frequency and prognosis of associated malignancies
in 504 patients with lymphomatoid papulosis. J Eur
Acad Dermatol Venereol 2020;34(2):260–6. https://
doi.org/10.1111/jdv.16065.

25. Oh Y, Stoll JR, Moskowitz A, et al. Primary cutaneous
T-cell lymphomas other than Mycosis Fungoides and
Sezary Syndrome – Part II: Prognosis and Management. J Am Acad Dermatol 2021. https://doi.org/10.
1016/j.jaad.2021.04.081. Published online.

26. Pulitzer M, Ogunrinade O, Lin O, et al. ALK-positive
(2p23 rearranged) anaplastic large cell lymphoma
with localization to the skin in a pediatric patient.
J Cutan Pathol 2015;42(3). https://doi.org/10.1111/
cup.12446.

27. Brown RA, Fernandez-Pol S, Kim J. Primary cutaneous anaplastic large cell lymphoma. J Cutan
Pathol 2017;44(6). https://doi.org/10.1111/cup.
12937.

28. Kempf W, Pfaltz K, Vermeer MH, et al. EORTC, ISCL,
and USCLC consensus recommendations for the
treatment of primary cutaneous CD30-positive lymphoproliferative disorders: lymphomatoid papulosis
and primary cutaneous anaplastic large-cell lymphoma. Blood 2011;118(15). https://doi.org/10.
1182/blood-2011-05-351346.

29. Fernández-de-Misa R, Hernández-Machín B,
Combalía A, et al. Prognostic factors in patients
with primary cutaneous anaplastic large cell lymphoma: a multicentric, retrospective analysis of the
Spanish Group of Cutaneous Lymphoma. J Eur
Acad Dermatol Venereol 2020;34(4):762–8. https://
doi.org/10.1111/jdv.16006.

30. Eberle FC, Song JY, Xi L, et al. Nodal involvement by
cutaneous CD30-positive T-cell lymphoma
mimicking classical Hodgkin lymphoma. Am J
Surg Pathol 2012;36(5). https://doi.org/10.1097/
PAS.0b013e3182487158.

31. Wada DA, Law ME, Hsi ED, et al. Specificity of IRF4
translocations for primary cutaneous anaplastic
large cell lymphoma: a multicenter study of 204
skin biopsies. Mod Pathol 2011;24(4):596–605.
https://doi.org/10.1038/modpathol.2010.225.

32. Parrilla Castellar ER, Jaffe ES, Said JW, et al. ALK-
negative anaplastic large cell lymphoma is a genetically heterogeneous disease with widely disparate
clinical outcomes. Blood 2014;124(9):1473–80.
https://doi.org/10.1182/blood-2014-04-571091.

33. Pham-Ledard A, Prochazkova-Carlotti M,
Laharanne E, et al. IRF4 gene rearrangements
define a subgroup of CD30-positive cutaneous
T-cell lymphoma: a study of 54 cases. J Invest Dermatol 2010;130(3). https://doi.org/10.1038/jid.2009.
314.

34. Gonzalez CL, Medeiros LJ, Braziel RM, et al. T-cell
lymphoma involving subcutaneous tissue. A clinicopathologic entity commonly associated with hemophagocytic syndrome. Am J Surg Pathol 1991;
15(1):17–27. https://doi.org/10.1097/00000478-
199101000-00002.

35. Goyal A, Goyal K, Bohjanen K, et al. Epidemiology of
primary cutaneous γδ T-cell lymphoma and subcutaneous panniculitis-like T-cell lymphoma in the
U.S.A. from 2006 to 2015: a Surveillance, Epidemiology, and End Results-18 analysis. Br J Dermatol
2019;181(4):848–50. https://doi.org/10.1111/bjd.
17985.

36. Willemze R, Jansen PM, Cerroni L, et al. Subcutaneous panniculitis-like T-cell lymphoma: definition,
classification, and prognostic factors: an EORTC
Cutaneous Lymphoma Group Study of 83 cases.
Blood 2008;111(2). https://doi.org/10.1182/blood-
2007-04-087288.

37. López-Lerma I, Peñate Y, Gallardo F, et al. Subcutaneous panniculitis-like T-cell lymphoma: Clinical
features, therapeutic approach, and outcome in a
case series of 16 patients. J Am Acad Dermatol
2018;79(5). https://doi.org/10.1016/j.jaad.2018.05.
1243.

38. Swerdlow S, Campo E, Lee Harris N, et al. WHO
classification of tumours of haematopoietic and
lymphoid tissues. WHO Press; 2008.

39. Takahashi Y, Takata K, Kato S, et al. Clinicopathological analysis of 17 primary cutaneous T-cell lymphoma of the γδ phenotype from Japan. Cancer Sci 2014;105(7). https://doi.org/10.1111/cas.12439.

40. Rodríguez-Pinilla SM, Ortiz-Romero PL, Monsalvez V, et al. TCR-γ expression in primary cutaneous T-cell lymphomas. Am J Surg Pathol 2013;37(3). https://doi.org/10.1097/PAS.0b013e318275d1a2.

41. Foppoli M, Ferreri AJM. Gamma-delta t-cell lymphomas. Eur J Haematol 2015;94(3). https://doi.org/10.1111/ejh.12439.

42. Daniels J, Doukas PG, Escala MEM, et al. Cellular origins and genetic landscape of cutaneous gamma delta T cell lymphomas. Nat Commun 2020;11(1): 1806. https://doi.org/10.1038/s41467-020-15572-7.

43. Goyal A, O'Leary D, Duncan LM. The significance of epidermal involvement in primary cutaneous gamma/delta (γδ) T-cell lymphoma: A systematic review and meta-analysis. J Cutan Pathol 2021;48(12): 1449–54. https://doi.org/10.1111/cup.14082.

44. Toro JR, Liewehr DJ, Pabby N, et al. Gamma-delta T-cell phenotype is associated with significantly decreased survival in cutaneous T-cell lymphoma. Blood 2003;101(9):3407–12. https://doi.org/10.1182/blood-2002-05-1597.

45. Küçük C, Jiang B, Hu X, et al. Activating mutations of STAT5B and STAT3 in lymphomas derived from γδ-T or NK cells. Nat Commun 2015;6. https://doi.org/10.1038/ncomms7025.

46. Merrill ED, Agbay R, Miranda RN, et al. Primary Cutaneous T-Cell Lymphomas Showing Gamma-Delta (γδ) Phenotype and Predominantly Epidermotropic Pattern are Clinicopathologically Distinct From Classic Primary Cutaneous γδ T-Cell Lymphomas. Am J Surg Pathol 2017;41(2):204–15. https://doi.org/10.1097/PAS.0000000000000768.

47. Yamaguchi M, Suzuki R, Oguchi M. Advances in the treatment of extranodal NK/T-cell lymphoma, nasal type. Blood 2018;131(23). https://doi.org/10.1182/blood-2017-12-791418.

48. Allen PB, Lechowicz MJ. Management of NK/T-Cell Lymphoma, Nasal Type. J Oncol Pract 2019; 15(10). https://doi.org/10.1200/JOP.18.00719.

49. Haverkos BM, Pan Z, Gru AA, et al. Extranodal NK/T Cell Lymphoma, Nasal Type (ENKTL-NT): An Update on Epidemiology, Clinical Presentation, and Natural History in North American and European Cases. Curr Hematol Malig Rep 2016;11(6). https://doi.org/10.1007/s11899-016-0355-9.

50. Tse E, Kwong YL. NK/T-cell lymphomas. Best Pract Res Clin Haematol 2019;32(3):253–61. https://doi.org/10.1016/j.beha.2019.06.005.

51. Rodríguez-Pinilla SM, Barrionuevo C, Garcia J, et al. EBV-associated cutaneous NK/T-cell lymphoma: review of a series of 14 cases from peru in children and young adults. Am J Surg Pathol 2010;34(12). https://doi.org/10.1097/PAS.0b013e3181fbb4fd.

52. Chan JK, Quintanilla-Martinez L, Ferry JA. Extranodal NK/T cell lymphoma, nasal type WHO classification of tumours of haematopoietic and lymphoid Tissues. International Agency for Research on Cancer; 2017. p. 368–71.

53. Horwitz SM, Ansell SM, Ai WZ, et al. NCCN Guidelines Insights: T-Cell Lymphomas, Version 2.2018. J Natl Compr Canc Netw 2018;16(2):123–35. https://doi.org/10.6004/jnccn.2018.0007.

54. Tse E, Chan TSY, Koh LP, et al. Allogeneic haematopoietic SCT for natural killer/T-cell lymphoma: a multicentre analysis from the Asia Lymphoma Study Group. Bone Marrow Transpl 2014;49(7):902–6. https://doi.org/10.1038/bmt.2014.65.

55. Goyal N, O'Leary D, Rubin N, et al. Localization patterns and survival of extranodal natural killer/T-cell lymphomas in the United States: A population-based study of 945 cases. J Am Acad Dermatol 2021;85(5):1318–21. https://doi.org/10.1016/j.jaad.2020.08.109.

56. Tolkachjov SN, Weenig RH, Comfere NI. Cutaneous peripheral T-cell lymphoma, not otherwise specified: A single-center prognostic analysis. J Am Acad Dermatol 2016;75(5). https://doi.org/10.1016/j.jaad.2016.06.011.

57. Kempf W, Mitteldorf C, Battistella M, et al. Primary cutaneous peripheral T-cell lymphoma, not otherwise specified: results of a multicentre European Organization for Research and Treatment of Cancer (EORTC) cutaneous lymphoma taskforce study on the clinico-pathological and prognostic features. J Eur Acad Dermatol Venereol 2021;35(3). https://doi.org/10.1111/jdv.16969.

58. Cardwell LA, Majerowski J, Chiu YE, et al. Post-transplant primary cutaneous peripheral T-cell lymphoma not otherwise specified in a pediatric patient. J Cutan Pathol 2021;48(5). https://doi.org/10.1111/cup.13967.

59. Peterson E, Weed J, Lo Sicco K, et al. Cutaneous T Cell Lymphoma: A Difficult Diagnosis Demystified. Dermatol Clin 2019;37(4). https://doi.org/10.1016/j.det.2019.05.007.

60. le Tourneau A, Audouin J, Molina T, et al. Primary cutaneous follicular variant of peripheral T-cell lymphoma NOS. A report of two cases. Histopathology 2010;56(4). https://doi.org/10.1111/j.1365-2559.2010.03498.x.

61. Uchiyama T, Yodoi J, Sagawa K, et al. Adult T-cell leukemia: clinical and hematologic features of 16 cases. Blood 1977;50(3):481–92.

62. Jain M, Goyal K, O'Leary D, et al. Improved survival for skin-primary presentation of adult T-cell leukemia/lymphoma (ATLL). J Am Acad Dermatol 2020;83(1). https://doi.org/10.1016/j.jaad.2019.11.034.

63. Sawada Y, Hino R, Hama K, et al. Type of skin eruption is an independent prognostic indicator for adult

T-cell leukemia/lymphoma. Blood 2011;117(15). https://doi.org/10.1182/blood-2010-11-316794.

64. Miyashiro D, Sanches JA. Cutaneous manifestations of adult T-cell leukemia/lymphoma. Semin Diagn Pathol 2020;37(2). https://doi.org/10.1053/j.semdp. 2019.07.010.

65. AbdullGaffar B, Abdulrahman S. Adult T-cell leukemia/lymphoma clinically confused with viral/drug skin eruptions and pathologically misinterpreted as mycosis fungoides/Sézary syndrome. J Cutan Pathol 2021;48(9). https://doi.org/10.1111/cup. 13789.

66. Bangham CRM, Ratner L. How does HTLV-1 cause adult T-cell leukaemia/lymphoma (ATL)? Curr Opin Virol 2015;14:93–100. https://doi.org/10.1016/j. coviro.2015.09.004.

67. Marchetti MA, Pulitzer MP, Myskowski PL, et al. Cutaneous manifestations of human T-cell lymphotrophic virus type-1-associated adult T-cell leukemia/lymphoma: a single-center, retrospective study. J Am Acad Dermatol 2015;72(2):293–301. https:// doi.org/10.1016/j.jaad.2014.10.006.

68. Ishida T, Fujiwara H, Nosaka K, et al. Multicenter Phase II Study of Lenalidomide in Relapsed or Recurrent Adult T-Cell Leukemia/Lymphoma: ATLL-002. J Clin Oncol 2016;34(34). https://doi.org/10. 1200/JCO.2016.67.7732.

69. Kchour G, Tarhini M, Kooshyar MM, et al. Phase 2 study of the efficacy and safety of the combination of arsenic trioxide, interferon alpha, and zidovudine in newly diagnosed chronic adult T-cell leukemia/lymphoma (ATL). Blood 2009;113(26). https://doi. org/10.1182/blood-2009-03-211821.

70. Cook LB, Fuji S, Hermine O, et al. Revised Adult T-Cell Leukemia-Lymphoma International Consensus Meeting Report. J Clin Oncol 2019;37(8):677–87. https://doi.org/10.1200/JCO.18.00501.

71. Walia R, Yeung CCS. An Update on Molecular Biology of Cutaneous T Cell Lymphoma. Front Oncol 2019;9: 1558. https://doi.org/10.3389/fonc.2019.01558.

72. Choi J, Goh G, Walradt T, et al. Genomic landscape of cutaneous T cell lymphoma. Nat Genet 2015; 47(9):1011–9. https://doi.org/10.1038/ng.3356.

73. Ungewickell A, Bhaduri A, Rios E, et al. Genomic analysis of mycosis fungoides and Sézary syndrome identifies recurrent alterations in TNFR2. Nat Genet 2015;47(9):1056–60. https://doi.org/10.1038/ng. 3370.

74. Pérez C, González-Rincón J, Onaindia A, et al. Mutated JAK kinases and deregulated STAT activity are potential therapeutic targets in cutaneous T-cell lymphoma. Haematologica 2015;100(11):e450–3. https://doi.org/10.3324/haematol.2015.132837.

75. Mirza AS, Horna P, Teer JK, et al. New Insights Into the Complex Mutational Landscape of Sézary Syndrome. Front Oncol 2020;10. https://doi.org/10. 3389/fonc.2020.00514.

76. Phyo ZH, Shanbhag S, Rozati S. Update on Biology of Cutaneous T-Cell Lymphoma. Front Oncol 2020; 10. https://doi.org/10.3389/fonc.2020.00765.

77. Machan S, Rodríguez M, Alonso-Alonso R, et al. Subcutaneous panniculitis-like T-cell lymphoma, lupus erythematosus profundus, and overlapping cases: molecular characterization through the study of 208 genes. Leuk Lymphoma 2021;62(9):2130–40. https://doi.org/10.1080/10428194.2021.1901098.

78. Gayden T, Sepulveda FE, Khuong-Quang DA, et al. Germline HAVCR2 mutations altering TIM-3 characterize subcutaneous panniculitis-like T cell lymphomas with hemophagocytic lymphohistiocytic syndrome. Nat Genet 2018;50(12):1650–7. https:// doi.org/10.1038/s41588-018-0251-4.

79. Polprasert C, Takeuchi Y, Kakiuchi N, et al. Frequent germline mutations of HAVCR2 in sporadic subcutaneous panniculitis-like T-cell lymphoma. Blood Adv 2019;3(4):588–95. https://doi.org/10.1182/ bloodadvances.2018028340.

80. Sonigo G, Battistella M, Beylot-Barry M, et al. HAVCR2 mutations are associated with severe hemophagocytic syndrome in subcutaneous panniculitis-like T-cell lymphoma. Blood 2020; 135(13):1058–61. https://doi.org/10.1182/blood. 2019003811.

SUPPLEMENTARY

CTCLs that fall within the category of "provisional diagnoses" in the 2018 WHO-EORTC classification for Primary Cutaneous Lymphomas are summarized in **Table 7**.[3] Features of Adult T-cell Leukemia/Lymphoma (ATLL) are summarized in **Table 8**.[18,25,61–70] Recent diagnostic and therapeutic advances in CTCL are summarized in **Table 9**.[42,71–80]

Preventative Options and the Future of Chemoprevention for Cutaneous Tumors

Jane Margaret Anderson, BSA[a,b], Lauren Moy, MD[a], Ronald L. Moy, MD[a,*]

KEYWORDS

- Chemoprophylaxis • Nonmelanoma skin cancer prevention
- Cutaneous malignancy chemoprevention

KEY POINTS

- NMSC prevention should be considered in high-risk patients and individualized based on risk factors.
- Therapies with proven benefits and little harm, including nicotinamide and topical DNA repair enzymes, can be used in patients who have had a single occurrence of NMSC, patients with a strong family history of NMSC, or in patients who show extensive actinic damage.
- Newer chemoprophylactic agents offer greater protective capabilities than traditional sunscreen, and some combinations may work synergistically to be even more efficacious.

INTRODUCTION

Chemoprophylaxis is defined as the use of drugs, vitamins, or other agents to prevent against or to slow the development of cancer. Treatment of nonmelanoma skin cancer (NMSC) can be invasive and associated with significant morbidity despite advances in treatment options. Chemoprophylaxis should be considered in patients who are at high risk of developing multiple or invasive NMSC, those with extensive actinic damage, or those with a history of NMSC (Box 1).[1] Current options for chemoprevention range from topical therapies to oral supplements (Table 1). Therapies like DNA repair enzymes, nicotinamide, nonsteroidal anti-inflammatory drugs (NSAIDs), sunscreen, and systemic retinoids have been proved to be effective in reducing the incidence of skin cancer, whereas other therapies have not yet been shown to definitively decrease the risk of NMSC. These therapies include the numerous therapeutic options that target actinic keratoses (AKs), which have less than a 3% chance of evolving into skin cancer, as well as capecitabine, difluoromethylornithine (DFMO), hedgehog inhibitors, metformin, polyphenolic antioxidants, and other nutritional factors.

PROVEN CHEMOPROPHYLAXIS THERAPIES

Sunscreen

Sunscreen has historically been the only form of prevention against skin cancer with multiple studies showing efficacy in preventing squamous cell carcinoma (SCC) and decreasing the amount of AKs.[1,4,5] However, a recent meta-analysis found there to be no association with the incidence of skin cancer, NMSC or melanoma, and sunscreen use.[6] This finding may be because studies on sunscreen are difficult to conduct because the effects are not seen until many years later. In addition, new evidence suggests that sunscreens targeting UV-B may not provide adequate coverage and

[a] Research Department, Moy-Fincher-Chipps Facial Plastics & Dermatology, 421 North Rodeo Drive #T-7, Beverly Hills, CA 90210, USA; [b] The University of Texas Health Science Center San Antonio, 7703 Floyd Curl Drive, San Antonio, TX 78229, USA
* Corresponding author. 421 North Rodeo Drive T-7, Beverly Hills, CA 90210.
E-mail address: ronmoymd@gmail.com

Dermatol Clin 41 (2023) 231–238
https://doi.org/10.1016/j.det.2022.07.020

UV-A may play a role especially in darker skin.[7] Although there is no emphasis on these rays and increased risk of NMSC, more research needs to be conducted.

Sunscreen has been a topic of controversy lately for being linked to carcinogens and ingredients with unclear safety profiles.[8,9] In addition, the US Food and Drug Administration has claimed there are insufficient data to deem commonly found sunscreen ingredients as safe and effective. As a result, the general population has become more skeptical of sunscreen despite continued FDA and American Academy of Dermatology backing.

With fewer people eager to apply sunscreen daily and ongoing questions regarding the safety of available products, it may be time to emphasize other, more effective agents of skin cancer chemoprophylaxis.

DNA Repair Enzymes

DNA repair enzymes were the topic of the 2015 Nobel Prize in Chemistry winner and since then, have been a subject of interest for skin cancer prevention. Several clinical studies composed of several hundred subjects have shown that enhanced DNA repair is associated with the prevention of AKs and skin cancer.[10] Topical DNA repair enzymes, specifically topical liposomal T4 endonuclease V and photolyases, target this mechanism and have been shown to decrease the risk of skin cancers in certain high-risk patients.[10] These enzymes function by repairing damage to DNA induced by UV exposure, especially cyclobutane pyrimidine dimers (CPDs), which have been associated with the development of AKs and NMSC.[10] Liposomal T4 endonuclease V was originally derived from a T4 bacteriophage-infected *Escherichia coli* and when applied topically has been shown to reduce the incidence of basal cell carcinoma (BCC) by 30% in patients with xeroderma pigmentosum (XP), a disease of defective DNA repair enzymes.[11] Photolyase is derived from algae and works by repairing CPDs and pyrimidine-pyrimidone photoproducts that are caused by UV radiation.[12] This effect has been demonstrated when applied topically by reducing the amount of CPDs in UV-irradiated skin by 40% to 45%.[10] Further supporting this study, a randomized control trial (RCT) found photolyase to reduce UV-induced CPDs by 61% when used in combination with sunscreen at 6 months compared with 35% when sunscreen was used alone.[10] DNA repair enzymes have also been found to reduce the number of AKs in healthy individuals with moderate to severe photodamage.[10] Adding to their appeal, topical DNA repair enzymes have a desirable safety profile with no serious adverse effects reported by any studies to date.[10] Although larger clinical trials are needed to definitively establish the usefulness of topical DNA repair enzymes outside of patients with XP, the in vitro data and the data on AKs support the observations that topical DNA repair enzymes prevent BCC and SCC in all patients.

Nicotinamide

Oral nicotinamide, a form of vitamin B_3, has been shown to effectively treat AKs and has been proved to decrease the rate of NMSC.[1,13] These

Table 1
Therapies for chemoprophylaxis

	Proven Chemopreventive Agents	Potential Chemopreventive Agents
Topical	Sunscreen DNA repair enzymes	Actinic keratosis treatments Difluoromethylornithine Nicotinamide Polyphenolic antioxidants
Systemic	Nicotinamide Isotretinoin & acitretin Celecoxib	Capecitabine Difluoromethylornithine Hedgehog inhibitors Metformin Polyphenolic antioxidants Nutritional factors

effects are largely due to nicotinamide's ability to increase DNA excision repair by preventing the depletion of cellular energy and immunosuppression resulting from UV radiation.[13] The accepted dose resulting in reduction of NMSC is 500 mg twice a day based on a phase 3 RCT, which found nicotinamide to be associated with a 23% reduction in the incidence of NMSC as well as of AKs at 12 months (P = .001).[1] The reduction was seen equally in BCC and SCC. At very high doses it has been reported to cause nausea but otherwise has minimal side effects.[13]

Topical nicotinamide is less studied than the oral form but has been associated with prevention of UV-induced immunosuppression, a mechanism that has been linked to the progression of skin cancer. One study found that topical 5% nicotinamide was associated with an increase in enzymes involved in p53 and cell metabolism and protected against UV-A- and UV-B-induced local immunosuppression when applied immediately after UV exposure.[14] Another study found that application of nicotinamide to UV-irradiated mice led to a decreased incidence of cutaneous tumors.[13] Unlike oral nicotinamide, topical nicotinamide is not a proven measure to prevent the incidence of NMSC in humans but is a promising candidate that needs to be researched in clinical trials.

Nonsteroidal Anti-inflammatory Drugs

NSAIDs have shown promising results as chemoprevention for various malignancies, but there has been inconsistent data on the association of NSAIDs and skin cancer. The proposed mechanisms by which NSAIDs could reduce the risk of skin cancer are through restoration of normal apoptosis and reduction of cell proliferation via inhibition of cyclooxygenase 2 (COX-2).[15] COX-2 is upregulated by UV radiation and is often overexpressed in keratinocyte skin cancers.[15] COX has

been shown to have increased expression and activity in NMSC and a significant impact on the regulation of cell growth.[15] The studies done on NSAIDs to date are difficult to compare due to different standards of analgesic use, patient-reported dosages, types of NSAIDs used, geographic factors, and other potentially confounding variables.

One review found that long-term use of aspirin and NSAIDs reduces the incidence of skin cancer, as well as other types of cancer, based on several epidemiologic, clinical, and experimental studies.[16] However, several population-based case-control studies found conflicting data with some supporting a relationship between NSAID use and decreased risk of BCC or SCC and others finding no relationship. These studies differed on the definition of NSAID use and were carried out in different geographic regions. In addition, different variables were taken into consideration in each study including the individual type of NSAID, high- versus low-risk populations, and location of NMSC among others.[15,17]

Despite the mixed results for overall NSAID use, distinctly targeting only COX-2 has shown promising effects in the reduction of NMSC. Celecoxib, a COX-2-specific inhibitor, has been shown to prevent NMSC tumor formation in mice.[18] In humans, it has been shown to reduce the number of BCC in high-risk patients with basal cell nevus syndrome.[18] Elmets and colleagues[19] looked at the effects of 200 mg celecoxib twice daily for 9 months on AKs and NMSC in patients with a history of extensive AKs. The investigators found a significant decrease in both SCC and BCC in the group assigned to celecoxib compared with placebo at 11 months after adjustment for confounding variables (Rate ratio [RR], 0.41; 95% confidence interval [CI], 0.23–0.72, P = .002).

Taken together, the evidence for generalized systemic NSAID use as chemoprophylaxis against skin cancer is not compelling, but celecoxib has shown efficacy in chemoprevention. One downfall of NSAIDs is their safety profile, and the risk of toxicity may offset the benefit in low-risk individuals. Celecoxib specifically is known to have cardiovascular effects, which may limit its generalized use.[18] However, it has been shown to be safe in RCT and has not increased the rate of cardiovascular events in participants.[19] Topical celecoxib is also being investigated as a means to increase efficacy and minimize side effects.[20] In response to the risk of toxicity with NSAIDs, nitric oxide (NO)-releasing NSAIDs were developed to both increase efficacy and minimize gastrointestinal and cardiovascular effects. Topical NO-sulindac has shown promise in mice studies by reducing tumor incidence and inhibiting UV-B-induced inflammatory responses.[21] However, to our knowledge no studies have been done in humans.

Systemic Retinoids: Acitretin and Isotretinoin

Retinoids are vitamin A analogues that are thought to decrease the incidence of SCC in high-risk patients through their influence on epithelial maturation and cellular differentiation as well as induction of growth arrest and apoptosis of tumor cells. Low-dose systemic retinoids are a well-studied form of chemoprevention and have been documented to decrease the risk of NMSC in high-risk patients through multiple studies.[22] This method of chemoprevention should be considered in patients who have developed a significant amount of SCC, usually an average of 5 to 10 SCCs per year.[22] Systemic retinoids that are currently available in the United States are acitretin, the drug of choice, and isotretinoin.[1] Acitretin is preferred due to more substantial data, but isotretinoin is preferred in women of childbearing age due to a shorter half-life and the contraindication of systemic retinoids in pregnancy. Multiple RCTs have cited a significant decrease in SCC development following initiation of therapy.[1,22] A reduction in the incidence of both BCC and SCC has been shown in patients with XP.[22] The main downfall of retinoids is the tendency for patients to experience a rebound effect with a relapse in tumor development following termination of treatment; this necessitates long-term and possibly lifelong use of low-dose retinoids, which increases the risk of adverse effects because of the direct correlation with the drug dosage.[1] Some of the reported adverse effects seen with longer-term use or higher dose include mucocutaneous xerosis, alopecia, musculoskeletal complications, hypertriglyceridemia and hypercholesterolemia, and hepatotoxicity. These effects may warrant a decrease in dosage if severe.

THERAPIES TARGETING PRECANCEROUS LESIONS

Treatment of AK through various modalities has historically been seen as preventative measures against NMSC. However, the risk of progression from AK to SCC has been cited to be anywhere from 0.025% to 20%, with an approximated overall risk of 2% and an estimated greater than 50% chance of spontaneous regression.[23] Furthermore, the management of AKs carries a large financial burden with an estimated more than $1 billion spent each year in the United States.[23] With it being nearly impossible to predict which lesions will progress to SCC, and a higher chance of the lesion regressing than progressing, it is questionable whether targeted AK treatment effectively prevents SCC and even more so, BCC. Nonetheless, limited data suggest that some AK therapies may slightly decrease the risk of SCC including cryotherapy, laser resurfacing, 5-fluorouracil, imiquimod, photodynamic therapy, tirbanibulin, and ingenol mebutate (**Table 2**).

POTENTIAL CHEMOPROPHYLAXIS THERAPIES
Capecitabine

Capecitabine is a prodrug of 5-fluorouracil and is metabolized by thymidine phosphorylase, an enzyme that is overexpressed in some malignancies.[1,24] One case series looked at the use of oral capecitabine as a monotherapy in 3 high-risk organ transplant patients.[24] All 3 patients demonstrated a significant reduction in SCC development 6 months after initiation. Another study in 10 solid organ transplant recipients found that low-dose oral capecitabine significantly reduced the incidence of new SCCs during treatment.[24] The use of capecitabine is contraindicated in patients with dihydropyrimidine dehydrogenase deficiency due to the risk of severe toxicity.[1] Therefore, patients should always be screened before initiating therapy. Adverse effects include hand-foot syndrome, erythema, pain, mild fatigue, diarrhea, stomatitis, and muscle aches.[24] Side effects are seen in up to 30% of patients but are largely dose related. Although capecitabine shows promise as a chemoprophylactic agent for both SCC and BCC, it has only shown usefulness in a small population and needs to be studied in a larger RCT to truly determine its efficacy.

Hedgehog Inhibitors: Vismodegib and Sonidegib

Mutations in genes involved in the hedgehog signaling pathway can lead to increased cell growth and proliferation and have been linked to

Table 2
Chemopreventative agents and dosing[1,19,41]

	Agent	Dose	Treatment Regimen
Treatment of AKs	Cryotherapy	10 s	Target center of lesion and complete 2 freeze-thaw cycles
	Laser resurfacing	Varies	Varies
	5-Fluorouracil	5% cream	Apply bid for 2–4 wk
	Imiquimod	12.5 mg or 1 single dose packet of 5% cream	Apply for 8 h then remove with soap and water
			Use twice per week for 16 wk
	Ingenol mebutate	0.015%, 0.05%	Apply qd for 2–3 d
	Tirbanibulin	1 single dose packet	Apply qd for 5 d
	PDT	ALA with blue light	Apply to area for 1–4 h without occlusion before illumination
		ALA with red light	Apply to area for 3 h with occlusion before illumination
			Repeat in 3 mo as needed
		MAL with red light[a]	Apply to area for 3 h with occlusion
			May repeat in 3 mo if no response
Proven chemopreventative agents	Nicotinamide	500 mg	po bid
	DNA repair enzymes	T4 endonuclease cream & photolyase cream	Apply qd
	Sunscreen	SPF 30+	Apply qd
	Isotretinoind and acitretin	Target dose of 20–25 mg/d	Start at 10 mg/d and increase by 10-mg increments every 2–4 wk as tolerated
	Celecoxib	200 mg	po bid

Abbreviations: ALA, aminolevulinic acid; BCC, basal cell carcinoma; bid, twice daily; EGCG, epigallocatechin3-gallate; GTP, green tea polyphenols; MAL, methyl-esterified ALA; po, by mouth; qd, every day.

[a] Only available in the European Union.

BCC in UV-damaged skin.[12,25] Vismodegib and sonidegib are approved for treatment of advanced BCC and more recently, vismodegib has been suggested to have a potential preventative effect on NMSC, particularly BCC.[26] However, adverse effects including muscle spasms, alopecia, weight loss, and loss of taste are common and may lead to the discontinuation of treatment[25]; this may limit the broad use of sonic hedgehog inhibitors as a means of chemoprevention by challenging patient compliance and safety in certain populations.

Difluoromethylornithine

DFMO is an irreversible inhibitor of ornithine decarboxylase.[27] Ornithine decarboxylase is the rate-limiting enzyme in a pathway that produces polyamines, which has been implicated in cutaneous malignancies when at increased levels.[12] DFMO has been associated with a reduction in the incidence of skin cancer and AKs. One study involving 48 patients with actinic damage found that topical 10% DFMO over a 6-month period reduced the number of AKs by 23.5%.[27] When taken orally, DFMO has been associated with a decrease in BCC but not SCC with no rebound effect once it is discontinued.[28,29] Inflammatory effects are not uncommon with topical DFMO and can be severe enough to warrant a dose reduction.[27] However, oral DFMO has a much better side effect profile with a documented compliance in greater than 90% of patients in 1 RCT.[28] The reported side effects of oral DFMO are gastrointestinal upset and reversible ototoxicity that is more prominent at higher doses.[30] No long-term adverse effects from systemic DFMO have been documented to date.[29] Both topical and oral DFMO are promising chemoprophylactic agents, but more studies need to be done to fully understand the association with NMSC.

Metformin

Metformin, a biguanide used to treat diabetes, has been associated with a decrease in overall cancer incidence as well as a reduction in mortality from cancer.[31] It is thought that metformin reduces the risk of cancer by decreasing protein synthesis and cell proliferation.[31] Metformin also has inhibitory effects on the sonic hedgehog pathway, which may play an additional role in chemoprevention.[32] Based on recent studies, metformin reduces the incidence of various cancers including prostate, colon, pancreas, and breast cancer.[31] However, it is unclear whether this translates to cutaneous malignancies, and there are mixed results on the effects of metformin on skin cancer. In fact, a recent meta-analysis found that there was no significant reduction in NMSC or melanoma skin cancer.[33] A retrospective cohort study found a decreased risk of keratinocyte carcinoma that was emphasized at higher doses of metformin.[34] A later retrospective cohort study re-examined the potential benefit of metformin on a second occurrence of NMSC and found no effect over a 3-year period.[35] The main limitation of both these studies is that there was no differentiation between BCC and SCC. A more recent, larger population-based case-control study evaluated the relationship between first-time NMSC and metformin with a differentiation between BCC and SCC.[32] The investigators found an overall decreased risk of developing BCC (odds ratio [OR], 0.71; 95% CI, 0.61–0.83) even when taken at low doses. There was no association between metformin and SCC reduction. These data suggest that metformin is a drug with minimal side effects that potentially prevents BCC in addition to other cancers.

Polyphenolic Antioxidants

Polyphenolic antioxidants, found in green tea derived from *Camellia sinensis* species, have been cited to have photoprotective properties.[12] The main contributor to polyphenol's photoprotective effects is the most abundant polyphenol, epigallocatechin-3-gallate (EGCG). Multiple studies have shown the ability of green tea polyphenols (GTPs) to inhibit carcinogenesis when applied topically or consumed. Polyphenols were first found to have potential chemopreventive properties when consumed by mice. It was later discovered that EGCG could be isolated and applied topically to achieve an equivalent effect. In humans, GTPs have been seen to decrease the erythema response induced by UV radiation, reduce the number of sunburn cells histologically, and reduce the formation of CPDs.[12,36] Furthermore, a mice study demonstrated that oral GTPs lead to a reduction in UV-B-induced skin tumor formation and a decrease in COX-2 and prostaglandin E_2 levels, markers of UV-B-induced inflammation.[37] Studies have also shown the ability of polyphenols to reduce UV-induced immunosuppression and oxidative stress.[12] Although more research needs to be done to determine the relationship between GTPs and the incidence of skin cancer in humans, polyphenols are an attractive option for prevention because they are natural, readily available, cost effective, and have little, if any, adverse effects.

Other nutritional factors that have been suggested to have a chemopreventive effect on NMSC include genistein from soybeans, lycopene, caffeine, and a low-fat diet.[1,12]

SUMMARY

Skin cancer prevention with options other than sunscreen is still relatively new. Sunscreen was first shown to be safe and effective in 1956, whereas nicotinamide was not proven to be safe and effective until 2015, almost 60 years after the introduction of UV-B sunscreen. A 2018 global review on skin cancer knowledge in medical students demonstrated that students were largely uneducated in sunscreen use and had little knowledge of UV radiation.[38] If future physicians are unknowledgeable about sunscreen use, the original method of NMSC chemoprevention, it is expected that their patients will also lack knowledge about skin cancer prevention, especially the newer preventative therapies.

Specialists in cutaneous malignancies have a larger base of knowledge when it comes to chemoprevention of NMSC. A recent article assessed the NMSC prevention recommendations of surgeons practicing Mohs surgery.[39] Of the 85 responses received, 95.3% recommended some type of NMSC prevention including nicotinamide, acitretin, and topical retinoids. However, it is often not until patients present with multiple skin cancers that they learn of these preventative strategies because the knowledge base is limited to highly specialized physicians. Primary care physicians and general dermatologists should be educated in the preventative options available so that they may also educate patients on how to reduce the risk of NMSC.

There are various options for chemoprevention of NMSC that should be customized to the individual patient (see **Table 2**). Therapies with proven benefits and little harm can be used in patients with a lower threshold to treat. Examples of these are nicotinamide and topical DNA repair enzymes, which can be considered after a single occurrence of NMSC, a family history of NMSC, or extensive actinic damage. Sunscreen should continue to be recommended to all patients. Other therapies that have more severe side effects should be reserved for the highest risk patients.

Complementary modalities of chemoprevention can be combined to offer greater protective capabilities to patients and may even work synergistically in some combinations. In the future, therapies may be highly individualized based on the patient and could prove to not be "one size fits all." Genomic studies like noninvasive tape stripping biopsies and pigmented lesion assays developed by Dermtech, may be able to predict the development of skin cancer on an individual basis.[40] The future of chemoprevention is promising and shifting away from the sole use of traditional sunscreen and toward therapies that are individualized and highly effective with few side effects.

CLINICS CARE POINTS: BULLETED LIST OF EVIDENCE-BASED PEARLS AND PITFALLS RELEVANT TO THE POINT OF CARE

- NMSC chemoprevention should be considered in high-risk populations
- The available agents for NMSC chemoprevention are continually expanding and can be used in conjunction to achieve a broader range of coverage
- The specific type of chemoprevention used should be individualized to the patient
- Proven therapies for NMSC chemoprevention include sunscreen, nicotinamide, DNA repair enzymes, celecoxib, and systemic retinoids

DISCLOSURE

The authors have nothing to disclose.

REFERENCES

1. Nemer KM, Council ML. Topical and Systemic Modalities for Chemoprevention of Nonmelanoma Skin Cancer. Dermatol Clin 2019;37(3):287–95.

2. Soltani-Arabshahi R, Tristani-Firouzi P. Chemoprevention of nonmelanoma skin cancer. Facial Plast Surg 2013;29(5):373–83.

3. Prado R, Francis SO, Mason MN, et al. Nonmelanoma skin cancer chemoprevention. Dermatol Surg Off Publ Am Soc Dermatol Surg [et al] 2011; 37(11):1566–78.

4. Thompson SC, Jolley D, Marks R. Reduction of solar keratoses by regular sunscreen use. N Engl J Med 1993;329(16):1147–51.

5. Green A, Williams G, Neale R, et al. Daily sunscreen application and betacarotene supplementation in prevention of basal-cell and squamous-cell carcinomas of the skin: a randomised controlled trial. Lancet (London, England) 1999;354(9180): 723–9.

6. Silva ES da, Tavares R, Paulitsch F da S, et al. Use of sunscreen and risk of melanoma and non-melanoma skin cancer: a systematic review and meta-analysis. Eur J Dermatol 2018;28(2):186–201.

7. Rigel DS, Taylor SC, Lim HW, et al. Photoprotection for skin of all color: Consensus and clinical guidance from an expert panel. J Am Acad Dermatol 2022; 86(3S):S1–8.

8. Downs CA, DiNardo JC, Stien D, et al. Benzophenone Accumulates over Time from the Degradation of Octocrylene in Commercial Sunscreen Products. Chem Res Toxicol 2021;34(4):1046–54.

9. Light D, Kucera K, Wu Q. Valisure Citizen Petition on Benzene in sunscreen and after-Sun care products.; 2021.

10. Yarosh DB, Rosenthal A, Moy R. Six critical questions for DNA repair enzymes in skincare products: a review in dialog. Clin Cosmet Investig Dermatol 2019;12:617–24.

11. Cafardi JA, Elmets CA. T4 endonuclease V: review and application to dermatology. Expert Opin Biol Ther 2008;8(6):829–38.

12. Camp WL, Turnham JW, Athar M, et al. New agents for prevention of ultraviolet-induced nonmelanoma skin cancer. Semin Cutan Med Surg 2011;30(1): 6–13.

13. Snaidr VA, Damian DL, Halliday GM. Nicotinamide for photoprotection and skin cancer chemoprevention: A review of efficacy and safety. Exp Dermatol 2019;28(Suppl 1):15–22.

14. Damian DL, Patterson CRS, Stapelberg M, et al. UV radiation-induced immunosuppression is greater in men and prevented by topical nicotinamide. J Invest Dermatol 2008;128(2):447–54.

15. Torti DC, Christensen BC, Storm CA, et al. Analgesic and nonsteroidal anti-inflammatory use in relation to nonmelanoma skin cancer: a population-based case-control study. J Am Acad Dermatol 2011; 65(2):304–12.

16. Rao CV, Reddy BS. NSAIDs and chemoprevention. Curr Cancer Drug Targets 2004;4(1):29–42.

17. Reinau D, Surber C, Jick SS, et al. Nonsteroidal anti-inflammatory drugs and the risk of nonmelanoma skin cancer. Int J Cancer 2015;137(1):144–53.

18. Elmets CA, Ledet JJ, Athar M. Cyclooxygenases: mediators of UV-induced skin cancer and potential targets for prevention. J Invest Dermatol 2014; 134(10):2497–502.

19. Elmets CA, Viner JL, Pentland AP, et al. Chemoprevention of nonmelanoma skin cancer with celecoxib: a randomized, double-blind, placebo-controlled trial. J Natl Cancer Inst 2010;102(24):1835–44.

20. Quiñones OG, Pierre MBR. Cutaneous Application of Celecoxib for Inflammatory and Cancer Diseases. Curr Cancer Drug Targets 2019;19(1):5–16.

21. Chaudhary SC, Singh T, Kapur P, et al. Nitric oxide-releasing sulindac is a novel skin cancer chemopreventive agent for UVB-induced photocarcinogenesis. Toxicol Appl Pharmacol 2013;268(3):249–55.

22. Otley CC, Stasko T, Tope WD, et al. Chemoprevention of nonmelanoma skin cancer with systemic retinoids: practical dosing and management of adverse effects. Dermatol Surg Off Publ Am Soc Dermatol Surg [et al] 2006;32(4):562–8.

23. Siegel JA, Korgavkar K, Weinstock MA. Current perspective on actinic keratosis: a review. Br J Dermatol 2017;177(2):350–8.

24. Schauder DM, Kim J, Nijhawan RI. Evaluation of the Use of Capecitabine for the Treatment and Prevention of Actinic Keratoses, Squamous Cell Carcinoma, and Basal Cell Carcinoma: A Systematic Review. JAMA Dermatol 2020;156(10):1117–24.

25. Dinulos J. Premalignant and malignant nonmelanoma skin tumors. In: Habif's clinical Dermatology. 2021. p. 815–62.

26. Tang JY, Mackay-Wiggan JM, Aszterbaum M, et al. Inhibiting the hedgehog pathway in patients with the basal-cell nevus syndrome. N Engl J Med 2012;366(23):2180–8.

27. Alberts DS, Dorr RT, Einspahr JG, et al. Chemoprevention of human actinic keratoses by topical 2-(difluoromethyl)-dl-ornithine. Cancer Epidemiol Biomarkers Prev A Publ Am Assoc Cancer Res Cosponsored By Am Soc Prev Oncol 2000;9(12):1281–6.

28. Bailey HH, Kim K, Verma AK, et al. A randomized, double-blind, placebo-controlled phase 3 skin cancer prevention study of {alpha}-difluoromethylornithine in subjects with previous history of skin cancer. Cancer Prev Res (Phila) 2010;3(1):35–47.

29. Kreul SM, Havighurst T, Kim K, et al. A phase III skin cancer chemoprevention study of DFMO: long-term follow-up of skin cancer events and toxicity. Cancer Prev Res (Phila) 2012;5(12):1368–74.

30. Meyskens FLJ, Gerner EW. Development of difluoromethylornithine (DFMO) as a chemoprevention agent. Clin Cancer Res 1999;5(5):945–51.

31. Saraei P, Asadi I, Kakar MA, et al. The beneficial effects of metformin on cancer prevention and therapy: a comprehensive review of recent advances. Cancer Manag Res 2019;11:3295–313.

32. Adalsteinsson JA, Muzumdar S, Waldman R, et al. Metformin is associated with decreased risk of basal cell carcinoma: A whole-population case-control study from Iceland. J Am Acad Dermatol 2021; 85(1):56–61.

33. Chang MS, Hartman RI, Xue J, et al. Risk of Skin Cancer Associated with Metformin Use: A Meta-Analysis of Randomized Controlled Trials and Observational Studies. Cancer Prev Res (Phila) 2021;14(1):77–84.

34. Tseng C-H. Metformin is associated with decreased skin cancer risk in Taiwanese patients with type 2 diabetes. J Am Acad Dermatol 2018;78(4):694–700.

35. Ravishankar A, Zhang T, Lindgren BR, et al. The effect of metformin on the risk of recurrent nonmelanoma skin cancers. Int J Dermatol 2020;59(8): e303–5.

36. Katiyar SK, Perez A, Mukhtar H. Green tea polyphenol treatment to human skin prevents formation of ultraviolet light B-induced pyrimidine dimers in DNA. Clin Cancer Res 2000;6(10):3864–9.

37. Meeran SM, Akhtar S, Katiyar SK. Inhibition of UVB-induced skin tumor development by drinking green tea polyphenols is mediated through DNA repair and subsequent inhibition of inflammation. J Invest Dermatol 2009;129(5):1258–70.

38. Nahar VK, Wilkerson AH, Ghafari G, et al. Skin cancer knowledge, attitudes, beliefs, and prevention practices among medical students: A systematic search and literature review. Int J Women's Dermatology 2018;4(3):139–49.

39. Arzeno J, Leavitt E, Lonowski S, et al. Current Practices for Preventative Interventions for Nonmelanoma Skin Cancers Among Dermatologic Surgeons. Dermatol Surg 2021;47(7):995–7.

40. Dorrell DN, Strowd LC. Skin Cancer Detection Technology. Dermatol Clin 2019;37(4):527–36.

41. Tirbanibulin. Am J Health Pharm 2021;78(8):656–7.

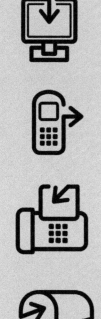

Printed and bound by CPI Group (UK) Ltd, Croydon, CR0 4YY

08/05/2025

01864721-0001